PUBLIC HEALTH IN THE 21ST CENTURY

OBESITY AND SYNDROME X

A GLOBAL PUBLIC HEALTH BURDEN

PUBLIC HEALTH IN THE 21ST CENTURY

Additional books and e-books in this series can be found on Nova's website under the Series tab.

PUBLIC HEALTH IN THE 21ST CENTURY

OBESITY AND SYNDROME X

A GLOBAL PUBLIC HEALTH BURDEN

MITHUN DAS
AND
KAUSHIK BOSE
EDITORS

nova
science publishers
New York

Library of Congress Cataloging-in-Publication Data

ISBN: 978-1-53614-669-1
Library of Congress Control Number: 2018962185

Published by Nova Science Publishers, Inc. † New York

CONTENTS

Foreword	*Partha P. Majumder*	**ix**
Preface		**xi**
Part I:	**Epidemiological Aspect**	**1**
Chapter 1	Associations with Obesity in Sub-Saharan Africa *Yackoob K. Seedat*	**3**
Chapter 2	Metabolic Syndrome in the Philippines and Asia: Concepts and Concerns *Gabriel V. Jasul, Jr., Rosa Allyn G. Sy and Rodolfo F. Florentino*	**13**
Chapter 3	Body Mass Index, Percent Body Fat and Fat Mass Index as Screening Tools for General Obesity among Adult Females of Amritsar (Punjab) *Ramanpreet Randhawa and Sharda Sidhu*	**39**
Chapter 4	The Association of Central Adiposity with Metabolic Syndrome among the Bhutias of Sikkim, India *Sovanjan Sarkar and Barun Mukhopadhyay*	**73**

Chapter 5	Bisexual Differences in the Association of Adiposity Measures with the Risk of Hypertension among the Tribes of Gujarat, India *Gautam K. Kshatriya*	**89**
Part II:	**Analytical Aspect**	**119**
Chapter 6	Obesity as an Important Predictor of Hypertension among Rajshahi University Students in Bangladesh: A Cross-Sectional Study *Md. Golam Hossain, Sadekur Rahman, Suhaili Mohd, Saw Aik, Rashidul Alam Mahumud, Premananda Bharati and Pete E. Lestrel*	**121**
Chapter 7	Increasing Incidence of Macrosomia: The Impact of Maternal Somatic and Behavioral Parameters on Newborn Weight Status *Sylvia Kirchengast*	**143**
Chapter 8	Metabolic Disorder and Type-2 Diabetes Associations with Anthropometric Measures among Adult Asian Indians *Sampriti Debnath, Nitish Mondal and Jaydip Sen*	**167**
Chapter 9	C-Reactive Protein and Family History: A Future Threat towards Diabetes and Syndrome X *Riddhi Goswami, Mithun Das and Indrani Lodh*	**201**
Chapter 10	Sensitivity and Specificity of Body Mass Index to Assess Excess Adiposity *Jyoti Ratan Ghosh*	**215**
Part III:	**Global Public Health Aspect**	**227**
Chapter 11	Framing Obesity and Undernutrition as Problems for Governments *Stanley Ulijaszek*	**229**

Chapter 12 Modernization and Obesity: A Pandemic Issue **249**
Soibam Jibonkumar Singh and Thoudam Bedita Devi

Chapter 13 Obesity and Syndrome X **265**
Anup Adhikari

Chapter 14 Syndrome X: Some Common Determinants Worldwide **273**
Mithun Das and Kaushik Bose

About the Editors **291**

List of Contributors **293**

Index **297**

FOREWORD

We now know there is consistent association among dysregulation of multiple organs. In other words, diseases often occur as constellations of defects in multiple organs or multiple physiological sub-systems. Syndrome X the most prominent among such defect-constellations, in which minimally there is increased level of blood sugar and an adverse lipid profile leading to type 2 diabetes and heart disease. Perturbations of biological pathways that result in such constellations of abnormal phenotypes have not been completely mapped, but researchers are actively engaged with this task. Meanwhile, consistent risk factors are being identified. In respect of Syndrome X, obesity is undoubtedly the prime risk factor. The editors have brought together a set of researchers who are actively pursuing research on Syndrome X with particular focus on obesity and produced a compendium of their research findings. The articles in this volume vary from descriptive (epidemiological profiling) to analytical (dissection of causes). Some articles have emphasized the impact of such studies in understanding burden on public health, globally. The authors who have contributed are from varied backgrounds, because of which this collection of essays is refreshingly diverse in spite of being focused. I do hope that researchers from equally varied backgrounds benefit from this collection.

Partha P. Majumder, PhD, FNA, FASc, FNASc, FTWAS
J. C. Bose National Fellow
Distinguished Professor and Founder
National Institute of Biomedical Genomics, Kalyani, India
Professor
Translational Health Science and Technology Institute, Faridabad, India

PREFACE

Obesity and Syndrome X continues to be an important global public health burden. Obesity occurs as a natural consequence of over nutrition and sedentary lifestyle. It further dysregulates metabolic process, if persistent over a period, ultimately leading to a cluster of risk factors known as metabolic syndrome or syndrome X. Close association of syndrome X with type 2 diabetes, cardiovascular diseases, and its co-morbidities results to leading causes of death and disability worldwide.

The book is therefore intended for specific readers who are proactive and have the ability to engage in research on their own on a much deeper level. It is a way to raise interest in individuals related to this area of study. It is however not possible to cover every single aspect in one book. We may not have been able to do full justice in all the areas involved in this field of work. However, it is a sincere attempt to give our best effort to address a specific audience.

The topics discussed in the book are from authors of diverse background thereby making every topic extremely large in breadth and depth. There are fourteen chapters divided into three parts. The first part of the book comprises five chapters related to *Epidemiological Aspects* of obesity and syndrome X, the second part is comprised of five chapters related to *Analytical Aspects*, and the third part is comprised of four chapters dedicated to the *Global Public Health Aspects*.

We envision the audience of this book to comprise a broad spectrum of those involved in the field of public health, epidemiology, medicine, anthropology and other related disciplines of biological and social sciences. Even individuals who are just beginners in this field of research may find these chapters of much interest.

We sincerely acknowledge the chapter authors for their valuable contribution despite having tight schedule to create what we believe is a truly diverse and informative book. Their expertise and insights will not only be gift to all interested readers, but it will help to develop a common agenda in future for combating this global public health burden comprehensively.

Last but not least, we thank NOVA Science Publishers (New York) for all their help and kind cooperation without which the publication of this book would not have been possible.

Mithun Das, PhD (Visva-Bharati) and
Kaushik Bose, PhD (Panjab), PhD (Cantab), DSc (Vidyasagar)

PART I: EPIDEMIOLOGICAL ASPECT

In: Obesity and Syndrome X
Editors: M. Das and K. Bose
ISBN: 978-1-53614-669-1

Chapter 1

ASSOCIATIONS WITH OBESITY IN SUB-SAHARAN AFRICA

Yackoob K. Seedat*
Department of Internal Medicine,
University of KwaZulu-Natal, Durban, South Africa

HYPERTENSION

There is a strong association between obesity, hypertension, and obesity. About three-quarters of adult type II diabetics and some two-thirds of hypertensives are overweight (Modan et al., 1985). Obesity as defined as body weight 20% or more above average or standard weight appears to be the link between diabetes and essential hypertension in a large majority of cases. However about 15.0% of the study's hypertensive group were free of the other two conditions, and some 4.7% of the general population presented all three of them. Thus it can be estimated that nearly 1 out of 10 of those in middle age and having a Westernised lifestyle are heavier than

* Emeritus Professor of Medicine; Corresponding Author Email: seedaty1@gmail.com

normal weight, more or less glucose intolerant, and have systolic or diastolic hypertension (Ferranini & De Fronzo, 1989).

Hypertension is common in patients with diabetes. Studies within populations have shown that hypertension occurs more frequently in patients with diabetes than in nondiabetic individuals (Kannel & McGee, 1979). And it is more common for hypertensive patients to become diabetic than for diabetic patients to become hypertensive. Hypertension associated with diabetes may be of three types: a) systolic hypertension secondary to atherosclerosis, and about 2-5 times as prevalent in diabetes as in nonmatched nondiabetes; b) renal hypertension secondary to diabetic nephropathy; and c) essential hypertension.

Hyperinsulinaemia

Plasma insulin levels are consistently increased in obese subjects (Salans, 1981). Likewise, patients with impaired glucose tolerance usually are hyperinsulinaemic even if their body weight is normal. Thus it is possible that patients with impaired glucose tolerance usually are hyperinsulinaemic even if their body weight is normal (De Fronzo & Ferranini, 1982). Thus it is possible that hyperinsulinaemia could be one link between diabetes, obesity, and hypertension. The association between hyperinsulinism and hypertension was noted in a large Israeli Jewish population characterised by a high prevalence of glucose intolerance and diabetes. The patients were stratified for age and body mass. It was found that the prevalence of hypertension as well as the actual BP rose from normal to overt diabetes. They concluded that hypertension per se is associated with hyperinsulinaemia, and there is common ground for the cluster of diabetes, obesity, and essential hypertension (Modan et al., 1985).

INSULIN RESISTANCE

Insulin resistance is reduced or impaired response of target tissues to insulin stimulation (Salans, 1981; Ferranini & De Fronzo, 1989). Insulin resistance occurs in 25% of normal people (De Fronzo & Ferranini, 1982). The impact of insulin on glucose may be unrelated to impacts of insulin on carbohydrate, fat, protein, or electrolyte metabolism. Insulin resistance occurs in obesity and in noninsulin-dependent diabetes. The actions of insulin can be studied with the insulin clamp technique.

AETIOLOGY OF THE INSULIN-RESISTANT STATE

Several causes may be associated with the aetiology of the insulin-resistant state, including genetics, hyperinsulinaemia, increased level of androgen with central obesity, elevated levels of free fatty acid, ageing, physical inactivity, diabetes and/or obesity, pregnancy, oral contraceptive pill, glucocorticoids, growth hormone, alcohol, and smoking (Lundgren et al., 1988; Pollare, 1989)..

ROLE OF INSULIN IN CAUSING HYPERTENSION

Insulin can raise BP by increased sodium retention (De Fronzo, 1981), or insulin can stimulate the activity of the sympathetic nervous system. An increased concentration of noradrenaline leads to increase in heart rate, vasoconstriction, sodium retention, and elevated BP (Rowe et al., 1981). Insulin also affects the transport of positive ions across the cell membrane. This affects sodium, potassium, calcium, and magnesium. An altered salt concentration in the endothelial cell can reduce the contractility of skeletal and heart muscle (James et al., 1985; Hilton, 1986). In theory, elevated insulin levels can increase the contraction of the vascular wall, resulting in an elevated BP.

Obesity—The Harmful Male Type

Abdominal obesity, i.e., the male type of obesity, brings increased risk of cardiovascular disease, while female obesity of the hip and thigh is not associated with cardiovascular disease. Abdominal obesity is associated with the following features: a) higher fasting insulin levels, b) reduced glucose tolerance and an increased risk of hypertension and diabetes, c) reduced insulin sensitivity, d) blood lipid abnormalities, e) higher levels of free fatty acid, because adipose tissue is more sensitive to catecholamine lipolysis, and f) an increased number of fast-twitch, white muscle fibres in the thigh muscle. Abdominal obesity is associated with increased incidence of coronary heart disease (CHD) before ages 60-65 years.

Treatment

Treatment for obesity should be by weight reduction, a diet consisting of less fat and more fibre, and an increase in physical activity. Smokers should receive advice on how to stop. The entire cardiovascular profile can be improved with this regimen. Pharmacological agents that have no metabolic side effects should be considered. In the syndrome of hypertension, obesity, and diabetes, one should consider hypotensive agents that lower BP and enhance insulin sensitivity. In this setting, drugs should be considered that lower BP and improve insulin sensitivity, like angiotensin converting enzyme inhibitors. Of patients in one study who developed diabetes, 98% were treated with diuretics and/or beta blocking agents (Pollare et al., 1989).

Lifestyle

Two important low-cost measures are, first, a reduction of dietary salt and increased potassium intake, and second, a greater awareness of the serious implications of obesity. Increased exercise, decreased obesity, and cessation of smoking are all important in Blacks and whites in control of hypertension. Financial and cultural barriers constrain implementation of the DASH high-fruit, high-vegetable, low-salt diet which is very effective in U.S. Blacks. In Africa, one hypothesis is that the rural diet is relatively protective but is abandoned with urban exposure that entails less carbohydrate and higher fat intake. In West Africa, sodium restriction is feasible as a solitary measure, but to achieve general adoption, it requires persuasion at a governmental level and multiple messages from various sources, including rural clinics and television (Cappuccio et al., 2004). The major problem is how to get lifestyle messages across and how to implement them.

HYPERTENSION IN SUB-SAHARAN AFRICAN POPULATIONS

Hypertension in sub-Saharan African populations is a widespread problem of immense economic importance because of its high prevalence in urban areas, its frequent underdiagnosis, and the severity of its complications. Mass migration from rural to periurban and urban areas probably accounts at least in part for the high incidence of hypertension in urban black Africans. In semirural areas, inroads in lifestyle changes associated with "civilisation" may explain the apparently rising prevalence of hypertension. Significant segments of the African populations are still afflicted by severe poverty, famine, and civil strife, making the prevalence of hypertension difficult to determine. Black South Africans have a stroke rate twice as high as that of whites. Two lifestyle changes that are feasible and can help stem the hypertension epidemic in Africa are a decrease salt intake and a decrease in obesity, especially in women (Opie & Seedat, 2005).

Exact data are difficult to obtain in South African surveys. In 1983 our age-adjusted prevalence study (Seedat, 1983) of the adult population of Durban (World Health Organisation criteria $\geq$ 160 mm Hg) showed that hypertension was highest in urban Blacks of the Zulu tribe (25%), followed by whites (17%), ethnic Indians (14%), and lowest in rural Blacks (9%). The first Demographic and Health Survey in South Africa was conducted in 1998 in a random sample of 13,802 subjects aged 15 years or older, of whom 76% were Black, 13% of mixed ancestry, 8% white, and 3% Indian/Asiatic. The age-adjusted incidence of hypertension, namely BP ≥ 140/90 mm Hg on medication, measured automatically, for the predominantly Black South African population was 21% (equal rates among males and females). For those > 65 years of age, 50% to 60% were hypertensive (Steyn et al., 1998), a slightly higher rate than those of a similar age group in semi-urban West Africa (Cappuccio et al., 2004).

Increasing obesity has been associated with increasing BP levels in West African and U.S. Blacks. In the South African Demographic and Health Survey of 1998, the incidence of obesity (body mass index was about 30% in females and 8% in males) was as high as 40%-49% in females and 13% in men (Steyn et al., 1998). Abdominal obesity was particularly common in females. The more urbanised these communities were, the higher the rate of obesity and the less prudent their diets became. It is probable that the lower male prevalence relates in part to the higher rate of heavy manual labour.

Diabetes Mellitus in South African Indians

A dramatic increase in the prevalence of type 2 diabetes is observed in many parts of the Indian diaspora, which includes the United Kingdom, Mauritius, and Fiji. Whilst there are marked cultural and social differences within the Indian racial group, Indians have the unenviable distinction of achieving a high death rate from CHD. Much of this additional high risk of type 2 diabetes may be due to the increased risk of type 2 diabetes (four times that of Europeans), which develops in Indians about 10 years earlier than in South African whites (Seedat, 1999; Seedat, 2005).

In a community study (World Health Organization, 1985) to determine the prevalence and known risk factors for CHD of 778 subjects in the metropolitan area of Durban, diabetes mellitus was present in 15.8% (age and sex adjusted for 12.4% of the total sample).

INCIDENCE OF INSULIN RESISTANCE

Insulin resistance consists of glucose intolerance, hyperinsulinaemia, hypertension, dyslipidaemia, low plasma HDL cholesterol, and high triglyceride (Reaven, 1988).[21] We have found that important factors denoting insulin resistance were associated with hypertension; hypercholesterolaemia, low plasma HDL cholesterol, truncal obesity, diabetes, and hypertriglyceridaemia were clustered in Indians in Durban (Seedat et al., 1991).[22] The Indian population has been shown to have high plasma insulin levels with insulin glucose tolerance. Young Indian medical students develop metabolic risk factors for CHD at an early age, compared with young Black medical students (Morar et al., 1998). It has been suggested that insulin resistance in the South Asians of London, U.K., leads to a high incidence of CHD (McKeigue et al., 1991). We consider that this interesting concept could explain the high incidence of CHD in migrant Indians throughout the world.

Our study shows that diabetes mellitus is common in the South African Indian population. The aetiology may consist of insulin resistance, abnormal dietary patterns consisting of low energy intake, high intake of polyunsaturated fatty acids, low fibre intake, and physical inactivity (Wolmarans et al., 1999). Because of the higher risk of cardiovascular disease with diabetes, Indian patients should be treated, with lower thresholds for intervention, for hypertension, dyslipidaemia, and hyperglycaemia compared to white patients.

Coronary Heart Disease in Durban Blacks—Links in Urban Racial Groups

CHD is still relatively uncommon in the Black population of South Africa. We embarked on a study to determine the prevalence of risk factors leading to CHD in the Black population of Durban. A total of 458 patients attending a hospital dental clinic were studied. The prevalence of CHD was 2.4%. The prevalence of risk factors were as follows: hypertension (TSP ≥ 140 mm Hg systolic and/or ≥ 90 mm Hg diastolic), 28.0% (31.9% for males, 25.4% for females); protective levels of high-density lipoprotein / total cholesterol ≥ 20.0%, 81.3%; diabetes mellitus, 4.9% for males, 2.9% for females; smoking ≥ 10 cigarettes per day, 28.1% for males, 3.4% for females; obesity, 3.7% for males, 22.6% for females. We found the Minnesota Coding system for electrocardiographic changes and the Rose questionnaire to be unreliable for eliciting CHD in Blacks. Hypercholesterolaemia was found to be less common, and this may explain the low incidence of CHD in Blacks. Epidemics of CHD seen in Indian, Coloured, and white South Africans can still be prevented in the Black population, but preventive measures must be initiated rapidly (Seedat et al., 1992).

References

Cappuccio FP, Micah FB, Emmett L, Kerry SM, Anturi S, Martin-Peprah R, Phillips RO, Plange-Rhule J, Eastwood JB. 2004. Prevalence, detection, management and control of hypertension in Ashanti, West Africa. *Hypertension* 43; 1017-1022.

Christlieb AR. 1973. Diabetes and hypertensive vascular disease. Mechanisms and treatment. *Am J Cardiol* 59; 592-605.

De Fronzo RA. 1981. The effect of insulin on renal sodium metabolism. A review with clinical implications. *Diabetologia* 21; 165-171.

De Fronzo RA, Ferranini E. 1982. The pathogenesis of non-insulin-dependent diabetes. An update. *Medicine* 61; 121-160.

Ferranini E, De Fronzo RA. 1989. The association of hypertension, diabetes and obesity. A review. *J Nephrol* 1; 3-15.

Hilton PJ. 1986. Cellular sodium transport in essential hypertension. *N Engl J Med* 4; 222-229.

James DE, Jenkin AB, Kraegen EW. 1985. Heterogeneity of insulin action in individual muscle in vivo. Euglycemic clamp studies in rats. *Am J Physiol* 248; E567-E574.

Kannel WB, McGee DL. 1979. Diabetes and cardiovascular risk factors. The Framingham Study. *Circulation* 59; 8-13.

Lundgen H, Bjorkman L, Keiding P, Lundmark S, Bengtsson C. 1988. Diabetes in patients receiving pharmacological treatment. *Br Med J*; 297-1512.

McKeigue PM, Shah B, Marmot MG. 1991. Central obesity and cardiovascular risk in South Asians. *Lancet* 337: 382-386.

Modan M, Halkin H, Almog S, et al. 1985. Hyperinsulinemia. A link between hypertension, obesity and glucose intolerance. *J Clin Invest* 75; 809-817.

Morar N, Seedat YK, Naidoo D, Desai DK. 1998. Ambulatory blood pressure and risk factors for coronary heart disease in Black and Indian medical students. *J Cardiovasc Risk* 5; 313-318.

Opie LH, Seedat YK. 2005. Hypertension in Sub-Saharan African populations. *Circulation* 112; 3562-3568.

Pollare T. 1989. *Hypertension as part of a metabolic cardiovascular syndrome*. In: Waterson and Lungberg. Malmo, Sweden, p. 38.

Pollare T, Lithell H, Berne C. 1989. A comparison of the effects of hydrochlorothiazide and captopril on glucose and lipid metabolism in patients with hypertension. *N Engl J Med* 321; 868-873.

Reaven GM. 1988. Role of insulin resistance in human disease. *Diabetes* 37; 1595-1607.

Rowe JW, Young TB, Minaker KL, et al. 1981. Effect of insulin and glucose infusion on sympathetic nervous system in normal man. *Diabetes* 30; 219-225.

Salans LB. 1981. The obesities. In: Felig P, et al. (eds), *Endocrinology and Metabolism*. New York: McGraw-Hill, pp. 891-916.

Seedat YK. 1983. Race, environment and blood pressure. The South African experience. *J Hypertens* 1; 7-12.

Seedat YK. 1999. Coronary heart disease in South African Indians. *S Afr Med J suppl* 20; C76-C80.

Seedat YK. 2005. Epidemic of coronary heart disease in the migrant South African Indian population. In: Rav GHP, Thanikachalan S (eds), *Coronary Artery Disease: Risk Promoters, Pathophysiology and Prevention*. New Delhi: Jaypee Brothers, pp. 1-11.

Seedat YK, Mayet FGH, Joubert G. 1991. A study of coronary heart disease. *Cor Heart Dis* 2; 1089-1091.

Seedat YK, Mayet FGH, Latiff GH, Joubert G. 1992. Risk factors and coronary heart disease in Durban Blacks. The missing link. *S Afr Med J* 82; 251-256.

Steyn K, Gaziano TA, Bradshaw D. Laubscher R, Fourie J. 2001. *Hypertension in South African adults. Results from the Demographic and Health Survey 1998*; 1717-1725.

Wolmarans P, Seedat YK, Mayet FGH, Wentzel E. 1999. Dietary intake of Indians living in the metropolitan area of Durban. *Public Health Nutrition* 2; 55-60.

World Health Organisation. 1985. Diabetes mellitus. *WHO Technical Report Series No. 727.*

In: Obesity and Syndrome X
Editors: M. Das and K. Bose
ISBN: 978-1-53614-669-1

Chapter 2

METABOLIC SYNDROME IN THE PHILIPPINES AND ASIA: CONCEPTS AND CONCERNS

Gabriel V. Jasul[1,*], Jr., Rosa Allyn G. Sy[2,†] and Rodolfo F. Florentino[3,#]

[1]University of the Philippines College of Medicine,
Diabetes, Thyroid and Endocrine Center,
St. Luke's Medical Center, Quezon City, Philippines
[2]Research Development Innovation Division,
Ospital ng Makati, Metro Manila, and
Endocrinology, Diabetes, Metabolism and Nutrition Specialty Center,
Cardinal Santos Medical Center, San Juan, Metro Manila, Philippines

* Corresponding Author Email: Clinical Associate Professor, University of the Philippines College of Medicine, Head, Diabetes, Thyroid and Endocrine Center, St. Luke's Medical Center; Email: gjasul@yahoo.com.

† Director, Research Development Innovation Division, Ospital ng Makati, and Head, Endocrinology, Diabetes, Metabolism and Nutrition Specialty Center, Cardinal Santos Medical Center.

\# Chairman-President, Nutrition Foundation of the Philippines, Director, Food and Nutrition Research Institute, Department of Science and Technology.

[3]Nutrition Foundation of the Philippines, and
Food and Nutrition Research Institute, Department of Science
and Technology, Manila, Philippines

Metabolic syndrome is a clustering of interrelated risk factors namely, dysglycemia, increased blood pressure, elevated triglyceride levels, low high-density lipoprotein levels, and obesity, particularly central obesity. This syndrome has been known for decades now and has been observed with the rising prevalence of obesity and the modern-day sedentary lifestyle. Insulin resistance linked with central, essentially visceral, adiposity remains to be postulated as its underlying pathogenetic mechanism. It is significantly associated with increased risk for the development of cardiovascular disease, 2x and higher, and for type 2 diabetes mellitus, 5x and higher, in individuals fulfilling its diagnostic criteria (Alberti et al., 2009).

Defining the diagnostic criteria of the metabolic syndrome (MS) has been a major task of several health organizations representing major stakeholders in the fields of cardiovascular and metabolic diseases. Varying sets of diagnostic criteria have been recommended previously by different organizations such as the World Health Organization (WHO) in 1998, the European Group for the Study of Insulin Resistance (EGIR) in 1999, the National Cholesterol Education Program's Adult Treatment Panel III (ATP III) in 2001, the American Association of Clinical Endocrinologists (AACE) in 2003, the International Diabetes Federation (IDF) in 2005 and the American Heart Association (AHA) and National Heart, Lung and Blood Institute (NHLBI) also in 2005 (Sperling et al.,2015). The harmonized definition of the metabolic syndrome (summarized in Table 1) was issued in 2009 from the joint scientific statement of the International Diabetes Federation Task Force on Epidemiology and Prevention (IDF), National Heart, Lung and Blood Institute (NHLBI), American Heart Association (AHA), World Heart Federation (WHF), International Atherosclerosis Society (IAS) and the

International Association for the Study of Obesity (IASO) (Alberti et al., 2009, Sperling et al., 2015).

Metabolic syndrome evolved both as a public health and a clinical problem largely because obesity is at the core of this clustering that carries a very high cardiometabolic risk. The contribution of obesity is critical thus eliciting further examination of the nature of obesity, the phenotypic profile, including the age, gender, ethnicity of the individuals with this syndrome. It becomes evident that individual characteristics define the cardiometabolic profile of different populations that in turn define their cardiometabolic risk. Better measures of obesity, particularly central obesity, are necessary and hence, waist circumference as a simple and cost-effective measure of central obesity is a critical criterion in diagnosing metabolic syndrome. The important ethnic-specific and gender-specific cut-offs for waist circumference reflects the epidemiologic evidence of the differences in cardiometabolic risk between individuals and between populations (Bluher, 2014, Seo and Rhee, 2014).

Table 1. Criteria for the clinical diagnosis of metabolic syndrome (MS)

Measure	Categorical cut points
Elevated waist circumference	Population or country-specific definitions
Elevated triglycerides (drug treatment for increased triglycerides is an alternate indicator)	>150 mg/dl
Reduced HDL-cholesterol (drug treatment for low HDL is an alternate indicator)	Males: <40 mg/dl Females: < 50 mg/dl
Elevated blood pressure (antihypertensive drug treatment for elevated BP is an alternate indicator)	Systolic BP >130 mm Hg and/or Diastolic BP >85 mm Hg
Elevated fasting glucose (drug treatment for elevated blood sugar is an alternate indicator)	FPG >100 mg/dl

NOTE: The use of ethnic-specific cut-offs for waist circumference is recommended and thus applied. The Asian cut-offs, >90 cm for males and >80 cm for females are used for the Philippine data from 2008. The presence of 3 of 5 criteria in each individual fulfills the diagnosis of metabolic syndrome.

Given this general background on metabolic syndrome, the current discussion will now focus on the epidemiology of this syndrome among Filipino adults, the similarities in the cardiometabolic profile of other Asian and Asia-Pacific populations vis-à-vis their Caucasian and non-Asian counterparts. The increasing prevalence of overweight and obesity is apparently driving the global diabetes epidemic and the consequent rise in cardiovascular and related diseases. This chain of events in the face of nutrition and lifestyle transition in amidst Westernization in developing countries is further magnified in the Asia-Pacific region where the majority of people with new-onset type 2 diabetes reside. Approximately half of the 422 million adults with diabetes in 2014 are from the Southeast Asia and Western Pacific regions (WHO 2016). The magnitude of the obesity problem, while clearly on the rise as well in these regions, is not proportional to the staggering diabetes burden in these regions.

Table 2. Survey data used for Figure 1

	Survey year	Prevalence of overweight adults (%)*	Prevalence of obese adults (%)†	Prevalence of diabetes (%)
USA	1999-2000[53]	34·0	30·0	
	1999-2000[33]			8·2
India	1998-99[54]	10·0	2·2	
	2000[21]			12·1
Philippines	1998[55]	16·9	3·3	
	1996[56]			5·1
Taiwan	1993-96[57]	21·1	4·0	
	1996[34]			9·2
Hong Kong	1996-97[58]	25·1	3·8	
	1995-96[59]			9·8
China	1999-2000[53]	25·0	4·0	
	2000-2001[29]			5·5
Singapore	1998[60]	24·4	6·0	
	1992[32]			8·4
Korea	2001[61]	27·4	3·2	
	2001[24]			7·6
Thailand	1998[62]	28·3	6·8	
	1995[35]			11·9

*25 kg/m²≤BMI<30 kg/m². †BMI≥30 kg/m².

Source: Yoon, Lee, et al., *Lancet* 2006; 368: 1684.

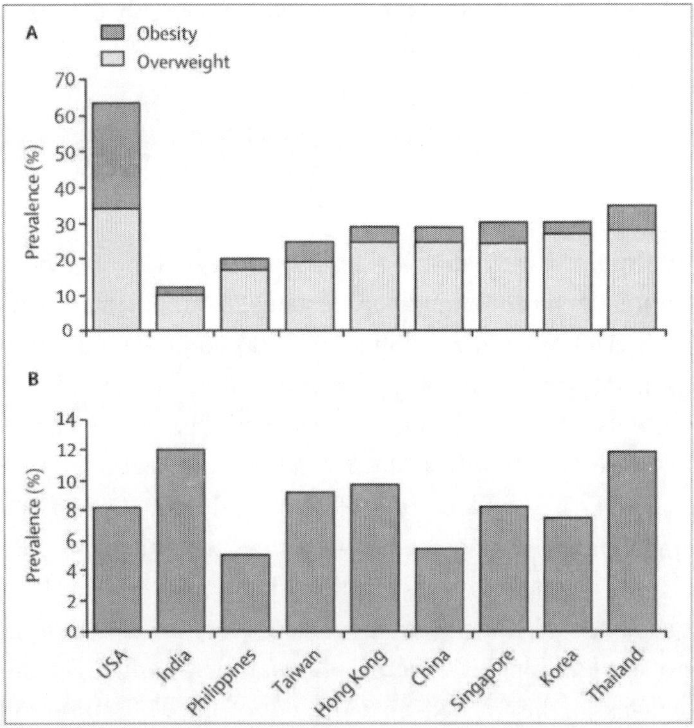

Source: Yoon, Lee et al. *Lancet* 2006; 368:1684.

Figure 1. International comparison of prevalence of adult obesity and diabetes. (A) Proportion of overweight and obese adults, (B) Prevalence of diabetes.

In an international comparison in 2003, with 34% and 30% of Americans being overweight and obese, respectively, the US national prevalence of diabetes was 8.2%. The overweight and obese Asians, on the other hand, ranged then from 10 to 28% and 2 to 6.8%, respectively in 7 countries (India, Philippines, Taiwan, Hong Kong, China, Singapore, Korea, and Thailand)and yet the average diabetes prevalence in these countries already ranged from 5 to 12% (Figure 1 and Table 2) (Yoon, Lee, et al., 2006). Diabetes, an important component of the metabolic syndrome, appears to develop among Asians, including Filipinos, at lower levels of obesity. It thus becomes important to examine closely the distinguishing characteristics of Filipinos, and Asians for that matter, with metabolic syndrome.

The Philippine Data on the Metabolic Syndrome

In the Philippines, the national nutrition survey (NNS) provides critical data on food intake, nutrition and health status of Filipinos as mandated by Executive Order 352 guiding policy and decision-making in both the government and private sectors. Since the first survey in 1978, this statistical activity has been done regularly by the Food and Nutrition Research Institute (FNRI) of the Department of Science and Technology (DOST). The NNS has evolved in 1998 during the 5th NNS to include the clinical component in collaboration with the Department of Health and various health agencies and groups including medical specialty organizations. The NNS has been conducted every 5 years throughout the 17 regions of the Philippines covering the National Capital Region (NCR) and 80 provinces. In the 8th NNS in 2013, out of the 97.7 million Filipinos, 45,047 households with 172, 323 persons were used for the multi-staged stratified sampling design. The 9th NNS will be undertaken this year (2018). The NNS is clearly a veritable source of health information including prevalence and trends of leading health problems including non-communicable diseases in the country. The Philippine data on metabolic syndrome under discussion are derived from various reports, published papers and unpublished data from the NNS. (FNRI-DOST reports/pdf files, www.fnri.dost.gov.ph>nutrition-statistic). A few published articles outside the NNS have been included to elucidate the problem of metabolic syndrome in the Philippines.

From the 5th NNS (1998), analysis of data from 4541 Filipino adults aged 20 years and over showed the proportion of subjects with co-morbid factors increased with high fasting blood sugar (FBS), except for high cholesterol. Having high body mass index (BMI $\geq$ 25), high waist-hip ratio (WHR $\geq$ 1.0 in males, $\geq$0.85 in females) and high waist circumference (WC $\geq$ 102 cm in males, $\geq$88 cm in females) in combination was associated with highest prevalence of high FBS in males (35.8%) and in females (14.5%) and with highest prevalence of hypertension in males (66.5%). Among females, the highest prevalence rate of hypertension (37.95) was seen among those with high FBS. This study indicated that waist circumference, with the higher cut-offs used, was the best predictor of metabolic risks, particularly of diabetes mellitus (Tanchoco et al., 2003).

Prevalence of metabolic syndrome among the same 4541 Filipino adults from the 5th NNS was determined using the NCEP and the IAS criteria in another study. For the IAS criteria, the Asian cut-offs for waist circumference, >90 cm in males and >80 cm in females, were used. Based on the NCEP criteria, the prevalence of metabolic syndrome was 14.2% and when stratified according to age, 6.6% (ages 20-39 years), 17.7% (ages 40-59 years), and 18.3% (ages 60 years and older). Using the IAS criteria, the prevalence of metabolic syndrome was 19.3% and with age stratification, 10.0%, 23.6%, and 24.1%, respectively. The study concluded that metabolic syndrome was common in this population and increased in prevalence with age. It was also noted that using NCEP criteria, instead of the IAS criteria, underestimated the prevalence of metabolic syndrome (Punzalan et al., 2004).

The 6th NNS, also called the National Nutrition and Health Survey (NNHeS) 2003-2004, also integrated the clinical component similar to the 5th NNS but also determined, for the first time, the national prevalence of 24 diseases and 11risk factors. Using 3 sets of definitions/criteria of the metabolic syndrome, namely, NCEP/ATP III (2001), IDF (2005) and NCEP/ATP III-AHA/NHLBI (2005), the prevalence of metabolic syndrome in the adult Filipinos aged 20 years and older was found to be 11.9%, 14.5%, and 18.6%, respectively. Low levels of high-density lipoprotein cholesterol (HDL-C), mean level of 41.3 mg/dL, were seen in 60.2% of men and 80.9% of women, making it the most common component of the syndrome in the population (70.2%), similarly observed in the previous 5th NNS with prevalence of 84%. The prevalence rates of the other MS components were as follows: blood pressure >130/≥85, 33.3%, abdominal obesity (WC ≥ 90 cm, male, ≥80 female), 26.1%, triglycerides ≥150 mg/dL, 20.6% and fasting blood sugar >100 mg/dL,

7.1%. Age-adjusted odds ratios showed that MS, by all 3 criteria, predisposed an individual to diabetes mellitus and stroke while MS using the IDF definition predisposed an individual to myocardial infarction (Morales et al., 2008).

In the analysis of data from the 7th NNS/ NNHeS 2008, the prevalence rate of MS utilizing the harmonized definition (Table 3) was 27.4%, significantly higher than the reported 18.6% in 2003. The prevalence rates of the individual components of MS similarly showed significant increases as follow: low HDL-C, 80.3%, abnormal BP, 39.3%, abdominal obesity, 29.8%, increased triglycerides, 30.1%, and elevated FBS, 12.2%. Both age and gender-related differences continued to be observed as in the previous NNS. Age-related increases in MS peaked in the age groups 50-59 years and 60-69 years, remaining high after age 70 years. Females had more abdominal obesity and lower HDL-C while men had higher BP and higher triglycerides (Table 4) (Jasul, unpublished data, 2008).

More rigorous analysis of the data from the 7215 Filipino adults from the 7th NNS/NNHeS 2008 concluded that the prevalence rates of measured variables, particularly the components of MS and the risk factors for atherosclerosis, were higher compared with values obtained in 2003.

Table 3. Prevalence of metabolic syndrome among Filipino adults aged 20 years and above, based on the harmonized definition of the IDF, NHLBI, AHA, WHF, IAS and IASO 2009: NNHeS 2008

Age (years)	Males % (SE)	Females% (SE)	Both sexes % (SE)
20 - 29	12.3 (1.27)	8.4 (1.14)	10.4 (0.86)
30 - 39	26.7 (1.79)	20.1 (1.61)	23.3 (1.22)
40 - 49	31.7 (1.97)	31.5 (1.80)	31.6 (1.40)
50 - 59	38.9 (2.42)	45.6 (2.20)	42.7 (1.74)
60 - 69	28.3 (2.87)	46.8 (2.85)	38.7 (2.13)
>70	15.8 (3.13)	38.3 (3.30)	29.3 (2.40)
All	**25.8 (0.87)**	**28.9 (0.92)**	**27.4 (0.67)**

Table 4. Prevalence of the individual components of metabolic syndrome (MS) among Filipino adults aged 20 years and above, by sex

MS Component	Male % (SE)	Female % (SE)	Total % (SE)
Waist circumference Male>=90 cm, Female >= 80 cm	17.8 (0.77)	41.0 (0.97)	29.8 (0.72)
Triglycerides.=150 mg/dl	37.9 (0.95)	23.2 (0.80)	30.1 (0.67)
HDL,Males < 40 mg/dl, Females < 50 mg/dl	71.6 (0.90)	88.1 (0.71)	80.3 (0.62)
Blood Pressure, >=130/>=85 mm Hg	44.4 (0.98)	35.0 (0.88)	39.3 (0.70)
Fasting Blood Sugar, >=100 mg/dl	11.9 (0.47)	11.6 (0.65)	12.2 (0.62)

Among adult Filipinos aged 20 years or older, the true prevalence of hypertension was 20.6% and the prevalence of diabetes was 3.9% based on fasting blood glucose (FBG), 5.2% by FBG and history, and 6.2% with 2-hour post-load plasma glucose was determined. Obesity, defined as BMI ≥ 30, was seen in 4.9% but obesity defined by abnormal waist-hip ratio (WHR) of 1.0 or higher in men and 0.85 in women, was seen in 10.2% and in 65.6%, respectively (Sy et al., 2012).

Table 5. Prevalence of blood glucose abnormalities among Filipino adults aged 20 years and above: NNHeS 2008

Glucose abnormalities	Male	Female	Total
Impaired Fasting Glucose (IFG) (FBG >100 and <125 mg/dl) (%)	7.9	6.7	7.2
Impaired Glucose Tolerance (IGT) (2-hr PPBG >140 and <199 mg/dl) (%)	6.7	7.3	7.0
Combined IFG/IGT (%)	0.4	0.6	0.5
Diabetes Mellitus, DM (FPG >126 and 2-hr PPBG >200 mg/dl)(%)	7.0	7.4	7.2

Patterns of glucose abnormalities were analyzed in a sub-study of the 7th NNS/NNHeS 2008 to address the contrasting data on prevalence and incidence rates reported from studies outside the NNS. Using FBS, 2-hour post-load glucose and DM questionnaire, the true diabetes prevalence was 7.2% and the prevalence of pre-diabetes was summed at 10.2%, with impaired fasting glucose (IFG), 2.7%, impaired glucose tolerance (IGT),

7.0% and both IFG/IGT, 0.5% (Table 5). Differences in the prevalence rates of diabetes between urban and rural populations were significant at 8.3% versus 5.8%, respectively (Jimeno et al., 2015).

From the results of the 8thNNS/NNHeS 2013, the burden of non-communicable diseases (NCDs) was reported and summarized as prevalence rates of selected risk factors. NCDs accounted for two-thirds (67%) of total deaths in the country in 2012. Obesity (BM I> = 30) was seen in 6.8% (males, 5.2%, females, 8.3%), with higher rates in urban areas (10.1%, National Capital Region (NCR)) than rural areas (around 4% in Ilocos Region, Cagayan Valley, Western Visayas, Autonomous Region in Muslim Mindanao (ARMM)). Combining overweight and obesity (BMI >=25) totaled 31.1% of adult population (males, 27.6%, females, 34.4%), simply put, three out of ten Filipinos were overweight or obese. Central or android obesity, based on high waist circumference (males, ≥102 cm, females, >88 cm), was seen in 3.8% of males and 23.1% of females and based on high waist-to-hip ratio (WHR) (males >1.0, females ≥0.85), was seen in 8% of males and 63.2% of females. Hypertension (SBP ≥ 140, DBP ≥ 90) was present in 22.3% of the adult population (males, 25.1%, females, 19.9%) while diabetes (fasting blood sugar (FBG) ≥ 126 mg/dl) was seen in 5.4% (males, 5.6%, females, 5.3%).

Abnormal cholesterol levels were reported as follows: total cholesterol (TC borderline 200-239 mg/dl to high >240 mg/dl), 46.9% (males, 41.5%, females, 51.4%), LDL cholesterol (LDL-C borderline 130-159 mg/dl to high >160 mg/dl), 47.2% (males, 40%, females, 53.6%) and triglycerides (TG borderline 150-199 mg/dl, high 200-399 mg/dl to very high >400 mg/dl), 38.6% (males, 46.4%, females, 31.8%). Low HDL cholesterol (HDL-C males, <40 mg/dl, females, <50 mg/dl) was seen in 71.3% (males, 63.2%, females, 78.2%). Insufficient physical activity (not meeting 3 or more days of vigorous-intensity activity of at least 20 minutes per day or 5 or more days of moderate-intensity activity or walking of at least 30 minutes per day) was seen in 45.2% (males, 36.7%, females, 52.7%) (FNRI DOST, 2013).

Prevalence of MS has not been reported from the 8th NNS/NNHeS 2013 data but clearly, the prevalence rates of the MS components remained significantly high. The trends in the prevalence rates of these important risk factors reflect continuing rise from 1993 (4th NNS) to 2013 (8th NNS). The accompanying figures (Figures 2-5) illustrate these alarming trends that point to unabated increasing cardiometabolic risk in the general adult Filipino population. While the prevalence of chronic energy deficiency has been slowly deceasing, the prevalence of overweight and obesity has almost doubled (Figure 2). The data on the pediatric age groups also show increasing trend but to a much lesser degree. Overweight in children below ten years of age was seen in around 2% and among adolescents, less than 5%. Central obesity has been similarly increasing and more markedly among females (Figure 3). Hypertension prevalence has been relatively steady in the 21-25% range (Figure 4) but the trends in high fasting glucose has been steadily increasing (Figure 5) (FNRI DOST 2013). The measures of glucose abnormality have varied in the different NNS and estimation of the true prevalence of diabetes mellitus may be limited by this variation, as addressed by Jimeno et al., (2015).

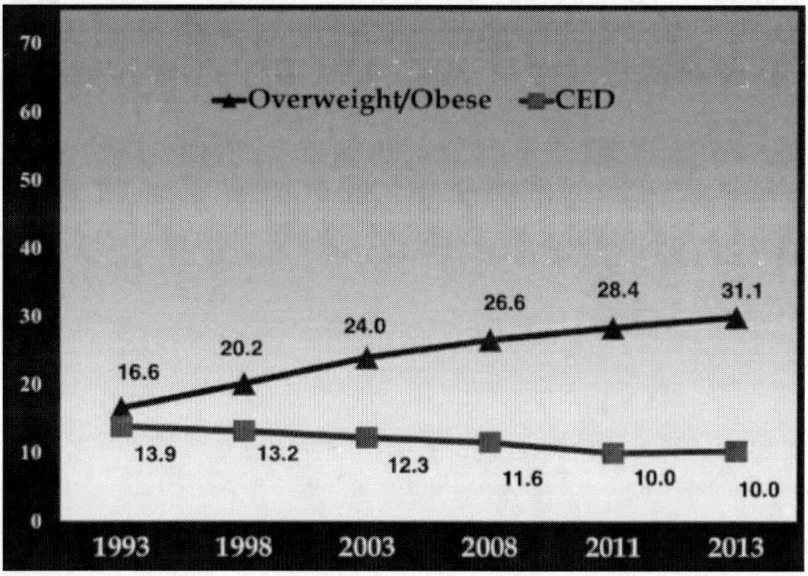

Figure 2. Prevalence of malnourished adults, >20 years old, Philippines, 1993-2013.

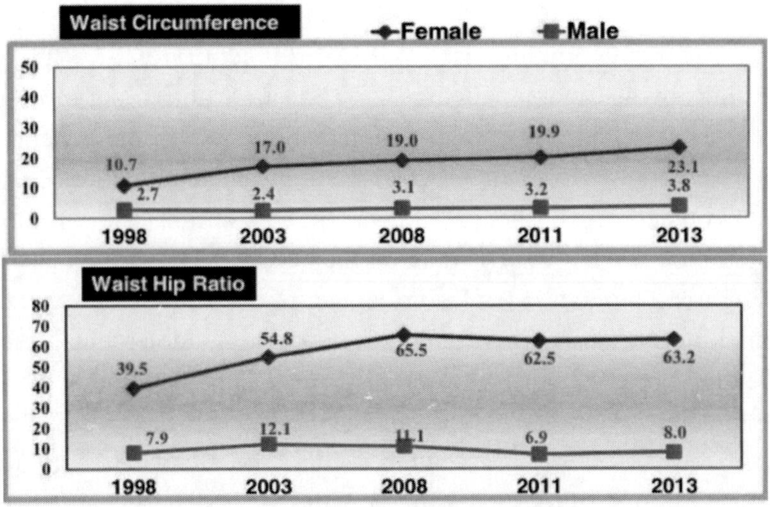

Figure 3. Trends in high waist circumference and high waist hip ratio prevalence among adults, 20 years old and over, Philippines, 1998-2013.

Differences in the cut-offs in the measured variables are common in published literature on obesity and metabolic syndrome. Determination of the cut-offs for BMI, WC and WHR that will help define levels of risk of co-morbidities was undertaken using data from the 6th NNS/NNHeS 2003. This sub analysis from the 2003 results emphasized that with increasing body fatness, there is an increasing risk of related co-morbidities among adult Filipinos. The tentative cut-offs associated with risk of co-morbidities were BMI of 23 for overweight and 27 for obesity, WC of 90 cm for males and 85 cm for women and WHR of 1.0 for males and 0.95 for females. These tentative cut-offs were closer to the recommended cut-offs for Asia-Pacific islanders and Asians from the International Obesity Task Force (AP/IOTF) and were considerably lower than the WHO cut-offs (Florentino and Duante, unpublished data, 2004).

Similar analysis was done using the 7th NNS/NNHeS 2008 results and concluded that the odds of developing 2 or more risk factors among adult Filipinos were noted even at a much lower BMI (18 kg/m2) in both males and females. The tentative cut-offs from the 2008 data were BMI of 22.5 for overweight and 27 for obesity, WC of 78 cm for both males and females and WHR of > = 0.92 for males and > = 0,88 for females. These cut-offs were almost similar to the 2003 tentative cut-offs of the AP/IOTF (Duante, unpublished data, 2008).

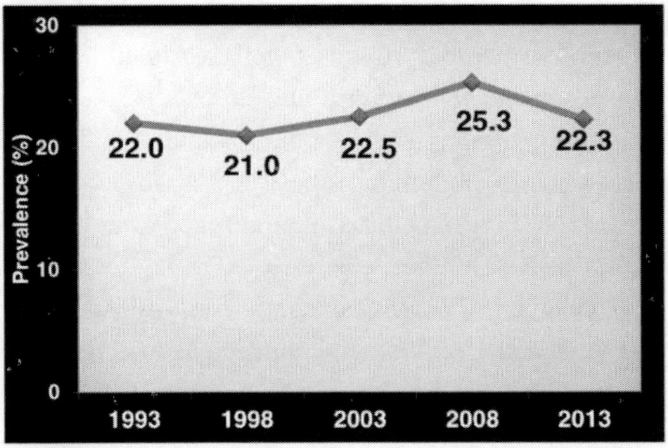

Based on single visit BP determination using the 7th Joint National Committee (JNC 7)
p-value< 0.0001

Figure 4. Trends in the prevalence of hypertension among adults >20 years old in the Philippines: 1993, 1998, 2003, 2008 and 2013.

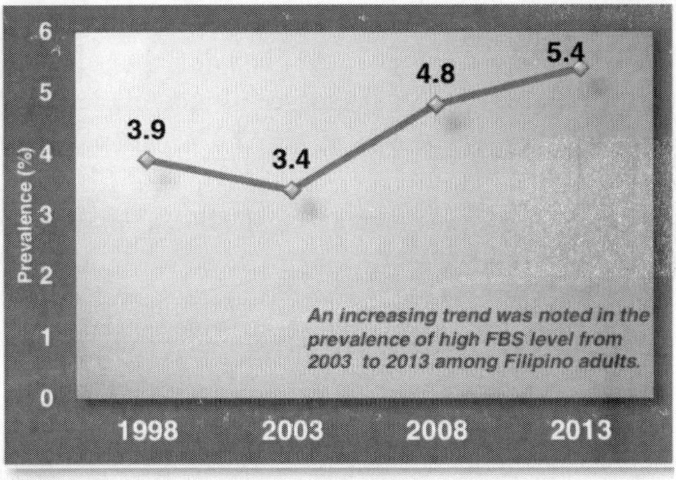

p-value: 0.0336

Figure 5. Trends in the prevalence of high fasting blood glucose among adults >20 years old, Philippines: 1998, 2003, 2008 and 2013.

Several studies independent of the NNS/NNHeS revealed similar findings of a very different profile of MS in Filipinos compared to Caucasians/non-Asians. In the Philippine cohort of the LIFECARE longitudinal study in Asia, 3,702 Filipinos aged 20 to 50 years old from Metro Manila and four nearby provinces were recruited. Prevalence of MS was 19.7%, based on the IDF criteria and 25.6%, based on the modified NCEP (mNCEP) or harmonized criteria (Table 1). The IDF criteria required the presence of abdominal obesity plus any 2 of the other risk factors while the mNCEP defined it as the presence of any 3 or more of the risk factors. This basic difference was reflected in higher MS prevalence in women by IDF, higher MS prevalence in men by mNCEP, with IDF missing 40% of men and 10% women identified as having MS by mNCEP. More males were categorized as having MS by mNCEP despite relatively normal waist circumference (mean WC 80.6 cm). MS was associated with increasing age, urban residence and employed status (Sy et al., 2014).

In the Cebu Longitudinal Health and Nutrition Survey (CLHNS), the community-based survey followed a cohort of infants born in 1983 to 1984 with surveys immediately after birth, bimonthly for two years, in 1991, 1994-5, 1998-99, 2002, and 2005. In 2005, fasting blood were drawn for CVD biomarkers and genetics and 1,621 individuals aged 20-21 years (889 men and 732 women) were included in the cluster analysis using biomarkers. The study identified 5 distinct sex-specific clusters: 1) healthy/high HDL (with the addition of high LDL-C in women), 2) healthy/low blood pressure, 3) high blood pressure, 4) insulin resistant/high triglycerides, and 5) high C-reactive protein. Low HDL-C was the most prevalent risk factor at 65%. Men had higher prevalence of elevated triglycerides and hypertension while women had higher prevalence of low HDL-C, elevated LDL-C and elevated HOMA-IR. Adiposity was most strongly associated with insulin-resistant/high triglyceride cluster. In this young (aged 20-21 years) and lean population (mean BMI 20-21, mean WC 72 cm (men), 68, (women), with 18% prevalence of overweight) with no significant clinical disease, cluster analysis identified patterns of cardiometabolic risk factors. Diet and environmental factors also influenced the predicted clustering of risk factors. The importance of screening both lean and overweight individuals for cardiometabolic risk was thus emphasized in such populations where the cardiometabolic risk is elevated even at lower BMI (Zubair et al., 2014).

In a rural community-based cross-sectional observational study in San Juan, Batangas, optimal cut-offs for BMI, WC and WHR for risk for cardiometabolic diseases were determined among 332 individuals, mean age of 48.4 years and 72% of whom were women. The optimal cut-offs for males and females were BMI of 24 and 23 kg/m^2, WC of 84 and 77 cm and WHR of 0.91 and 0.85, respectively. Similar to the analyses by Florentino and Duante and by Duante, lower indices of overweight and obesity, were associated with cardiometabolic diseases among Filipino adults in this rural community (Pagsisihan et al., 2016).

In a retrospective study of 1367 patient seen at the wellness center and the weight management center of a Philippine tertiary hospital, the prevalence of metabolic syndrome, defined by the mNCEP/harmonized criteria, and its individual components was determined across the different BMI categories. While the study population (mean age 53 years, mean BMI of 28 kg/m^2, and mean WC of 96.8 cm) did not reflect the general Filipino population, the finding of high prevalence of MS even in individuals with normal BMI (Table 6) suggests that cardiometabolic abnormalities are present even at lower and normal BMI levels (Mata and Jasul, 2017).

Table 6. Presence of metabolic syndrome in relation to different BMI categories and gender

BMI Category	Metabolic Syndrome		
	Male n (%)	Female n (%)	Total with Metabolic Syndrome n (%)
Normal (18.5-22.9 kg/m^2)	13 (21)	48 (33.3)	61 (29.6)
Overweight (23-24.9 kg/m^2)	41 (37.3)	59 (40.1)	100 (38.9)
Pre-obese (25-29.9 kg/m^2)	159 (60.5)	130 (53.1)	289 (56.9)
Obese (≥30 kg/m^2)	135 (64.6)	112 (69.9)	247 (62.4)
Overall			697 (51.0)

THE ASIAN DATA ON THE METABOLIC SYNDROME

In developing countries, the prevalence of obesity and metabolic syndrome is rapidly rising with the main causes all related to economic progress, namely, urbanization, nutrition transition and physical inactivity. This public health problem carries enormous burden of increased morbidity and mortality due to type 2 diabetes mellitus and cardiovascular disease and consequent effects on health expenditures and economic productivity. Nutrition transitioning led to a decrease in the undernourished population and an increase in the over nourished population. This development is mirrored in the Philippines as described in the previous section of this discussion. Since the 1980s, obesity rates have increased three-fold or more in the Middle East, the Pacific Islands, Australasia, and China. Compiled data from developing countries on obesity, defined using varying BMI and WC cut-offs, showed rates as low as 2.9% to as high as 68%. Differences were evident based on gender, urban versus rural residence, educational attainment, and socioeconomic status, among others. Reported rates of metabolic syndrome using different definitions ranged from 6.5% to 46.5% in developing countries (Misra and Khurana, 2008).

Surveys from East Asian and Southeast Asian populations consistently showed increase in the prevalence of metabolic abnormalities associated with abdominal adiposity with cited MS prevalence of 10 to 30% using Asian-adapted definitions of obesity (BMI $\geq$ 25 kg/m^2) and increased WC (males, $\geq$90 cm, females, >80 cm) (Nestel, et al., 2007). Defining obesity in the different Asian populations has become critical with the generally accepted observation that metabolic risks are greater in Asians than Caucasians at a given BMI. The inter-ethnic differences in percent body fat at a given BMI and in the metabolic responses to fatness have to be considered in setting which appropriate cut-offs to use for Asians in general and for individual ethnic groups (Pan and Yeh, 2008).

Considerations of the ethnic differences in abdominal and visceral fat distribution began early in the Asia-Pacific region. The influence of dietary patterns and physical activity on fat distribution and the development of MS even at lower or normal BMI supported the perspective that lower optimal cut-offs should be used not only for screening but also for strategies for intervention. Attention to lifestyle modification has been pushed early on in the Asia-Pacific region through public health initiatives to stem the tide of obesity and metabolic syndrome (Gill, 2001, Sullivan, 2001).

Recent systematic reviews however showed that the rising problem of MS in Asia remains staggering. Data from 15 Asia-Pacific countries showed the range of the prevalence rates of MS from a low of 11.9% in the Philippines to a high of 49% in urban Pakistan. Higher prevalence in women and in urban dwellers was consistent findings. Temporal trends were available for China, South Korea and Taiwan and all showed increasing prevalence for all three countries from 1993 to 2009. Despite differences in methodology, diagnostic criteria and age of subjects studied, MS is of epidemic proportion in the Asia-Pacific region, with nearly one-fifth of the adult population affected by MS in most countries (Ranasinghe et al., 2017).

Similar trends were reported in South Asia in a recent systematic review of 16 MS population-based prevalence studies from 5 countries. Four definitions of MS were used and the weighted mean prevalence rates of MS were 14.0% (WHO), 26.1% (ATPIII), 29.8% (IDF) and 32.5% (modified ATPIII). Half of the study population had low HDL-C levels and had hypertension. In general, females had a higher prevalence of MS and were more likely to have low HDL-C levels and central obesity. Males, on the other hand, were more hypertensive. These gender-based findings are consistent with the MS profile in Filipino and other Asian populations. Research remains limited despite the enormous burden of MS especially in Asian populations (Aryal and Wasti, 2006).

METABOLIC SYNDROME IN MIGRANT FILIPINOS AND MIGRANT ASIANS IN WESTERN COUNTRIES

Emerging data have shown that cardiometabolic diseases are common in Asian Americans despite mean lower BMI. Asian Americans are the fastest growing ethnic group in the US, numbering over 18 million in 2011. Filipino Americans (3.4 millions) are second only to the Chinese Americans (4.0 millions) and followed by Asian Indians (3.2 millions) and the rest of the migrant Asian population (Vietnamese, Korean and Japanese) (Hsu, et al., 2015). Striking differences in the risk of CVD, obesity, type 2 diabetes mellitus, hypertension, and other CVD risk factors are observed across the Asian-American population (Narayan et al., 2010). The large and the rising number of Asian Americans and their apparent high cardiometabolic risk present an important public health challenge needing better understanding and timely intervention (Palaniappan et al., 2011).

Seminal work by Araneta et al., showed that Filipina women aged 50 to 69 years, compared to Caucasian women, had larger WC and higher percentages of truncal fat, were less likely to be obese, less likely to smoke, consume alcohol, or take postmenopausal estrogen, and had lower HDL-C levels. Filipina women had higher prevalence of type 2 diabetes (36% vs 9%) and MS (34 vs. 13%). A total of 10% of Filipinas with diabetes were obese, compared with over 30% of Caucasians with diabetes. The high prevalence of diabetes in a non-obese ethnic group led to a realization that there is diversity in the development of diabetes across populations and that this high diabetes risk might be missed if Western standards of obesity were applied (Araneta et al., 2002).

Subsequent studies indicated that many Filipino Americans suffer from chronic illnesses, particularly type 2 diabetes, hypertension and dyslipidemia and central adiposity is a common. MS was seen in 18.3% of Filipino American men and women in Clark County, Nevada. Abdominal obesity was seen in 80.6%; hypertension in 47.7%; overweight in 36.7%; and type 2 diabetes in 11.7% (Dalusung-Angosta, 2013). Review of literature on the cardiovascular health of Filipinos in the US from 27 published studies concluded that Filipino Americans were at high risk for CVD, hypertension, type 2 diabetes and MS at lower BMI levels (Abesamis et al., 2015). A cross-sectional study of 335 Filipinos living in Rome, Italy similarly showed high prevalence of abdominal obesity (52.5%), BMI > 25 kg/m^2 (44.5%), diabetes (6%), and hypertension (9%). Age and WC were associated with both diabetes and hypertension (Gentilucci et al., 2008).

Patterns seen in Filipino and Asian populations manifested as well in Asian Americans, similarly requiring the need to define obesity indices to better predict risk of developing diabetes and hypertension. In the Filipino American women cardiovascular study, using Asian-specific thresholds for BMI, WC and WHR increased the accuracy of prediction (Battie, et al., 2016). The high incidence of type 2 diabetes in non-obese Asian Americans, particularly Asian Indian and Filipinos, led to the recommendation that screening for type 2 diabetes in these populations should start at BMI of 23kg/m^2 (Wang et al., 2011, Hsu et al., 2015). Differences in the body fat percentages and body fat distribution are evident not only between Asian Americans and other ethnic groups but also between Asian Americans and Asian immigrants. These differences may largely affect susceptibility to developing cardiometabolic diseases (Alpert and Thomason, 2016, Unjali et al., 2017). Better measures of obesity, lower cut-offs for BMI, WC and WHR as indices of cardiometabolic risk, and even newer indices such as triglyceride glucose (TyG), TyG waist circumference (TyG-WC), TyG-BMI and visceral adiposity index (VAI) may be helpful in predicting risk of developing cardiometabolic diseases, especially type 2 diabetes (Zheng, et al., 2016).

Conclusion and Recommendations

Metabolic syndrome, as a public health and a clinical problem, develops along with increasing obesity. Distinct characteristics between individuals and between populations dictate the attendant cardiometabolic risk in metabolic syndrome. Filipinos, like other Asians, appear to develop metabolic syndrome at lower or even normal BMI levels and this observation maybe explained by higher visceral fat percentages. Gene-environment interaction evidently happened when westernization altered the lifestyle, dietary and physical activity patterns that led to obesity and metabolic syndrome. However, the similarities in cardiometabolic features in Philippine-based Filipinos and migrant Filipinos, as well as Asian residents and migrant Asians, are evidences of strong genetic influences in the disease causation. Characterization of the genetic factors underlying metabolic syndrome will help towards its better understanding, prevention and management. Definition of the syndrome with a universally accepted set of criteria with adjusted cut-offs for ethnic groups should be a goal so that future studies have standardized definitions, making comparisons meaningful. Population-based surveys on metabolic syndrome should be continued along with intervention studies to minimize, if not prevent, the attendant cardiometabolic risk.

References

Abesamis CJ, Fruh S, Hall H, Lemley T. 2015. Cardiovascular health of Filipinos in the United States: A review of the literature. *J Transcultural Nursing*. 1-11.

Alberti KGMM, Eckel,RH, Grundy SM, Zimmet PZ, Cleeman JM, Donato KA, Fruchart JC, James PT, Loria CM, Smith Jr., SC. 2009. Harmonizing the metabolic syndrome: A joint statement of the International Diabetes Federation Task Force on Epidemiology and Prevention; National Heart, Lung, and Blood Institute; American Heart Association; World Heart Federation; International Atherosclerosis Society; and International Association for the Study of Obesity. *Circulation*. 120:1640-1645.

Alpert PT and Thomason D. 2016. Metabolic syndrome: Differences for Asian Americans is in their body fat percentages. *Asian/Pacific Island Nursing J*. 1(3): 70-81.

Araneta MRG, Wingard DL, Barrett-Connor E. 2002. Type 2 diabetes and metabolic syndrome in Filipina-American women: A high-risk nonobese population. *Diabetes Care*. 25: 494-499.

Aryal N and Wasti SP. 2016. The prevalence of metabolic syndrome in South Asia: a systematic review. *Int J Diabetes Dev Ctries*. 36(3):255-262.

Battie CA, Borja-Hart N, Ancheta IB, Flores R, Rao G, Palaniappan L. 2016. Comparison of body mass index, waist circumference, and waist to height ratio in the prediction of hypertension and diabetes mellitus: Filipino-American women cardiovascular study. *Prev Med Rep*. 4:608-613.

Bluhe, M. 2014. Are metabolically healthy obese individuals really healthy? *Eur J Endocrinol*. 171:R209-R219.

Dalusung-Angosta A. 2013. Prevalence of metabolic syndrome among Filipino-Americans: A cross-sectional study. *Appl Nurs Res*. 26(4): 192-197.

Duante CA for the *7th National Nutrition and Health Survey* (2008) Philippines. Unpublished data.

Eckel RH, Kahn SE, Ferrannini E, Goldfine AB, Nathan DM, Schwartz MW, Smith RJ, Smith SR. 2011. Obesity and type 2 diabetes: What can be unified and what needs to be individualized? *Diabetes Care*. 34: 1424-1430.

Florentino RF and Duante CA for the 6th National Nutrition and Health Survey (2003-2004) Philippines. Unpublished data.

Food and Nutrition Research Institute (FNRI) Department of Science and Technology (DOST). 2013. *Burden of selected risk factors to non-communicable diseases (NCDs) among Filipino adults from the results of the 8th National Nutrition Survey*. Available online at www.fnri.dost.gov.ph>nutrition-statistic.

Fuller-Thomson E, Roy A, Chan KT-K, Kobayashi KM. 2017. Diabetes among non-obese Filipino Americans: Findings from a large population-based study. *Can J Public Health*. 108(1): e36-e42.

Gentilucci UV, Picardi A, Manfrini S, Khazrai YM, Fioriti E, Altomare M, Guglielmi C, Di Stasio E, Pozzilli P. 2008. Westernization of the

Filipino population resident in Rome: obesity, diabetes and hypertension. *Diabetes Metab Res Rev*. 24: 364-370.

Gill TM. 2001. Cardiovascular risk in the Asia-Pacific region from a nutrition and metabolic point of view: abdominal obesity. *Asia Pac J Clin Nutr*. 10(2):85-89.

Hsu WC, Araneta MRG, Kanaya AM, Chiang JL, Fujimoto W. 2015. BMI cut points to identify at-risk Asian-Americans for type 2 diabetes screening. *Diabetes Care*. 38(1): 150-158.

Jasul GV for the Metabolic Syndrome Study Group of the 7th National Nutrition and Health Survey (2008) Philippines. Unpublished data.

Jih J, Mukherjea A Vittinghoff E, Nguyen TT, Tsoh JY, Fukuoka Y, Bender MS, Tseng W, Kanaya, AM. 2014. Using appropriate body mass index cut points for overweight and obesity among Asian Americans. *Prev Med*. 65: 1-6.

Jimeno, CA, Kho, SA, Matawaran, BJ, Duante, CA, Jasul, GV. 2015. Prevalence of diabetes mellitus and pre-diabetes in the Philippines: A sub-study of the 7th National Nutrition and Health Survey (2008). *Phil J Int Med*; 53(2): 1-8.

Mata, A and Jasul, GV. 2017. Prevalence of metabolic syndrome and its individual features across different (normal, overweight, pre-obese, and obese) body mass index (BMI) categories in a tertiary hospital in the Philippines. *J ASEAN Fed Endocr Soc*. 32(2): 117-122.

Misra A and Khurana L. 2008. Obesity and the metabolic syndrome in developing countries. *J Clin Endocrinol Metab*. 93:S9-S30.

Morales DD, Punzalan FER, Paz-Pacheco E, Sy RG, Duante CA for the National Nutrition and Health Survey (NNHES):2003 Group. 2008. Metabolic syndrome in the Philippine general population: prevalence and risk for atherosclerotic cardiovascular disease and diabetes mellitus. *Diabetes Vasc Dis Res*. 5:36-43.

Narayan KMV, Aviles-Santa L, Oza-Frank R, Pandey M, Curb JD, MCNeeley M, Araneta MRG, Palaniappan L, Rajpathak S, Barrett-Connor E for the Cardiovascular Disease in Asian and Pacific Islander Populations NHLBI Working Group. 2010. Report of a NHLBI

Workshop: Heterogeneity in cardiometabolic risk in Asian Americans in the US. *J Am Coll Cardiol*. 55: 966-973.

Nestel P, Lyu R, Low LP, Sheu WHH, Nitiyanant W, Saito I, Tan CE. 2007. Metabolic syndrome: recent prevalence in East and Southeast Asian populations. *Asia Pac J Clin Nutr*. 1692: 362-367.

Pagsisihan D, Sandoval MA, Paz-Pacheco E, Jimeno CA. 2016. Low indices of overweight and obesity are associated with cardiometabolic diseases among adult Filipinos in a rural community. *J ASEAN Fed Endocr Soc*. 31(2):97-105.

Palaniappan LP, Wong EC, Shin JJ, Fortmann SP, Lauderdale DS. 2011. Asian Americans have greater prevalence of metabolic syndrome despite lower body mass index. *Int J Obes (Lond)*. 35(3): 393-400.

Pan WH and Yeh WT. 2008. How to define obesity? Evidence-based multiple action points for public awareness, screening and treatment: an extension of Asia-Pacific recommendations. *Asia Pac J Clin Nutr*. 17(3): 370-374.

Pan WH, Yeh WT, Weng LC. 2008. Epidemiology of metabolic syndrome in Asia. *Asia Pac J Clin Nutr*. 17(S1):37-42.

Punzalan FER, Sy RG, Ty-Willing T. 2004. Prevalence of metabolic syndrome among adult Filipinos. *International Congress Series*. 1262:442-445.

Rakugi H and Ogihara T. 2005. The metabolic syndrome in the Asian population. *Current Hypertension Reports*. 7: 103-109.

Ranasinghe P. Mathangasinghe Y, Jayawardena R, Hills AP, Misra A. 2017. Prevalence and trends among adults in the Asia-Pacific region: a systematic review. *BMC Public Health*. 17:101.

Seo MH and Rhee E-J. 2014. Metabolic and cardiovascular implications of a metabolically healthy obesity phenotype. *Endocrinol Metab*. 29:427-434.

Sperling LS, Mechanick JI, Neeland IJ, Herrick CJ, Despres JP, Ndumele CE, Vijayaraghavan K, Handelsman Y, Puckrein GA, Araneta MRG, Blum QK, Collins KK, Cook S, Dhurandhar NV, Dixon DL, Egan BM, Ferdinand DP, Herman LM, Hessen SE, Jacobson TA, Pate RR, Ratner RE, Brinton EA, Forker AD, Ritzenhaller LL, Grundy SM.

2015. The CardioMetabolic Health Alliance: Working toward a new care model for the metabolic syndrome. *J Am Coll Cardiol*. 66: 1050-67.

Sullivan DR. 2001. Cardiovascular risk in the Asia-Pacific region from a nutrition and metabolic point of view: visceral obesity. *Asia Pac J Clin Nutr*. 10(2): 82-84.

Sy RG, Morales DD, Dans AL, Paz-Pacheco E, Punzalan FER, Abelardo NS, Duante CA. 2012. Prevalence of atherosclerosis-related risk factors and diseases in the Philippines. *J Epidemiol*. 22(5): 440-447.

Sy RG, Llanes EJB, Reganit PFM, Castillo-Carandang N, Punzalan FER, Sison OT, Khaing NEE, Poulton R, Woodward M, Shyong Tai E. 2014. Socio-demographic factors and the prevalence of metabolic syndrome among Filipinos from the LIFECARE cohort. *J Atheroscler Thromb*. 21:S19-S17.

Tanchoco CC, Cruz AJ, Duante CA, Litonjua AD. 2003. Prevalence of metabolic syndrome among Filipino adults aged 20 years and over. *Asia Pac J Clin Nutr*. 12(3): 271-276.

Unjali UP, Vittinghoff E, Mongraw-Chaffin M, Vaidya D, Kandula NR, Allison M, Carr J, Liu K, Narayan V, Kanaya AM. 2017. Cardiometabolic abnormalities among normal-weight persons from five racial ethnic groups in the United States. *Ann Intern Med*. doi: 10.7326/M16-1895.

Wang EJ, Wong EC, Dixit AA, Fortmann SP, Linde RB, Palaniappan LP. 2011. Type 2 diabetes: Identifying high risk Asian American subgroups in a clinical population. *Diab Res Clin Pract*. 93(2): 248-254.

World Health Organization. 2016. Global report on diabetes. *WHO*. Available online at: http://www.who.int.

Yoon K-H, Lee JH, Kim JW, Cho JH, Choi YH, Ko SH, Zimmet P, Son HY. 2006. Epidemic obesity and type 2 diabetes in Asia. *Lancet*. 368:1681-88.

Zheng S, Shi S, Ren X, Han T, Li Y, Chen Y, Liu W, Hou PC, Hu Y. 2016. Triglyceride glucose-waist circumference, a novel and effective predictor of diabetes in first-degree relatives of type 2 diabetes patients: cross-sectional and prospective cohort study. *J Transl Med.* 14:260.

Zubair N, Kuzawa CW, Lee NR, McDade TW, Adaur LS. 2014. Clustering and determinants of cardiometabolic risk factors among Filipino young adults. *Asia Pac J Clin Nutr*. 23(1):148-158.

In: Obesity and Syndrome X
Editors: M. Das and K. Bose
ISBN: 978-1-53614-669-1

Chapter 3

BODY MASS INDEX, PERCENT BODY FAT AND FAT MASS INDEX AS SCREENING TOOLS FOR GENERAL OBESITY AMONG ADULT FEMALES OF AMRITSAR (PUNJAB)

Ramanpreet Randhawa [*] ***and Sharda Sidhu***
Department of Human Genetics, Guru Nanak Dev University,
Amritsar, Punjab, India

INTRODUCTION

Obesity has emerged as a chronic nutritional disorder almost three decades ago and still continues to escalate its dimensions as one of the most serious considerable non-communicable public health hazard (WHO, 2013). It is now so common that in many environments it is replacing more traditional public health concerns such as undernutrition, infectious diseases, communicable diseases and recognised as a major risk factor for developing hypertension (Warren et al., 2012), lipid disorders (Brown et al., 2000;

[*] Corresponding Author Email: raman.randhawa19@gmail.com.

Sherwood, 2010), glucose intolerance (Kannel, 1987), T2DM (Kahn et al., 2006), heart disease (Taylor et al., 2010), stroke (Oeschet al., 2017), osteoarthritis (King et al., 2013), CVDs (Vangaal et al., 2006), certain cancers (Singhal et al., 2013) and all-cause morbidity and mortality (WHO, 2000; Dalton et al., 2003; Kopelman et al., 2006; Whitlock et al., 2009; Shukla et al., 2014). It is estimated that 2.8 million people die each year and 35.8 million of global disability-adjusted life years (DALYs) across the globe are caused by overweight and obesity (WHO, 2016). The worldwide prevalence of obesity nearly tripled between 1975 and 2016. Very recent data shows that globally 650 billion adults (≥18 years) were observed to be obese. In other words, 13% of the world's adult population was diagnosed as obese, out of which 11% of males and 15% of females manifested obesity (WHO, 2016; Behl and Misra, 2017; Meharda et al., 2017). Obesity can be measured in two ways i.e., general obesity and central/abdominal obesity. The accumulation of fat to that extent that can impair health is known as general obesity. It is prime most important health concern especially among women (Amugsi et al., 2017). It is a critical force behind the progression of an asymptomatic cluster of non-communicable diseases called as metabolic syndrome (Grundy, 2004). However, obesity is not only pivotal cause for the occurrence of metabolic and cardiovascular diseases but also responsible for social stigmatization, psychosocial stress and psychological morbidity (Geiss et al., 2001; Kraig and Keel, 2001). Furthermore, the prevalence of obesity is more pronounced among those residing in the urban areas as compared to rural areas (Bhadra et al., 2005; Senet al., 2013; Kamboj et al., 2017). Currently, the obesity has attained an alarming figures in our nation with approximately 30-65% of adult urban Indians is either overweight, or obese (Mondal and Sen, 2014; Pradeepa et al., 2015). Importantly, this predominance is due to rapid demographic transitions, nutrition transitions and socioeconomic transitions. India, especially Punjab, is a unique example of such transitions, because it has undergone such transitions at a rate much faster than other states of India. However, to the best of my knowledge, there is no published data illustrating the comparative picture of general obesity among adult women using anthropometric and body composition variables from Amritsar. Therefore, in the present study, an attempt has been made to generate baseline data about the prevalence of general obesity among adult females of Amritsar on applying Body Mass Index (BMI), Percent Body Fat (PBF) and Fat Mass Index (FMI) criteria.

MATERIALS AND METHODS

The data for the present cross-sectional study was collected from adult females ranging in age 40-65 years and residing in various urban and rural areas of Amritsar district during the period from June 2013 to September 2016 by using a convenient sampling method. The participants were found in their homes and data was collected from door to door. At each urban and rural area, a uniform protocol of recruitment was followed. Ethical clearance from the Institutional Ethics Committee of Guru Nanak Dev University, Amritsar was obtained prior to carrying out the study.

The study group included 1520 females, out of which, 800 females were urban and 720 females were rural. First of all, women were taken into confidence and then contacted for the study according to their convenience and prior appointment. After fully explaining the nature, procedure, aims and objectives of the study to all the females in Punjabi language, verbal as well as written informed consent was obtained. In person interaction provides an opportunity to the investigator to extract maximum information from the participant about socio-demographic characteristics (name, caste, age and type of family), socioeconomic status (education, occupation and income), lifestyle habits (dietary pattern, physical activity pattern and sedentary behaviour) and menstrual status (regular/irregular/ completely stopped) from each subject by investigator herself after ensuring confidentiality of the information. Anthropometric measurements (body weight, height) were taken on each subject using standard methodology given by Weiner and Lourie (1981) while subjects were lightly clothed and wore no shoes. Body weight was measured to the nearest 0.1 kg using automated calibrated electronic scale. Standing height was measured without shoes to the nearest 0.5centimetre using anthropometric rod. From height and weight measurements, BMI was calculated by dividing weight in kilograms with height in metre squared as follows:

BMI = Weight (kg)/ $(\text{Height})^2$ (m).

The suggested critical limits of BMI by WHO (2000) were used for the assessment of general obesity:

Category	WHO (2000) cut-offs
	BMI (kg/m^2)
Underweight	<18.5
Normal	18.5-22.9
Overweight	23.0-24.9
Obesity	≥25

Per cent Body Fat (PBF) is the percentage of total body weight that consists of fat only not fat-free mass (water, muscle, bone and vital organs). It is evident from the published literature that no criterion for the assessment of body composition has been recommended for South-Asians. Therefore, following criterion of PBF given by Gomez-Ambrosi et al. (2012) was used for the assessment of general obesity among adult females:

Category	PBF cut-offs
Normal	≤30
Overweight	30.1-34.9
Obese	≥35

Fat Mass Index (FMI) estimate or quantify fat stores accurately is the integral part of the prevention and treatment of obesity-related conditions. A potential, more simplified, accurate and highly useful indicator of body adiposity in field research is FMI. This index was first introduced in a study involving nutritional assessment (Van ltallie, 1990) and requires information on body height and fat mass content for calculations. It was calculated by dividing total body fat (kg) by square of height (m).

FMI = Fat mass (kg)/ $(\text{Height})^2$ (m).

In the present study, the prevalence of general obesity was determined using FMI levels divided into separate quartiles for females. Following FMI quartiles recommended by Liu et al. (2013) were used for the assessment of general obesity:

Quartiles	FMI cut-offs (kg/m^2)	Category
Q1	<5.25	Underweight
Q2	5.25-6.32	Normal
Q3	6.33-7.93	Overweight
Q4	≥ 7.93	Obese

The data was analysed using the Statistical Package for Social Sciences (SPSS Inc, Chicago, IL, USA version 21). Mean and standard deviations were calculated for continuous variables and percentage for categorical variables. In order to test the level of significance of differences between the baseline characteristics of urban and rural women, Student's t-test was applied. The Chi-square test was applied to compare differences between the proportions.

RESULTS

The results of the present study have been arranged in tabular form as well as graphical form, wherever possible, along with the statistical interpretation.

Distribution of Participants According to Place Ofresidence

Out of 1520 subjects, 52.6% (800) females were urban and 47.4% (720) females were rural (Table 1, Figure 1).

Table 1. Distribution of participants according to place of residence

Category	Adult Females
Urban	52.6 (800)
Rural	47.4 (720)
Total	100.0 (1520)

Figures in parentheses indicate the number of subjects.

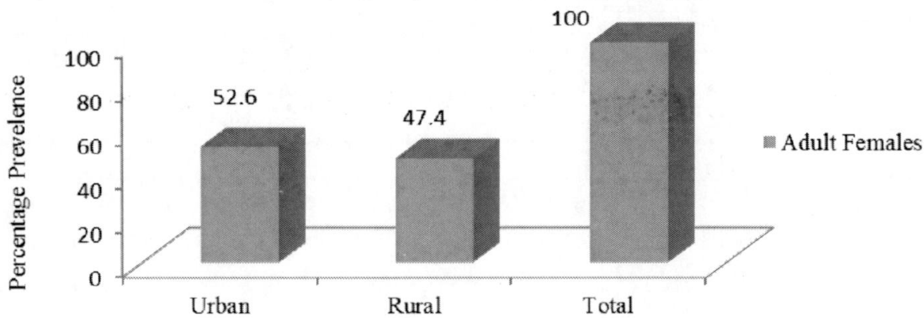

Figure 1. Histogram showing the distribution of adult females according to place of residence.

Anthropometricand Body Composition Variables Studied among Adult Females of Amritsar

Table 2 shows mean (±SD) values of anthropometric and body composition variables studied among adult Amritsar females after stratification of females according to the region. Considering anthropometric variables, among urban and rural females, it was noticed that urban females were having more weight (65.90±14.3 kg) than rural females (63.47±14.0 kg) whereas rural females were taller (155.98±6.0 cm) than urban females (154.91±5.9 cm) and the differences in weight ($p<0.01$) and height ($p<0.05$) were statistically significant between urban and rural females. Mean value of Body Mass Index (BMI) among urban and rural females was 27.45±5.7 kg/m^2 and 26.09±5.7 kg/m^2, respectively, and the difference in the mean values of BMI between the two groups was highly significant ($p<0.001$).

Table 2. Mean and standard deviation (±SD) values of anthropometric and body composition variables of Amritsar adult females studied

Variable	Total (1520)				
	Urban (800)		Rural (720)		't'-value
	Mean	SD	Mean	SD	
Weight (kg)	65.90	14.3	63.47	14.0	3.345**
Height (cm)	154.91	5.9	155.98	6.0	3.456*
BMI	27.45	5.7	26.09	5.7	4.632***
TBF	33.16	8.0	28.93	9.3	6.019***
PBF	44.44	10.9	43.82	9.7	1.164***
FFM	37.32	7.4	38.23	9.8	2.019*
FMI	13.92	5.4	12.54	4.3	5.754***

*Significant at p<0.05, **Significant at p<0.01, ***Significant at p<0.001.
BMI: Body Mass Index (kg/m^2), FFM: Fat-Free Mass (kg),
FMI: Fat Mass Index (kg/m^2), PBF: Percent Body Fat,
TBF: Total Body Fat (kg).

In context to body composition variables, compared to rural counterparts, higher mean value of total body fat (urban 33.16±8.0 kg vs. rural 28.93±9.3 kg, p<0.001) was observed in urban females. In addition to this, the differences were found to be highly significant (p<0.001 for both variables) in the mean values of per cent body fat (urban: 44.44±10.9 vs. rural: 43.82±9.7) and fat mass index (urban 13.92±5.4 kg/m^{2}vs. rural 12.54±4.3 kg/m^2) between the two groups. In contrast to this, rural females were found to have significantly (p<0.05) elevated levels of fat-free mass (urban 37.32±7.4 kg vs. rural 38.23±9.8 kg) than urban females.

Assessment of General Obesity

BMI criterion of WHO (2000): Table 3 and Figure 3 shows the percentage prevalence of obesity in the study females using WHO (2000) criterion of BMI for Asian populations. According to this classification, the overall prevalence of obesity was 61.4% whereas 12.8% females were overweight, 19.6% females were normal and only 6.2% females were underweight. After stratification of females according to region, it was noticed that the prevalence of obesity was 68.7% and 53.3% among urban and rural females, respectively. The difference in the percentage prevalence of obesity between urban and rural females was found to be statistically significant (χ^2=37.37, df=1; p<0.001). It is clear from the table that the prevalence of overweight, normal and underweight urban females was 10.6%, 15.4% and 5.3%, respectively, whereas the corresponding figures for rural females were 15.3%, 24.3% and 7.1%, respectively.

Table 3. Percentage prevalence of General Obesity according to Body Mass Index (WHO, 2000) criterion among adult females of Amritsar

Category	Adult Females			
	Urban (800)	Rural (720)	Total (1520)	χ^2-value
Underweight	5.3 (42)	7.1 (51)	6.2 (93)	1.91
Normal	15.4 (123)	24.3 (175)	19.6 (298)	18.61***
Overweight	10.6 (85)	15.3 (110)	12.8 (195)	6.93**
Obese	68.7 (550)	53.3 (384)	61.4 (934)	37.37***

Figures in parentheses indicate the number of subjects.
*Significant at p<0.05, **Significant at p<0.01, ***Significant at p<0.001.

Percent Body Fat (PBF)

It is defined as the proportion of total body fat mass of total body weight and it accurately predicts cardiovascular risks than BMI (Zenget al., 2012). Table 4 and Figure 4 depict the percentage prevalence of obesity assessed with the help of per cent body fat determined by Bioelectrical Impedance Analysis (BIA) among females according to per cent body fat criterion (Gomez-Ambrosiet al., 2012). The overall prevalence of obesity was 80.3% (urban 83.2% vs. rural 76.9%). On the other hand, 11.5% females were observed as overweight (urban 8.5% vs. rural 14.9%) and 8.2% as normal (urban 8.3% vs. rural 8.2%). The difference in the percentage prevalence of obesity between urban and rural females was statistically significant (χ^2=9.12, df=1; p<0.01).

Table 4. Percentage prevalence of General Obesity using Percent Body Fat (PBF) criterion as given by Gomez-Ambrosiet al. (2012) among adult females of Amritsar

Category	Adult Females			
	Urban (800)	Rural (720)	Total (1520)	χ^2-value
Normal	8.3 (66)	8.2 (59)	8.2 (125)	–
Overweight	8.5 (68)	14.9 (107)	11.5 (175)	14.43***
Obese	83.2 (666)	76.9 (554)	80.3 (1220)	9.12**

Figures in parentheses indicate the number of subjects.
*Significant at p<0.05, **Significant at p<0.01, ***Significant at p<0.001.

Fat Mass Index (FMI)

Fat mass index was first introduced by Van ltallie et al., (1990) and is calculated by taking the total body fat mass component from bioelectrical impedance analysis and dividing it by height squared. Table 5 and Figure 5 demonstrate the percentage prevalence of obesity among participants using fat mass index criterion (Liu et al., 2013). In the present sample, the overall prevalence of obesity was 88.5%. In addition to this, 5.8%, 2.9% and 2.8% females were encountered as overweight, normal and underweight, respectively. Region-wise prevalence of obesity in the study participants was almost similar (urban 88.7% vs. rural 88.4%) and the difference between the two groups was statistically non-significant. Further, it was noticed that 4.6% (urban) and 7.1% (rural) females were overweight, 3.8% (urban) and 1.9% (rural) were normal, and 2.9% (urban) and 2.6% (rural) were underweight.

Table 5. Percentage prevalence of general obesity using Fat Mass Index (FMI) quartiles as given by Liu et al. (2013) among adult females of Amritsar

Category	Urban (800)	Rural (720)	Total (1520)	χ^2-value
Underweight	2.9 (23)	2.6 (19)	2.8 (42)	0.02
Normal	3.8 (30)	1.9 (14)	2.9 (44)	3.79
Overweight	4.6 (37)	7.1 (51)	5.8 (88)	3.76
Obese	88.7 (710)	88.4 (636)	88.5 (1346)	0.03

Figures in parentheses indicate the number of subjects. *Significant at p<0.05, **Significant at p<0.01.

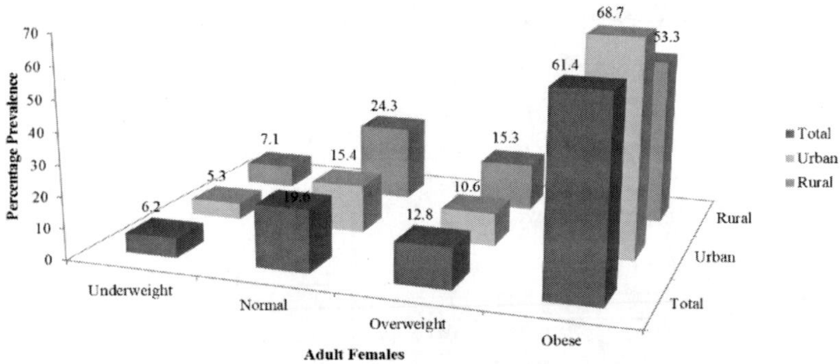

Figure 3. Histogram showing the percentage prevalence of underweight, normal, overweight and obese among adult females according to Body Mass Index (WHO, 2000) criterion.

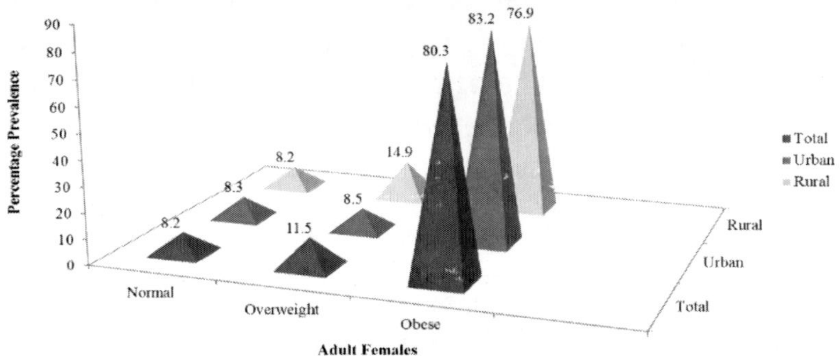

Figure 4. Histogram exhibiting the percentage prevalence of normal, overweight and obese among adult females using Percent Body Fat (PBF) criterion.

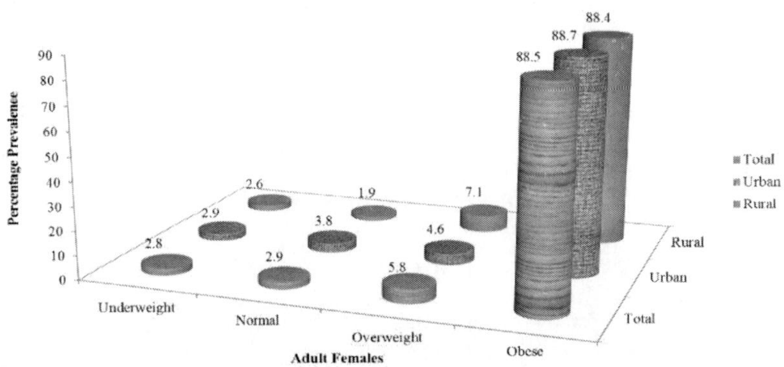

Figure 5. Histogram demonstrating the percentage prevalence of underweight, normal, overweight and obese among adult females using Fat Mass Index quartiles.

DISCUSSION

The anthropometry is pioneer in the series of obesity assessment methods in large field surveys and epidemiological studies. The measurement of anthropometric index known as Body Mass Index (BMI) is found as the simplest, easiest, non-invasive and cost-effective potential indicator of medical complications of obesity (Ouyang et al., 2015; Choi et al., 2017). In the nineteenth century, the mathematician and social statiscian Adolphe Quetelet observed that the weight of the average person was proportional to the square of the height. The ratio of body weight measured in kilograms divided by the square of the height measured in metres was termed as quetelet's index and later renamed as body mass index (Keys et al., 1972). The simplicity and ease of measurement have entrenched the widespread use of BMI as a marker of adiposity not only for epidemiological purposes but also in clinical practice. In the present study, the mean values of BMI observed in urban and rural females were 27.45±5.7 kg/m^2 and 26.09±5.7 kg/m^2, respectively and the difference in the mean values of BMI between urban and rural females was statistically significant ($p<0.001$).

WHO (2000) classification of BMI has been recommended for Asian population including lower cut-off of BMI for the assessment of obesity because Asian people depict substantial risk of T2DM and CVDs at lower weight or fat accumulation (WHO, 2004). The overall prevalence of obesity was found as 61.4% on applying BMI criterion of WHO (2000) in the females studied (Table 3). The difference in the prevalence of obesity between urban females (68.7%) and rural females (53.3%) was statistically significant (χ^2= 37.37, df= 1, p< 0.001). The results of the present study were compared with the general female populations of different parts of India to expedite a relative estimation of obesity prevalence. Table 6 presents the percentage prevalence of obesity according to BMI criteria of WHO (2000) among women residing in various urban regions of India. Nonetheless, the extent of obesity is not firmly comparable because of divergence in the methods of measurements, dissimilarity in sample size and study design, difference in age and socioeconomic status of subjects, ethnic variation, diverse food habits, their lifestyle and periodic dissimilarities in the studies. It is very clear from this table that the prevalence of obesity using BMI criterion of WHO (2000) among urban Indian females varies considerably from one region to another region with rates as high as 71.8% among females of West Bengal (Das and Bose, 2006) and as low as 15.6% among females of South Delhi (Misra et al., 2001) After three years in 2003, the prevalence of obesity was observed to be four times higher i.e., 66.7% in New Delhi females depicting a rising trend with the passage of time under similar geographical conditions (Misra et al., 2003). Apparently, the estimates of obesity in the present study were observed to be close to the females of New Delhi. In addition to this, Reddy et al. (2002) performed an epidemiological study among New Delhi females and examined 48.0% females as obese. In the western region, three cross-sectional studies were performed by Malshe and Udipi (2017), Rathi et al. (2014) and Senet al. (2009), and reported 43.6%, 40.5% and 29.3% females as obese residing in Mumbai city and Pune city of Maharashtra and Jalpaiguri, West Bengal, respectively. Moreover, 30.2% prevalence of obesity was assessed among adult females of Rajasthan by Gupta et al. (2002). In the Southern region, the most latest study for the assessment of obesity among 1000 Karnataka females ranging in age 15-64 years was accomplished by Nagendra et al. (2017) and revealed 34.9% obesity. In an earlier study carried out in Dharwad, Dandeli and Belgaum districts of Karanataka, 63.3% females yielded obesity (Goyal et al., 2012). Among Chennai females, Anuradha et al. (2011) observed the prevalence of obesity as 19.8% whereas 31.2% females were noticed as obese by Deepaet al. (2009). In the eastern region, a very recent cross-sectional study was executed by Senet al. (2017) and analysed 48.7% females falling in the category of obesity.

The prevalence of obesity among women of Punjab has also been studied by other investigators. Girdhar et al. (2016) and Singh et al. (2015) carried out two cross-sectional studies in Ludhiana on 324 females (20-60 years) and 618 females (25-64) of Ludhiana and diagnosed 29.6% and

28.8% females as obese according to BMI criterion of 2000 and 1998, respectively. On applying WHO (2000) criterion of BMI, the prevalence of obesity varied from 23.2 - 34.3% among 1088 females of Punjab ranging in age 45-69 years and 18-44 years, respectively (Tripathy et al., 2016). In Amritsar, the figures of obesity were found to be 56.4% on investigating 172 females by Randhawa and Sidhu (2014). One of the large sample size (N=3000) study conducted in Punjab by Sidhu and Randhawa (2014) reported 33.4% females as obese using Asian BMI cut-offs ($\geq$25 kg/ m^2). In another study on Punjabi urban females, Sidhu et al. (2005) found 21.1% obese females as per BMI (WHO, 1998) criterion of obesity. Sidhu and Prabhjot (2004) performed a study on 500 Punjabi women and reported 15.0% prevalence of obesity. Sidhu and Tatla (2002) studied adult Punjabi females and reported 25.3% of them as obese (BMI$\geq$30.0 kg/m^2). It can be deciphered from this table that Amritsar females were noticed to be more obese as compared to females residing in other districts of Punjab.

Table 7 presents a compilation of studies demonstrating the prevalence of obesity reported in rural females of India. A recent study performed by Bharali et al. (2017) involving adult Nyishi tribal females in Arunachal Pradesh found 9.5% prevalence of obesity according to WHO (2000) criterion of BMI. In addition to this, two cross-sectional studies were carried out among tribal females hailing from Assam (Mondal et al., 2016) and Manipur (Mungreiphy and Kapoor, 2008) and examined 15.2% and 27.1% females as obese (BMI $\geq$25 kg/m^2). Furthermore, 36.9% females of Haryana aged $\geq$20years were categorized as obese (BMI $\geq$ 25 kg/m^2) during a population-based study attempted by Verma et al. (2016). An another study, among rural females of Tamil Nadu, the prevalence of obesity was found to be 21.2% by the WHO (2000) classification of BMI (Little et al., 2016). Assessment of obesity among females of union territory named as Puducherry was accomplished by Shrivastava et al. (2015) and findings of the study revealed that 27.3% females were obese as per BMI (2000) classification.

Table 6. Percentage prevalence of general obesity among urban Indian females reported in various studies using BMI criteria of WHO (2000)

Place/Area/State	Age group (years)	No. of females	Percentage prevalence using BMI cut-offs	Investigator
			≥25 kg/m²	
Other than Punjab				
Meerut	≥18	567	---	Kamboj et al. (2017)
Mumbai	21-45	1500	43.6	Malshe and Udipi (2017)
Agartala, Tripura	25-65	388	48.7	Senet al. (2017)
Karnataka	15-64	1000	34.9	Nagendra et al. (2017)
Udipi and Manipal areas of Karnataka	40-70	140	42.1	Ranasinghe et al. (2017)
Aligarh, Uttar Pradesh	15-65	2002	---	Khayyam et al. (2015)
Town in Central India	≥17	267	---	Jain et al. (2015)
Delhi	18-50	123	---	Duaet al. (2014)
Pune, Maharshtra	20-45	518	40.5	Rathiet al. (2014)
Ahmedabad, Gujarat	20-60	200	---	Sabooet al. (2014)
Pantnagar, Uttarakhand	18-28	629	---	Raguvanshi and Singhal (2013)
Jalpaiguri, West Bengal	20-60	300	29.3	Senet al. (2009)
Dharwad, Dandeli and Belgaum districts, Karnataka	41-50	30	63.3	Goyalet al. (2012)
Bhopal, Madhya Pradesh	>20	177	---	Naharet al. (2012)
Tirupati, Andhra Pradesh	20-70	772	---	Reddy et al. (2012)
Salem, Tamil Nadu	20-59	262	---	Kanniyappanet al. (2011)
Urban slum Chennai	≥ 20	520	19.8	Anuradha et al. (2011)
Salem, Tamil Nadu	19-49	540	---	Aarthiet al. (2010)
Warangal, Andhra Pradesh	20-90	639	---	Eshtari et al. (2009)
Gwalior, Madhya Pradesh	≥30	755	---	Tiwari et al. (2009)
Chennai	≥ 20	2350	31.2	Deepa et al. (2009)
West Bengal	>20	110	71.8	Das and Bose (2006)
Hindu Bengali Females	20-50	854	---	Bhadra et al. (2005)
Punjabi Bhatia family, Jaipur	20-60	232	---	Gupta et al. (2004)
New Delhi	15-58	60	66.7	Misra et al. (2003)
Jaipur, Rajasthan	≥ 20	573	30.2	Gupta et al. (2002)
New Delhi	35-64	1456	48.0	Reddy et al. (2002)
South Delhi	>18	362	15.6	Misra et al. (2001)
Kashmir	≥ 40	2587	---	Zargar et al. (2000)
Punjab				
Ludhiana	20-60	324	29.6	Girdhar et al. (2016)

Place/Area/State	Age group (years)	No. of females	Percentage prevalence using BMI cut-offs	Investigator
			≥25 kg/m2	
Punjab	18-44 45-69	1088	34.3 23.2	Tripathy et al. (2016)
Ludhiana	25-64	618	---	Singh et al. (2015)
Adult Amritsar females	30-50	172	56.4	Randhawa and Sidhu (2014)
Middle class females	20-50	3000	33.4	Sidhu and Randhawa (2014)
Punjabi females	20-45	900	---	Sidhu et al. (2005)
Punjab	≥ 18	500	---	Sidhu and Prabhjot (2004)
Adult Punjabi females	≥ 20	1000	---	Sidhu and Tatla (2002)
Urban areas of Amritsar district	40-65	800	68.7	Present study

In the same year, a community-based study was conducted in Kerala by Bindhu et al. (2014) revealed 44.7% females as obese using BMI (≥25 kg/m^2) cut-offs. The prevalence of obesity among Tamil Nadu females was studied by Chauhanet al. (2015) and found 23.8% females as obese (BMI≥25 kg/m^2). Almost similar prevalence of obesity was encountered among females of Uttar Pradesh (22.0%) and Maharashtra (22.7%) on employing WHO (2000) classification of BMI (Kumar et al., 2014; Rathi et al., 2014). The higher rates of obesity (40.0%) were observed in Delhi females by Reddy et al. (2002) using BMI (≥25 kg/m^2) cut-offs. Other than this, very few studies have been performed in rural areas of Punjab to assess obesity.

Comparison of three major studies conducted by National Family Health Survey (a multicentric study; NFHS-2 during the period from 1998-1999; conducted on 90,000 women in the age group of 15-49 years in 26 states), NFHS-3 (2005-2006, conducted on 1,24,385 women in the age group of 15-49 years in 29 states) and NFHS-4 (2015-2016, conducted on 6,99,686 women in 29 states and 7 union territories) was done. NFHS-2 and NFHS-3 used BMI≥25 kg/m^2 criterion for the assessment of overweight and obese individuals while in NFHS-4, BMI≥25 kg/m^2 criterion was applied for the assessment of obese individuals only.

Table 7. Percentage prevalence of general obesity among rural Indian females using BMI criteria of WHO (2000)

Place/Area/State	Age group (years)	No. of females	Percentage prevalence using BMI cut-offs ≥25 kg/m²	Investigator
Other than Punjab				
Tribal females, Arunachal Pradesh	15-44	543	9.5	Bharaliet al. (2017)
Tribal females, Assam	20-49	544	15.2	Mondal et al. (2016)
Haryana	≥ 20	540	36.9	Verma et al. (2016)
Krishnagiri, Tamil Nadu	20-80	412	21.2	Little et al. (2016)
Hazratbal, Srinagar	≥ 18	2267	---	Nazki et al. (2015)
Rural Puducherry	>25	534	27.3	Shrivastava et al. (2015)
Tamil Nadu	≥ 15	143	23.8	Chauhan et al. (2015)
Meerut, Uttar Pradesh	≥ 18	656	22.0	Kumar et al. (2014)
Trivandrum, Kerala	≥ 18	---	44.7	Bindhu et al. (2014)
Pune, Maharashtra	20-45	545	22.7	Rathi et al. (2014)
Bhalwal, Jammu & Kashmir	≥ 30	1135	---	Raina and Jamwal (2009)
Tribal females, Manipur	20-70	346	27.1	Mungreiphy and Kapoor (2008)
Chittor, Andhra Pradesh Kammas Kailaka Malas	≥20	T= 394 146 101 147	---	Venkatrama et al. (2005)
New Delhi	35-64	1417	40.0	Reddy et al. (2002)
Punjab				
Punjabi females	≥ 20	800	10.2	Sidhu et al. (2005)
Rural areas of Amritsar district	40-65	720	53.3	Present study

According to these national reports, the prevalence of obesity has elevated among Indian women from 10.6% in NFHS-2 to 12.6% in NFHS-3 and to 20.7% in NFHS-4. This data shows that the prevalence of obesity has increased 10.1 percentage points higher during the period from 1998 to 2016. The prevalence of obesity is dramatically increasing among urban and rural females. It has been reported by NFHS-4 that 31.3% of urban women were obese as compared to 23.5% in NFHS-3 and 9.4% in NFHS-2. In rural areas, the prevalence of obesity has also risen from 2.6% in NFHS-2 to 7.4% in NFHS-3 and to 15.0% in NFHS-4. These figures depict that the prevalence of obesity has increased 21.9 percentage points and 12.4 percentage points higher among urban and rural females, respectively from NFHS-2 to NFHS-4.

Table 8. Prevalence of obesity among Indian females according to National Family Health Survey (NFHS-4, 2015-2016) report

States	Obesity		
	Urban	Rural	Total
Andhra Pradesh	45.6	27.6	33.2
Arunachal Pradesh	25.7	16.3	18.8
Assam	26.1	10.9	13.2
Bihar	23.5	9.7	11.7
Chhattisgarh	24.4	7.8	11.9
Goa	36.3	28.5	33.5
Gujarat	34.5	15.4	23.7
Haryana	24.3	18.8	21.0
Himachal Pradesh	38.4	27.6	28.6
Jammu & Kashmir	40.6	24.1	29.1
Jharkhand	21.7	5.9	10.3
Karnataka	31.8	16.6	23.3
Kerala	33.5	31.5	32.4
Madhya Pradesh	23.8	9.1	13.6
Maharashtra	32.4	14.6	23.4
Manipur	31.2	22.4	26.0
Meghalaya	18.4	10.2	12.2
Mizoram	6.0	9.2	7.2
Nagaland	20.7	13.2	16.2
Odisha	32.0	30.6	31.3
Punjab	32.4	30.6	36.7
Rajasthan	23.7	10.7	14.1
Sikkim	34.1	23.1	26.7
Tamil Nadu	36.2	25.4	30.9
Telangana	39.5	18.5	28.1
Tripura	23.5	12.8	16.0
Uttar Pradesh	27.1	12.6	16.5
Uttarakhand	28.4	16.0	20.4
West Bengal	30.6	15.0	19.9
Andaman & Nicobar	38.3	26.6	31.8
Chandigarh	NA	NA	41.5
Delhi	34.9	29.2	34.9
Dadra and Nagar Haweli	34.2	6.9	19.2
Daman and Diu	32.7	29.0	31.6
Lakshadweep	42.4	28.2	41.4
Puducherry	38.1	33.6	36.7

Among Punjabi women, according to NFHS-2 report, the prevalence of obesity was 31.3%, it was 29.9% as per NFHS-3 report but in NFHS-4 report the estimates of obesity were noticed as 31.2%. This shows that there is decline in the prevalence of obesity among Punjabi females from NFHS-2 to NFHS-3 but in NFHS- 4 it was almost similar to the prevalence of obesity reported by NFHS-2. It is evident from these studies that the extent of obesity reported in these studies is not strictly comparable because of the variation in criteria of BMI used. Some of the states and union territories where the prevalence of obesity among women was found to be higher than national prevalence (20.7% in NFHS-4, Table 8) includes Puducherry (36.7%), Punjab (36.7%), Delhi (34.9%), Goa (33.5%), Andhra Pradesh (33.2%), Kerala (32.4%), Daman and Diu (31.6%), Odisha (31.3%), and Tamil Nadu (30.9%).

Among urban and rural areas of Punjab, the epidemic of obesity has also increasing rapidly. NFHS-4 conducted field work on 19,484 urban and rural females during the period from 28 January, 2016 to 20 June, 2016 and observed that the prevalence of obesity was 32.4% in urban females and 30.6% in rural females. It is concluded from the present study that prevalence of obesity in Amritsar females is about 1.9 times and 2.9 times higher than the prevalence of obesity in Punjabi females and Indian females reported in NFHS-4, respectively.

Results from the 2011–2012 National Health and Nutrition Examination Survey (NHANES) among adults aged 20 and over, documented 35.1% prevalence of obesity (Fryar et al., 2014) which is far less than reported in the present study of adult Jat-Sikh females of Amritsar. A total of 2,50,651 women (aged 15–49 years) from 32 Sub-Saharan countries were studied between January 2005 and December 2013 under Demographic and Health Survey (DHS), nationally representative cross-sectional study revealed 23.0% as the highest obesity estimates in Swaziland women (Neupane et al., 2016) which is no doubt less than assessed in the present study adult females. Ellulu et al. (2014) quoted that obesity is one of the most glaring body condition which increase the chances of a person to be the victim of various other non-communicable diseases and reported that in Europe, the figures of obesity among females were 22.0%, 17.0%, 16.0%, 7.0% and 6.0% residing in Germany, Latvia, Ireland, Sweden and Norway, respectively which are very less than present findings. Evidences of obesity from Pacific Islands put forward 79.0% obesity among females of Nauru which is higher than obesity found in Amritsar females. Moreover, 50.0% obesity was yielded by Cook Islands females which are in concordance with the current study estimates. Amugsi et al. (2017) elucidated increase in obesity among women hailing from urban settings of 24 African countries. The results documented that Egypt country, earlier ranked among the countries in the world with the most obese people reported 39% females as obese followed by Ghana (22%). The findings of the present study depicted that urban females had even higher prevalence of obesity than Egypt females residing in urban settings. It is absolutely marked from the comparative profile of Indian literature (Table 6) that obesity assessed in the adult urban Amritsar females in the present study is quite high as compared to most of the other national studies.

The present study investigated that obesity estimates were higher among urban dwellers than rural inhabitants. The overindulgence in high calorie diet and indoor sedentary leisure activities may contribute the higher risk of obesity among urban dwellers. The present findings are in agreement with urban-rural disparity study of Yangon region, Myanmar (Htet et al. 2016). They performed two cross-sectional studies in urban and rural regions of Yangon region including 379 (urban) and 362 (rural) females ranging in age 25 to 74 years between September and November of 2013 and 2014, respectively, and published results demonstrated that urban women had significantly higher prevalence of obesity (urban: 17.3% vs. rural: 11.5%) than rural women. In accordance with few other researchers (Sophal et al., 2010; Benjakul et al., 2013), the estimates of obesity are generally worse for urban populations than rural populations. Duda et al. (2007) also postulated that obesity was found to be more prevalent in the urban rather than rural areas. Data from the 2000–2001 Behavior Risk Factor Surveillance System (BRFSS) and the 1997–1998 National Health Interview Survey (NHIS) contradict present findings by revealing obesity prevalence higher in rural regions compared to urban counties (Patterson et al., 2004; Jackson et al., 2005). Similarly, National Center for Health Statistics (NHANES 2005-2008) included 7,325 urban and 1,490 rural adults ranging in age 20 to 75 years to assess the health and nutritional status of US population and demonstrated that rural regions significantly affected with higher rates of obesity than urban counterparts (Befortet al., 2012). It is striking to know that the prevalence of obesity among adult urban and rural females of Amritsar is tremendously higher than developed nation US, urban and rural populations (CDC, 2011; Hill et al., 2014). Disparity comes into existence from ethnic, nutritional, demographical and socioeconomic population dissimilarities.

With the advancement in technologies in digital age; more sophisticated measurement tools for the assessment of body composition rather than body mass is increasingly used to study obesity-associated health risks (Atanas and Georgi, 2011; Krachler et al., 2013). These health conditions are attributed to distribution and pattern of fat in the body constituting total body weight. The true body fatness may be better evaluated by assessment of per cent body fat and fat-free mass (Thibault and Pichard, 2012). Therefore, obese individuals can be examined precisely by measuring body composition which has been considered as a better approach in the evaluation of nutritional and health status (Willet et al., 2006; Peppa et al., 2012; Zeng et al., 2012; Bintvibok et al., 2013). Body composition methods measure tissue conductivity of a body segment under stable conditions which is directly proportional to the amount of electrolyte-rich fluid present. Fat is anhydrous and their all body water and fluids are found in fat free mass body component (Heymsfield et al., 1996). Recent development in modern anthropology provided Computed Tomography (CT) scan, Dual-Energy X-ray Absorptiometry (DEXA) and Bioelectrical Impedance Analysis (BIA) devices for body fat measurement. CT scan and DEXA equipment estimates per cent fat mass with suitable accuracy and have emerged as the reference method for estimating body composition (Heymsfield et al., 1996). However, both these procedures drawbacks are radiation exposure, relatively high cost, non-portable and limited approachability for epidemiological studies. BIA depicted excellent correlation with CT scan and DEXA in assessing per cent body fat and is believed to be best replacement for these high-priced techniques to screen large group of individuals (Ryo et al., 2005; Jeong et al., 2006; Xu et al., 2011). Bioelectrical Impedance Analysis (BIA) has been extensively recognised as one of the simplest, safest, valid, portable and non-invasive procedure to determine the individual's body composition, particularly body fat (Houtkooper et al., 1996; Kyle et al., 2004; Rana and Sidhu, 2012; Rani and Gupta, 2014; Randhawa and Sidhu, 2014) and Percent Body Fat (PBF) is the percentage of total body weight that is only fat.

In the present study, the mean values of percent body fat observed in urban and rural females were 44.44±10.9 kg/m^2 and 43.82±9.7 kg/m^2, respectively and the difference in the mean values of percent body fat between urban and rural females was statistically significant ($p<0.001$). According to menstrual status, among urban and rural females, it was noticed that postmenopausal females had significantly ($p<0.001$) higher mean value of percent body fat than premenopausal females (Table 2). The overall prevalence of obesity according to percent body fat criterion was 80.3% (urban: 83.2% vs. rural: 76.9%) in the study population (Table 4). The difference in the prevalence of obesity between urban and rural females was statistically significant (χ^2=9.12, df=1, $p<0.01$).

Table 9. Percentage prevalence of general obesity among females reported in various Indian studies using PBF cut-offs

Place/Area/State	Age group (years)	No. of females	PBF cut-offs used	Percentage prevalence	Investigator
Urban					
Mumbai	21-45	1500	>30	59.5	Malshe and Udipi (2017)
Raipur, Chhattisgarh	25-50	70	>30	70.0	Vermaet al. (2015)
Amritsar	30-50	172	≥35	60.4	Randhawa and Sidhu (2014)
Amritsar	20-25	150		36.0	Rana and Sidhu (2012)
Hindu Bengali Females	20-50	854	≥30	36.5	Bhadraet al. (2005)
New Delhi	≥18	362		40.2	Misraet al. (2001)
Urban areas of Amritsar district	40-65	800	≥35	83.2	Present study
Rural					
Haryana	≥ 20	540	>30	43.1	Vermaet al. (2016)
Rural areas of Amritsar district	40-65	720	≥35	76.9	Present study

National studies for the assessment of obesity using PBF criterion was very scarce or may be unpublished in the literature. It is evident from Table 9 that adult Jat-Sikh urban females of Amritsar reported two times more PBF as compared to females of capital city of nation (Misra et al., 2001). It is worth mentioning that even rural counterparts of the present study reflected humongous accumulation of body fat than other female populations of country. This shows that Punjabi females have more propensity of amassing body fat due to their dietary habits and sedentary lifestyle pattern. Malshe and Udipi (2017) exhibited 59.5% females of Mumbai as obese (PBF >30). The females studied by Verma et al. (2015) yielded 70.0% obesity according to >30 criterion of PBF. In Amritsar, two studies were attempted within a gap of two years and to our surprise estimates of obesity regarding deposition of body fat in the concerned area females raised two fold from 36.0% (Rana and Sidhu, 2012) to 60.4% (Randhawa and Sidhu, 2014) with the passage of time. Among Hindu Bengali females, the figures of obesity were 36.5% on applying ≥ 30 cut-offs of PBF (Bhadra et al., 2005). With respect to rural dwellers, only one study was available which was performed by Verma et al. (2016) in Haryana and estimated that 43.1% females were inclined towards the excess building-up of body fat when >30 PBF criterion was incorporated. It is evident that both urban and rural females of Amritsar manifested quite high prevalence of general obesity using PBF cut-offs.

Furthermore, in the studied population, the difference was found to be highly significant ($p<0.001$) for fat mass index (urban 13.92±5.4 kg/m^2 vs. rural 12.54±4.3 kg/m^2) between urban females and rural females (Table 2). In the present sample, the overall prevalence of obesity was 88.5% using FMI criterion (Table 5). Region-wise prevalence of obesity in the study participants was almost similar and the difference between the two groups was statistically non-significant. Unfortunately, there is no report in the current literature regarding the prevalence of obesity on the basis of FMI on Indian females. The outcome drawn by the results of the present study with respect to the assessment of general obesity confirms that adult Jat Sikh females of Amritsar were observed to be more obese using body composition method than the most frequently used diagnostic tool i.e.,

BMI. In other words, FMI assessed the highest prevalence of obesity followed by PBF and BMI. However, despite of the common usage of BMI among clinical settings and large scale field studies still its facing criticism in the terms of its diagnostic precision (Romero-Corral et al., 2008; Paniagua et al., 2013; Gurunathan and Myles, 2016).

BMI is not reliable to discriminate between total body fat and fat free mass. Even though BMI is the most commonly used index, it does not correspond to fatness uniformly in all populations, and inter-ethnic extrapolations are not possible (Deurenberg et al., 1998). The overestimation of adiposity in muscular body build and underestimation of obesity in the elderly is the evident shortcoming of using BMI (Kyle et al., 2004; Pasco et al., 2012; Liu et al., 2013). Therefore, it introduces misclassification problem by not providing information about fat free components (bone mass, muscle mass, mineral content and body fluids) for a given BMI across age, gender and ethnicity (Whitlock et al., 2009). Thus, resulting in variability in different individuals and populations (Gomez-Ambrosi et al., 2012). Various scientists (WHO, 1998; Raji et al., 2001; Deurenberg et al., 2002; Rush et al., 2004; Kagawa et al., 2006) reported that Asians like Indians have a smaller body frame and body mass index classification of obesity based on large framed Europid populations may be inappropriate for them. In fact, BMI of 30 kg/m^2 among Europeans correlate with about 25% of percent body fat content in males and 30% of percent body fat in females, while for same age, gender and BMI; South Asians have an increased percent body fat and lesser fat free mass predicting higher risks for cardiovascular diseases (Bagry et al., 2008; Abdullah et al., 2010). Elucidating from the accumulating results set forth by influential researchers (Raji et al., 2001; Joshi, 2003; Lorenzo et al., 2003; Gupta et al., 2004) that for similar value of BMI, Asian Indians illustrate so called "Asian Indian Phenotype" characterized by less of general obesity as measured by BMI but have significantly large percentages of body fat and greater total abdominal and visceral fat area (McGee, 2005; Darokar et al., 2016) compared with white Caucasians resulting in metabolic disorders at much lower levels of BMI. Therefore, the BMI, usually used in population studies to diagnose obesity is unreliable and necessitate the screening of individuals for distribution of body fat rather than simply measuring the increase of body weight. Soni and Verma (2013) described BIA is the best option to measure body composition in field surveys.

Notably, BIA is dependent not only on body composition (fat mass and fat free mass components) but also on body size (cross-sectional areas in trunk and limbs). Since the proportions of body segments depend not only on weight, age and gender but also on race and ethnicity. Therefore, the estimation equations of percent body fat need to be population-specific and revalidated when applied in population that differs from the one in which original method was developed (Krachler et al., 2013). This seemingly obvious step is often overlooked by researchers (Heymsfield et al., 1996). Moreover, there is inadequacy of literature on population-specific studies to validate these equations. Further studies were warranted to generate consensus on the exact, usable and population-specific cut-offs for both PBF and FMI which can be used to counsel females of different races or ethnicity about their actual risk of morbidity based on their body fat distribution. For instance, to reduce the risk of obesity allied morbidity, White and Hispanic obese women could be advised to reduce their BMI levels 28-29 kg/m^2 as they have more deposition of body fat for a given BMI ($\geq$30 kg/m^2) than black women (Rahman et al., 2009). Similarly, ethnic-specific cut-offs of PBF and FMI are required to facilitate the assessment of obesity associated co-morbidities across the globe.

ACKNOWLEDGMENTS

We would like to express our profound gratitude to all the females for their cooperation and contribution towards this study. We are wholeheartedly thankful to Miss Jaspreet Kaur for her assistance in the collection of data. The authors deeply acknowledge the funding received from the Guru Nanak Dev University under the scheme University with Potential for Excellence (UPE) and Centre with Potential for Excellence in Particular Area (CPEPA).

REFERENCES

Abdullah, A., Peeters, A., Courten, M. and Stoelwinder, J. (2010). The magnitude of association between overweight and obesity and the risk of diabetes: a meta analysis of prospective cohort studies. *Diabetes Research and Clinical Practice* 89 (3): 309-319.

Amugsi, D. A., Dimbuene, Z. T., Mberu, B., Muthuri, S. and Alex, C. (2017). Prevalence and time trends in overweight and obesity among urban women: an analysis of demographic and health surveys data from 24 African countries, 1991–2014 *BMJ Open*. 7(10): e017344.

Atanas, B. and Georgi, B. (2011). Assessment of body composition of male patients with Type 2 diabetes by bioelectrical impedance analysis. *Folia Medica* 53(3): 52-57.

Bagry, H., Raghavendran, S. and Carli, F. (2008). Metabolic Syndrome and insulin resistance. *Anaesthiology* 108: 506-523.

Befort, C. A., Nazir, N. and Perri, M. G (2012). Prevalence of Obesity Among Adults From Rural and Urban Areas of the United States: Findings From NHANES (2005–2008). *J Rural Health* 28(4): 392-397.

Benjakul, S., Termsirikulchai, L., Hsia, J., Kengganpanich, M., Puckcharern, H., Touchchai, C., Lohtongmongkol, A., Andes, L. and Asma, S. (2013). Current manufactured cigarette smoking and roll-your-own cigarette smoking in Thailand: findings from the 2009 global adult tobacco survey. *BMC Public Health* 13: 277.

Bhadra, M., Mukhopadhyay, A. and Bose, K. (2005). Overweight and obesity among adult Bengaleehindu women of Kolkata, India. *Journal of Human Ecology* 13: 77-83.

Bintvibok, W., Cbaikittisilpa, S., Panyakamlerd, K., Jaisamrarn, U. and Taecbakraicbana, N. (2013). Cut-off value of body fat in association with metabolic syndrome in Thai peri- and postmenopausal women. *Climacteric* 16: 1-5.

Brown, C. D., Higgins, M., Donato, K. A., Rohde, F. C., Garrison, R., Oberzanek, E., Ernst N. D. and Horan, M. (2000). Body mass index and the prevalence of hypertension and dyslipidemia. *Obesity* 8(9): 605-619.

Centers for Disease Control and Prevention (CDC) (2011). *Behavioral Risk Factor Surveillance System Survey Data.* Atlanta, Georgia: U.S: Department of Health and Human Services, Centers for Disease Control and Prevention.

Choi, D., Hur, Y., Kang, J., Kim, K., Cho, Y., Hong, S. and Cho, E. (2017). Usefulness of the Waist Circumference-to-Height Ratio in Screening for Obesity and Metabolic Syndrome among Korean Children and Adolescents: Korea National Health and Nutrition Examination Survey, 2010–2014. *Nutrients* 9(256): doi:10.3390/nu 9030256 www.mdpi.com/journal/nutrients.

Dalton, M., Cameron, A. J., Zimmet, P. Z., Shaw, J. E., Jolley, D. et al. (2003). Waist circumference, waist-hip ratio and body mass index and their correlation with cardiovascular disease risk factors in Australian adults *Journal of International Medicine* 254: 555-563.

Darokar, A. G., Phatak, M. S., Thobani, B. A. and Pate, A. K. (2016). Assessment of Body Composition by Bioelectrical Impedance Analysis in Type 2 Diabetes Mellitus Women of Central India *Int. J. Life. Sci. Res.* 2(4): 457-461.

Das, M. and Bose, K. (2006). Presence of high rates of overweight and obesity among adult Marwaris of Howrah, West Bengal, India. *Collegium Anthroplogium* 30: 81-86.

Deepa, M., Farooq, S., Deepa, R., Manjula, D. and Mohan, V. (2009). Prevalence and significance of generalized and central body obesity in an urban Asian Indian population in Chennai, India (CURES: 47). *European Journal of Clinical Nutrition* 63(2): 259-267.

Deurenberg, P., Deurenberg-Yap, M. and Guricci, S. (2002). Asians are different from Caucasians and from each other in their body mass index/body fat per cent relationship. *Obes Rev.* 3: 141–6.

Deurenberg, P., Yap, M. and Staveren, W. A. (1998). Body mass index and percent body fat: a meta-analysis among different ethnic groups. *Int J Obes Relat Metab Disord.* 22: 1164–71

Duda, R. B., Darko, R., Seffah, J., Adanu, R. M. K., Anarfi, J. K. and Hill, A. G. (2007). Prevalence of obesity in women of Accra, Ghana. *Afr J Health Sci* 14: 154-5.

Ellulu, M., Abed, Y., Rahmat, A., Ranneh, Y. and Ali, F. (2014). Epidemiology of obesity in developing countries: challenges and prevention. *Glob Epidemi Obes.* 2: 2. http://dx.doi.org/10.7243/2052-5966-2-2

Fryar, C. D., Carroll, M. D. and Ogden, C. L. (2014) *Prevalence of Overweight, Obesity, and Extreme Obesity among Adults: United States, 1960–1962 Through 2011–2012 Division of Health and Nutrition Examination Surveys.* CDC. http://www.cdc.gov/nchs/nhanes/survey_methods.htm.

Geiss, H. C., Parhofer, K. G. and Schwandt, P. (2001). Parameters of childhood obesity and their relationship to cardiovascular risk factors in healthy prepubescent children. *Int. J. Obes* 25: 830-37.

Gomez-Ambrosi, J., Silva, C., Galofre, J. C., Escalada, J., Santos, S., Millan, D., Villa, N., Ibanez, P., Gil, M. J., Valenti, V., Rotellar, F., Ramirez, B., Salvador, J. and Fruhbeck, G. (2012). Body Mass Index classification misses subjects with increased cardiometabolic risk factors related to elevated obesity. *International Journal of Obesity* 36: 286-294.

Grundy, S. M. (2004). Obesity, metabolic syndrome and cardiovascular disease. *J Clin Endocrinol Metab* 89: 2595-2600.

Gupta, R., Deedwania, P. C., Gupta, A., Rastogi, S., Panwar, R. B. and Kothari, K. (2004). Prevalence of metabolic syndrome in an Indian urban population. *Int J Cardiol.* 97: 257–261.

Gupta, R., Deedwania, P. C., Gupta, A., Rastogi, S., Panwar, R. B. and Kothari, K. (2004). Prevalence of metabolic syndrome in an Indian urban population. *Int J Cardiol.* 97: 257–261.

Gupta, R., Gupta, V. P., Sarna, M. et al. (2002). Prevalence of coronary heart disease and risk factors in an urban Indian population: Jaipur Heart Watch -2. *Indian Heart J* 54: 59-66.

Heymsfield, S. B., Wang, Z. M. and Withers, R. T. (1996). Multicomponent molecular level model of body composition analysis.

In: Roche, AF.; Heymsfield, SB.; Lohman, TG., editors. *Human Body Composition.* Human Kinetics; IL, Champaign: p. 129-47.

Hill, L., You, W. and Zoellner, J. M. (2014). Disparities in obesity among rural and urban residents in a health disparate region *BMC Public Health* 14:1051. doi:10.1186/1471-2458-14-1051.

Houtkeeper, L. B., Lohman, T. G., Going, S. B. and Howell, W. H. (1996). Why bioelectrical impedance analysis should be used for estimating adiposity. *Am. J. Clin. Nutr.* 64: 436S-448S.

Htet, A. S., Bjertness, M. B., Sherpa, L. Y., Meyer, H. E., Stigum, H. and Bjertness, E. (2016). Urban-rural differences in the prevalence of non-communicable diseases risk factors among 25–74 years old citizens in Yangon Region, Myanmar: a cross sectional study. *BMC Public Health* 16: 1225 DOI 10.1186/s12889-016-3882-3.

Jackson, J. E., Doescher, M. P., Jerant, A. F. and Hart, L. G. (2005). A national study of obesity prevalence and trends by type of rural county. *J Rural Health.* 21(2):140–148.

Jain, J., Rao, T., Desmukh, P. and Bnait, S. (2015). Prevalence and Correlates of Metabolic Syndrome in Young Population: A Cross Sectional Study. *J Diabetes Metab* 6 (3): 1-5.

Jain, J., Rao, T., Desmukh, P. and Bnait, S. (2015). Prevalence and Correlates of Metabolic Syndrome in Young Population: A Cross Sectional Study. *J Diabetes Metab* 6 (3): 1-5.

Jeong, D. L. S., Min, H., Kim, Y., Choi, S. and Kim, Y. (2006). Measuring performance evaluation of body fat measuring instrument applying body measuring value method. *Korean J Health Promot Dis Prev* 6: 79-87.

Joshi, R. (2003). Metabolic Syndrome –Emerging clusters of the Indian phenotype. *J Assoc Physicians India* 51: 445-6.

Kagawa, M., Kerr, D., Uchida, H. and Binns, C. W. (2006). Differences in the relationship between BMI and percentage body fat between Japanese and Australian-Caucasian youths. *Br J Nutr.* 95: 1002-1007.

Kahn, S. E., Hull, R. L. and Utzscneider, K. M. (2006). Mechanisms linking obesity to insulin resistance and Type 2 Diabetes Mellitus. *Nature* 444: 840-846.

Kamboj, A. K., Chopra, H., Singh, J. V., Garg, S. K and Bajpai, S. K. (2017). Overweight and Obesity above 18 years of Age in An Urban Population. *Indian J Comm Health* 29(2): 151-155.

Kannel, W. B. (1987). Metabolic risk factors for coronary heart disease in women: perspective from the Framingham study. *Am Heart J.* 114(2): 413-9.

Keys, A., Fidanza, F., Karvonen, M. J., Kimura, N. and Taylor, H. L. (1972). Indices of relative weight and obesity. *J Chronic Dis.* 25: 329-343.

King, L. K., March, L. and Anandacoomarasamy, A. (2013). Obesity and osteoarthritis. Indian. *J Med Res.* 138: 185-193.

Kopelman, P. G., Caterson, I. D. and Dietz, W. H. (2006). *Clinical obesity in Adults and Children.* New Delhi: Blackwell Publishing.

Krachler, B., Volgyi, E., Savonen, K., Tyllavsky, M. A. and Cheng, S. (2013). BMI and an anthropometry based estimates of fat mass percentage are both valid discriminators of cardiometabolic risk: a comparison with DXA and bioimpedance. *Journal of Obesity* http://dx.doi.org/10.1155/2013/862514.

Kraig, K. A. and Keel, P. K (2001). Weight based stigmatisation in children. *Int. J. Obes.* 25: 1661-1666.

Kyle, U. G., Bosaeus., I., De Lorenzo, A. D., Deurenberg, P. E., Luisa, M. G. et al. (2004). Bioelectrical impedanceanalysis—part I: review of principles and methods. *Clinical Nutrition* 23 (5): 1226–43.

Little, M., Humphries, S., Patel, K., Dodd, W. and Dewey, C. (2016). Factors associated with glucose tolerance, pre-diabetes, and type 2 diabetes in a rural community of south India: a cross-sectional study. *Diabetol Metab Syndr.* 8: 21.

Liu, P., Ma, F., Lou, H. et al. (2013). The utility of fat mass index vs. body mass index and percentage of body fat in screening of metabolic syndrome. *BMC Public Health* 13: 629.

Lorenzo, C., Okoloise, M., Wiliams, K., Stern, M. P. and Haffner, S. M. (2003). The metabolic syndrome as predictor of type 2 diabetes mellitus: the San Antonio heart study. *Diabetes Care* 26(11): 3153-9.

McGee, D. L. (2005). Diverse Populations Collaboration. Body mass index and mortality: a meta-analysis based on person-level data from twenty-six observational studies. *Ann Epidemiol.* 15: 87-97.

Meharda, B., Sharma, S. K., Singhal, G. and Kumar, D. (2017). Overweight and Obesity: a rising problem in India. *International Journal of Community Medicine and Public Health.* 4(12): 4548-4552.

Misra, A., Pandey, R. M., Devi, J. R. and Baitule, M. N. (2001). High prevalence of diabetes, obesity and dyslipidaemia in urban slum population in northern India. *Int J Obes.* 25: 1722–9.

Mondal, N. and Sen, J. (2014). Role of anthropometry in assessment of excess adiposity and metabolic disorder in Asian Indians. In: *Health Consequences of Human Central Obesity.* Nova Science Publishers, New York, Chapter- V, pp. 71-83.

National Family Health Survey-3 (2005-2006). http://rchiips.org/nfhs/NFHS-3%20Data/VOL 1/India_volume_I_corrected_17oct08.pdf.

National Family Health Survey-4 (2015-2016). Available at http://www.rchiips.org/ NFHS/pdf/NFHS4/India.pdf. Accessed on 15 August 2017.

Neupane, D., McLachlan, C. S., Sharma, R. et al. (2014). Prevalence of hypertension in member countries of South Asian Association for Regional Cooperation (SAARC): systematic review and meta-analysis. *Medicine* (Baltimore). 93: e74.

Oesch, L., Tatlisumak, T., Arnold, M. and Sarikaya, H. (2017) Obesity paradox in stroke – Myth or reality? A systematic review. *PLoS ONE* 12 (3): e0171334.

Ouyang, X., Q. Lou, L. Gu, G. T. Ko, Y. Mo, H. Wu and Bian, R. 2015. Anthropometric parameters and their associations with cardio-metabolic risk in Chinese working population. *Diabetology and Metabolic Syndrome* 7: 37.

Pasco, J. A., Nicholson, G. C., Brennan, S. L. and Kotowicz, M. A (2012). Prevalence of obesity and the relationship between body mass index and per cent body fat: cross-sectional, population based data. *PLoS One* 7: e29580.

Patterson, P. D., Moore, C. G., Probst, J. C. and Shinogle, J. A. (2004). Obesity and physical inactivity in rural America. *J Rural Health* 20(2): 151–159.

Peppa, M., Koliaki, C. and Raptis, S. A. (2012). Body composition as an important determinant of metabolic syndrome in postmenopausal women. *Endocrinol Metab Syndrome* doi: 10.4172/2161-1017.S1-009.

Pradeepa, R., Anjana, R. M., Joshi, S. R., Bhansali, A., Deepa, M., Joshi, P. P., Dhandania, V. K., Madhu, S. V., Rao, P. V., Geetha, L., Subashini, R., Unnikrishnan, R., Shukla, D. K., Kaur, T., Mohan, V., Das, A. K. and the ICMR-INDIAB Collaborative Study GroupPrevalence of generalized & abdominal obesity in urban & rural India- the ICMR - INDIAB Study (Phase-I) [ICMR - INDIAB-3]. (2015). *Indian J Med Res.* 142(2): 139–150.

Raina, D. J. and Jamwal, D. S. (2009). *Prevalence study of overweight/obesity and hypertension among rural adults.* www.jkscience.org 11(1): 20-23.

Raji, A., Seely, E. W., Arky, R. A. and Simonson, D. C. (2001). Body fat distribution and insulin resistance in healthy Asian Indians and Caucasians. *The Journal of Clinical Endocrinology and Metabolism* 86: 5366-5371.

Ranasinghe, C., Shettigar, P. G. and Garg, M. (2017). Dietary Intake, Physical Activity and Body Mass Index among Postmenopausal Women. *J Mid-life Health* 8: 163-9.

Randhawa, R. and Sidhu, S. (2014). Assessment of Obesity from Body Mass Index and Percent Body Fat among Adult Females of Amritsar, Punjab. *South Asian Anthropologist* 14(2): 181-186.

Rani, S. and Gupta, N. (2014). Body Composition Analysis of Staff members of College Using Bioelectrical Impedance Analysis Method. *International Journal of Chemical Engineering and Applications* 5(3): 259-265.

Reddy, K. S., Prabhakaran, D., Shah, P. and Shah, B. (2002). Differences in body mass index and waist-to-hip ratio in north Indian rural and urban populations. *Obesity Reviews*. 3: 197-202.

Rush, E., Plank, L. D., Chandu, V., Laulu, M., Simmons, D., Swinburn, B and Yajnik, C. (2004). Body size, body composition and fat distribution: a comparison of New Zealand men of Europeans, Pacific island and Asian Indian ethnicities. *Med Journal* 117: U1203.

Ryo, W., Maeda, K., Onda, T. et al. (2005). A new simple method for the measurement of visceral fat accumulation by bioelectrical impedance. *Diabetes Care* 28(2): 451-453.

Sen, J., Mondal, N. and Dutta, S. (2013). Factors affecting overweight and obesity among urban adults: a cross-sectional study. *Epidemiology Biostatistics and Public Health* 10 (1): 1-6.

Sen, P., Sandeep, D., Hore, S., Bhattacharjee, S. and Choudhuri, D. (2017). Obesity and associated cardiometabolic risk among women from Tripura- A northeastern state of India. *Journal of Mid-Life Health* 110-117.

Sherwood, L. (2010). *Human Physiology 7th edition*, Brooks/Cole Cengage Learning, Morgantown, WV, USA.

Shukla, A., Kumar, K. and Singh, A. (2014). Association between Obesity and Selected Morbidities: A Study of BRICS Countries. *PLoS ONE* 9(4): e94433. https://doi.org/10.1371/journal.pone.0094433.

Singh, V., Sahu, M., Yadav, S. and Harris, K. K. (2012). Incidence of obesity among the pre-menopausal and post-menopausal workingwomen of Raipur district (Chhattisgarh State). *World Journal of Science and Technology* 2(6): 83-86.

Singhal, M., Vishnu, V. R. M., Raju, S. V. R and Upadhyay, Y (2013). Interrelationship between Obesity and Cancer (A Review). *Academic Journal of Cancer Research* 6 (1): 13-20.

Soni, A. and Verma, V. (2013). Anthropometric indicators of obesity and percent body fat- A measure for weight management. *International Journal of Science and Research* 4(4): 2229-2233.

Sophal, O., Mey, V., Aim, S., Bounchan, Y., Cin, S., Pen, L. and Loun, S. (2010). *Prevalence of Noncommunicable risk factors in Cambodia; STEPS Survey, Country Report 2010.* Kingdom of Cambodia: The University of Health Sciences and the Preventive Medicine Department of the Ministry of Health.

Taylor, A. E., Ebrahim, S., Ben-Shlomo, Y., Martin, R. M., Whinchup, P. H., Yarnell, J. W. et al. (2010). Comparisons of the associations of body mass index and measures of central adiposity and fat mass with coronary heart disease, diabetes and all-cause: a study using data from 4 UK cohorts. *Am J ClinNutr* 91(3): 547-556.

Thibault, R., Genton, L. and Pichard, C. (2012). Body composition: why, when and for who? *Clinical Nutrition* 31(4): 435-447.

Tripathy, J. P., Thakur, J. S., Jeet, G., Chawla, S., Jain, S., Pal, A., Prasad, R. and Saran, R. (2017). Prevalence and risk factors of diabetes in a large community-based study in North India: results from a STEPS survey in Punjab, India. *Diabetol Metab Syndr* 9: 8 doi.10.1186/s13098-017-0207-3.

Vangaal, L., Rillaerts, E., Creten, W. and Leeuw, I. (1988). Relationship of body fat distribution pattern to atherogenic risk factors in NIDDM: Preliminary Results. *Diabetes Care* 11: 103-106.

Vanltallie, T. B., Yang, M., Heymsfield, S. B., Funk, R. C. and Boileau, R. A. (1990). Height-normalized indices of the body's fat free mass and fat mass: Potentially useful indicators of nutritional status. *Am. J. Clin. Nutr.* 52: 953-959.

Verma, M., Rajput, M., Sahoo, S. S., Kaur, N. and Rohilla, R. (2016). Correlation between the percentage of body fat and surrogate indices of obesity among adult population in rural block of Haryana. *Journal of Family Medicine and Primary Care* 5: 154-9.

Weiner J. S., Lourie J. A. (1981). *Practical Human Biology*. Landon: Academic Press.

Whitlock, G., Lewington, S., Sherliker, P., Clarke, R., Emberson, J., Halsey, J., Qizilbash, N., Collins, R. and Peto, R (2009). Body-mass index and cause-specific mortality in 900 000 adults: collaborative analyses of 57 prospective studies. *Lancet* 373: 1083-1096.

Whitlock, G., Lewington, S., Sherliker, P., Clarke, R., Emberson, J., Halsey, J., Qizilbash, N., Collins, R. and Peto, R (2009). Body-mass index and cause-specific mortality in 900 000 adults: collaborative analyses of 57 prospective studies. *Lancet* 373: 1083-1096.

WHO (World Health Organization) (2000). *Obesity: Preventing and managing the global epidemic. Report of a WHO consultation. (WHO Technical Report Series 894).*

Willet, K., Jiang, E., Lenart, D. and Willet, W. (2006). Composition of bioelectrical impedance and BMI in predicting obesity-related medical conditions. *Obesity* 14: 480-490.

World Health Organization (2004). Expert consultation: appropriate body-mass index for Asian populations and its implications for policy and intervention strategies *Lancet* 363(9403): 157–63.

World Health Organization (2013). Controlling the global obesity epidemic-The Challenge. Geneva: *WHO.* http://www.who.int/nutrition accessed March 15, 2013.

World Health Organization (2016). Obesity. Situation and trends: Global Health Observatory (GHO) data. *WHO.* http://www.who.int/gho/ncd/risk_factors/obesity_text/en/ (accessed 1 Feb 2017).

World Health Organization. (1998). Obesity: Preventing and managing the global epidemic, 1997. *Report of a WHO Consultation on Obesity. Geneva, June 3-5*, Geneva: WHO.

Xu, L., Cheng, X., Wang, J., Cao, Q., Sato, T., Wang, M. et al. (2011). Comparisons of body-composition prediction accuracy. A study of 2 bioelectric impedance consumer devices in healthy Chinese persons using DXA and MRI as criteria methods. *J Clin Densitom.* 14: 458-464.

Zargar, A. H., Khan, A. K., Masoodi, S. R., Laway, B. A., Wani, A. I., Bashir, M. I. et al. (2000). Prevalence of type 2 diabetes mellitus and impaired glucose tolerance in the Kashmir Valley of the Indian subcontinent. *Diabetes Res Clin Pract.* 47: 135–46.

Zeng, Q., Dong, S. Y., Sun, X. N., Xie, J. and Cui, Y. (2012) Percent body fat is a better predictor of cardiovascular risk factors than body mass index. *Braz J Med Biol Res.* 45: 591-600.

In: Obesity and Syndrome X
Editors: M. Das and K. Bose
ISBN: 978-1-53614-669-1

Chapter 4

THE ASSOCIATION OF CENTRAL ADIPOSITY WITH METABOLIC SYNDROME AMONG THE BHUTIAS OF SIKKIM, INDIA

Sovanjan Sarkar*[1,*]*, PhD
and Barun Mukhopadhyay*[2,†]*, PhD
[1]Department of Anthropology,
Vidyasagar University, Midnapore, West Bengal, India
[2]Biological Anthropology Unit,
Indian Statistical Institute, Kolkata, India

ABSTRACT

Metabolic syndrome (MetS) or Syndrome – X is considered to be a major public health problem in the developed as well as developing countries. Present study has attempted to evaluate the plausible relationship between central adiposity and MetS, among the Bhutias of

---

* Assistant Professor; Corresponding Author Email: sovanjan@mail.vidyasagar.ac.in.
† Professor.

Sikkim, India. 428 adult Bhutias, an Indian tribe, were systematically chosen from urban and rural areas of the Himalayan State of Sikkim. Blood pressures and anthropometrics along with fasting glucose and lipid profile were recorded from all the participants (aged ≥ 20 years). Data on sociodemographic aspects and selected lifestyle related variables were collected by using pre-tested questionnaires. Prevalence of MetS was found to be significantly higher among the individuals with sedentary lifestyle, those who are engaged in less active job and those who regularly consume alcohol than their corresponding counterparts. After adjusting for significant lifestyle related predictors, abdomen circumference was found to predict MetS significantly. This small scale cross-sectional study evidently found the positive association of central adiposity related measures with MetS.

INTRODUCTION

The World Health Organization (WHO) has considered the Metabolic Syndrome (MetS) as one of the most burning issues pertaining to health research in both developed and developing countries since decades (Alberti and Zimmet 1998). The MetS is a group of several risk factors such as excess body fat or obesity, higher lipid, blood pressure and glucose level, i.e, dyslipidaemia, hypertension and hyperglycaemia, respectively (Reaven 1988; Timer et al. 2000). Later, International Diabetes Federation (IDF) redefined MetS, where central obesity as measured by waist circumference (WC) is considered as the essential constituent (Alberti et al. 2005). Reaven (1988) coined the term 'Syndrome X', while for the first time he draw attention to this clustering of physiological abnormalities, mainly in overweight individuals.

The prevalence of MetS and cardiovascular disease (CVD) have radically risen in parallel with the global obesity epidemic (Zimmet et al. 2001; Ford et al. 2002). Study has shown that the development of MetS is based on certain complex interaction between genetics, lifestyles and other metabolic factors (Groop 2000). US population shows a prevalence of MetS of more than 20% (Park et al. 2003), while that of Australia is 35.8% (Vaughan et al. 2009) and of China is 21.3% (Xi et al. 2013). In addition to the developed countries, MetS becomes a burning issue in the health research of the developing countries. Transition from rural way of life to comparatively complex urban lifestyle was frequently reported to be a major causal factor pertaining to this abrupt increase in the prevalence of MetS in the developing nations. Since last two decades, many researchers of different countries have reported the prevalence of MetS. The prevalence of MetS is found to be 28.4% in Indonesia (Soweondo et al. 2010), 16.5% in Japan (Hao et al. 2007), 34.8% in Pakistan (Hydrie et al. 2009), 31.3% in South Korea (Park et al. 2015), 24.3% in Sri Lanka (Katulanda et al. 2012) and 24.6% in India (Ravikiran et al. 2010).

The association of dietary habits and physical activity pattern with MetS has been shown in developing countries (Solomons and Gross 1995). Study among urban population also shows sedentary lifestyle and physical inactivity as imperative factors in developing MetS (Torjensen et al. 1997). It is widely and universally accepted that central obesity in terms of waist circumference (WC) happens to be one of the most important and essential components in identifying MetS (NCEP and IDF). Many studies have reported the association between lifestyle related factors, including psychosocial factors and MetS, along with hypertension, obesity, hypertriglyceridaemia (Everson et al. 2002; Wardle et al. 2002; Brunner et al. 2002).

Among the north Indian population the prevalence of MetS was found to be 22.9% in males, 39.9% in females and 31.6% in total sample considering all ages (Gupta et al. 2004). Study pertaining to MetS among the Indian ethnic populations is almost lacking. However, comparison has been made between the Bhutias of Sikkim and Totos of West Bengal pertaining to MetS and its lifestyle related correlates (Sarkar et al. 2005). The aforementioned data prompted us to carry the present study on examining the association of central adiposity with MetS among the Bhutias, an ethnic group inhabiting the eastern Himalayan State of Sikkim. Specifically, attempt has been made to find out the set of adiposity related variables that are responsible for MetS in this population.

Materials and Methods

The Bhutias, inhabiting the town of Gangtok, and also those residing in the rural villages under Ralong Revenue Block of South District were selected as study participants. The individuals of this ethnic group bear Mongoloid features. Agriculture, service in different Government and private sectors, business are their principal ways of earning. Other behavioural and population features can be found elsewhere (Sarkar and Mukhopadhyay 2008).

428 Bhutia individuals of both sexes aged 20 years and above were considered for the study. All the households were considered in case of Ralong Revenue Block and from Gangtok, 100 households were systematically selected. One male and one female, preferably the household head and his wife, were chosen to participate in the present study. Those who were under medication for any chronic disease(s), were excluded from the study. All the parameters pertaining to MetS, viz. blood pressures, lipid profiles, fasting blood glucose, skinfold thicknesses and circumferences were recorded from all the study participants following standard methods and techniques (Lohman et al. 1988). In addition, conicity index was deduced as per universally accepted formula. Summation of six skinfold thicknesses (biceps, triceps, sub-scapular, supra-iliac, abdominal and calf) was used as one of the overall adiposity measures. Bioelectrical impedance was used to know the percent body fat and fat mass of each study participant. Data on socioeconomic and lifestyle related variables (socioeconomic status, alcohol consumption, dietary practices, physical activity pattern) were collected from each study participant with the help of pre-tested questionnaires.

The categorization of the socioeconomic status variables were mentioned in an earlier study among the Bhutias of Sikkim (Mukhopadhyay and Sarkar 2018). Blood pressure (BP) measurements of each study participant were recorded following standard technique (Pickering et al. 2003). The average of two consecutive measurements was used in statistical analysis. Fasting blood glucose was examined by one drop of whole blood with the help of "Accutrend Alfa" glucometer. 2ml. blood sample was collected after 12 hours of fasting for estimating the lipid levels of the study participants. Present study follows the recommended criteria of the International Diabetes Federation (Alberti et al. 2005) for the diagnosis of the MetS (WC: > 94cm for males and > 80cm for females; TG: ≥ 150mg/dL; HDL: < 40mg/dL for males and < 50mg/dL for females; SBP ≥ 130 mm Hg and/or DBP ≥ 85mm Hg; Fasting blood glucose ≥ 100mg/dL). Individuals, who satisfied WC cut-off and any two other conditions from the rest four criteria, were considered as having MetS. Informed consent was obtained from all the study participants before collecting any data.

Statistical Analyses

All statistical analyses have been done with the help of SPSS 16.0 for windows software. Test of equality of proportion and t-tests were performed to test the significance of difference between percentage and mean values of lifestyle related variables, respectively. Logistic regression analysis was used to evaluate the maximum odds ratios (ORs) of the prevalence of MetS. Multiple logistic regression analyses were performed to estimate the age adjusted ORs using lifestyle related variables as covariates. Further, multiple logistic regression analysis was performed to find out the maximum odds of MetS after adjusting for significant lifestyle related variables. Level of significance was considered at $p < 0.05$.

RESULTS

Table 1 depicts the prevalence of MetS of the study participants. Irrespective of sex and total sample, significantly higher ($z = 3.79$, 2.92

and 4.76 respectively for males, females and total sample, $p < 0.05$) prevalence of metabolic syndrome has been noticed in case of urban study participants than that in case of rural participants. Considering urban habitat, markedly high prevalence of metabolic syndrome is found among males (43.75%), females (47.47%) and also in total sample (45.64%). Fact remains that the prevalence of metabolic syndrome is found to be alarmingly high among the rural females (27.27%), too.

Table 2 shows the mean and percentage values of different lifestyle related variables. Significant rural-urban differences are evident for almost all the quantitative and qualitative variables, irrespective of sex.

Table 3 shows the prevalence of MetS according to education, occupation and media exposure status by sex and total sample. It is evident that participants with lower level of education have lower prevalence of MetS. As expected, sedentary jobholders show significantly higher prevalence of MetS than those with non-sedentary jobs in males, females and in total sample ($z = 2.96$, 10.47 and 4.11, respectively, $p < 0.01$). Considering both males and females, more than 30% of the sedentary jobholders are shown to have MetS. Irrespective of sex, participants exposed to mass media, show significantly higher prevalence of MetS compared to their media non-exposed counterparts. Media exposed females show a prevalence of 45.56% as against 34.62% for the male media exposed participants.

Table 4 depicts the prevalence of MetS according to activity level. As expected, irrespective of sex, less active participants show significantly higher prevalence (34.55% for males, 41.57% for females) of MetS compared to more active participants (16.35% for males, 28.00% for females) ($z = 3.13$, $p < 0.01$ for males; $z = 2.06$, $p < 0.05$ for females). Similar trend has also been noticed in case of total sample ($z = 3.40$, $p < 0.01$).

Table 1. Prevalence of MetS, by sex and habitat group

Trait	Male (%)			Female (%)			Total (%)		
	Urban (n = 96)	Rural (n = 94)	z (df = 1)	Urban (n = 99)	Rural (n = 88)	z (df = 1)	Urban (n = 195)	Rural (n = 182)	z (df = 1)
MetS	43.75	19.15	3.79*	47.47	27.27	2.92*	45.64	23.08	4.76*

* Significant at < 0.01 level.

Table 2. Lifestyle related variables, by habitat and sex

Lifestyle related variable	Male			Female		
	Urban (100)	Rural (114)	P	Urban (100)	Rural (114)	P
Cereals	67.28 ± 13.65	66.26 ± 12.54	> 0.05	67.85 ± 13.73	68.19 ± 13.80	> 0.05
Pulses	28.42 ± 22.69	9.82 ± 10.77	< 0.0001	25.65 ± 23.40	9.58 ± 9.17	< 0.001
Tubers	39.83 ± 24.36	13.19 ± 19.04	< 0.0001	45.75 ± 20.59	8.99 ± 14.33	< 0.0001
Vegetables	95.22 ± 32.38	60.49 ± 13.16	< 0.0001	92.35 ± 23.76	58.09 ± 14.46	< 0.0001
Red meats	37.95 ± 22.48	29.01 ± 20.58	< 0.01	34.26 ± 21.90	26.61 ± 21.62	< 0.05
Lean meat	3.46 ± 4.93	1.47 ± 2.01	< 0.001	3.37 ± 4.28	1.49 ± 3.51	< 0.001
Eggs	10.23 ± 12.87	5.03 ± 6.07	< 0.001	10.53 ± 13.80	5.05 ± 6.65	< 0.001
Fish	2.59 ± 3.06	1.15 ± 1.96	< 0.001	2.42 ± 2.87	1.13 ± 2.16	< 0.001
Milk products	75.55 ± 30.32	24.03 ± 20.45	< 0.0001	80.05 ± 30.52	21.01 ± 16.97	< 0.0001
Fruits	16.80 ± 18.67	1.10 ± 6.44	< 0.0001	18.85 ± 22.22	1.02 ± 6.50	< 0.0001
PSSI	0.48 ± 0.06	0.22 ± 0.07	< 0.0001	0.48 ± 0.07	0.20 ± 0.05	< 0.0001
Energy Expenditure (Kcal)	2416.87± 554.25	3559.96± 1219.05	< 0.0001	2142.18± 419.69	23.6.64± 409.93	< 0.05

Table 2. (Continued)

Lifestyle related variable	Male			Female		
	Urban (100)	Rural (114)	P	Urban (100)	Rural (114)	P
Activity level						
More active	20.00	73.68	< 0.0001	33.00	80.70	< 0.0001
Less active	80.00	26.32		67.00	19.30	
Education level						
Upto primary	20.00	64.91	< 0.0001	45.00	79.82	< 0.001
Above primary	80.00	35.09		55.00	21.18	
Occupation						
Non-sedentary	20.00	73.68	< 0.0001	12.00	19.30	> 0.05
Sedentary	80.00	26.32		88.00	80.70	
Household income						
< INR 10,000/m	28.00	82.45	< 0.0001	25.00	80.70	< 0.0001
≥ INR 10,000/m	72.00	17.55		75.00	19.30	
Media exposure						
Non-exposed	17.00	78.10	< 0.0001	18.00	91.60	< 0.0001
Exposed	83.00	21.90		82.00	8.40	
Alcohol intake						
Non-drinker	75.00	53.43	< 0.01	90.00	61.06	< 0.001
Drinker	25.00	47.57		10.00	38.94	
Media exposure						
Non-exposed	17.00	78.10	< 0.0001	18.00	91.60	< 0.0001
Exposed	83.00	21.90		82.00	8.40	
Alcohol intake						
Non-drinker	75.00	53.43	< 0.01	90.00	61.06	< 0.001
Drinker	25.00	47.57		10.00	38.94	

[Source: Mukhopadhyay and Sarkar 2018].

Table 3. Prevalence of MetS according to education, occupation and media, exposure status, by sex and total sample

Socioeconomic status variables including media exposure	Category	MetS (%)		
		Male	Female	Total
Education	Upto primary	20.43	33.58	28.26
	Above primary	29.75	33.77	31.31
	z	1.58	0.03	0.69
Occupation	Sedentary	32.31	34.29	33.53
	Non-sedentary	15.48	0.00	14.77
	z	2.96**	10.47**	4.11**
Media exposure	Exposed	34.62	45.56	39.69
	Non-exposed	18.48	23.81	21.32
	z	2.61**	3.25**	4.02**

* Significant at 0.05 level; ** Significant at < 0.01 level.

Table 4. Prevalence of MetS according to activity level, by sex and total sample

Activity level	MetS (%)		
	Male	Female	Total
More active	16.35	28.00	22.71
Less active	34.55	41.57	37.69
z	3.13**	2.06*	3.40**

* Significant at 0.05 level;
** Significant at < 0.01 level.

Table 5 shows the prevalence of MetS according to substance use. It is evident from the table, that irrespective of sex, smokers and smokeless tobacco users show lower prevalence of MetS, and the difference between these two groups in each sex is not statistically significant. On the other hand, prevalence of MetS is found to be significantly higher in the alcohol drinker group compared to non-drinker group for males, females and total sample, while the difference is significant in females ($z = 2.90$, $p < 0.01$) and in total sample ($z = 2.26$, $p < 0.05$). While drinker females have a prevalence of 46.08%, non-drinker females show a prevalence of 26.60%.

Table 5. Prevalence of MetS according to tobacco use and alcohol consumption, by sex and total sample

Substance use	Category	MetS (%)		
		Male	Female	Total
Smoking status	Smoker	20.83	33.33	23.33
	Non-smoker	29.03	36.76	33.24
	z	1.19	0.24	1.64
Smokeless tobacco use	User	25.00	30.43	26.26
	Non-user	28.35	37.36	33.55
	z	0.53	0.67	1.40
Alcohol consumption	Drinker	28.46	46.08	36.21
	Non-drinker	24.66	26.60	25.75
	z	0.59	2.90**	2.26*

* Significant at 0.05 level; ** Significant at 0.01 level.

Table 6. Multiple logistic regression analysis using significant lifestyle variables adjusted MetS as dependent and adiposity related measures as independent variables

Adiposity related variable	Wald	df	Sig.	Exp(B)	95.0% C.I.for EXP(B)	
					Lower	Upper
Abdomen circumference	4.737	1	.030	.951	.908	.995
Waist circumference	.613	1	.434	1.052	.926	1.195
Percent body fat	1.256	1	.262	.965	.906	1.027
BMI	1.639	1	.200	.848	.658	1.092
WHR	1.371	1	.242	24.347	.116	5.101E3
Conicity index	2.651	1	.104	.001	.000	4.002
Sum of skinfold	.127	1	.722	1.002	.991	1.014

Discussion and Conclusion

In the developing nations, including India, the forces of modernization play an important role in changing the lifestyle of the people. Availability of high fat rich food and accessibility to low cost vehicle are simultaneously affecting the health of the individuals in accumulating excess body fat, specifically at the central region of the body. This eventually increases the risk of certain CVD risk factors and MetS.

The present study portrayed a very high prevalence of MetS among the Bhutias, an ethnic group residing in the Himalayan State of Sikkim. Previously, in a different set of Bhutias, the present authors studied the MetS epidemiology (Mukhopadhyay and Sarkar 2018), where females showed a significantly higher prevalence of MetS which corroborates with the present study and the study among the US (Freiberg et al. 2004). On the other hand, higher prevalence of MetS among the males has been found elsewhere (Dallongeville et al. 2005).

It has been observed that the female study participants are mostly housewives and usually spend most of their times in doing household works. Bhutias were fond of fat and fiber rich food items like *chhurpi* (product made from buffalo milk), beef, pork and so on. Frequent consumption of fast food available in the market was also evident among them. Again, the energy expenditure was found to be very less due to availability of low cost transportation. This double effect of high fat rich food and less energy expenditure accumulates fat in their body and gradually harms their cardio-metabolic health. It can be intuitively stated that the transition from a rural traditional lifestyle to an urbanized modern lifestyle leads to a substantial change in socioeconomic and demographic changes. That in turn may change education level, occupational status and income level of the population. The changes in these attributes can have influence on dietary habits, behaviors and physical activity level that in turn affects the MetS.

Adjusted multiple logistic regression analysis showed the importance of central obesity in predicting MetS than overall obesity measured by BMI and bioelectrical impedance. Present study has uniquely found abdomen circumference as the most significant predictor of MetS, even after adjustment for significant lifestyle related variables. Abdomen circumference as a significant predictor of different CVD risk factors was shown in a previous study among the Bhutias of Sikkim (Sarkar 2013). The central adiposity by means of abdomen circumference might be of interest in future in predicting chronic illnesses like CVD, MetS, diabetes, dyslipidaemia and so on.

ACKNOWLEDGMENT

Authors are grateful to the study participants for their cooperation to conduct the study successfully. Indian Statistical Institute is acknowledged for financial and other logistic supports.

REFERENCES

Alberti, K. G., Zimmet, P. J. (1998). Definition, diagnosis and classification of diabetes mellitus, provisional report of a WHO consultation. *Diabet. Med.,* 15: 539 - 553.

Alberti, K. G., Zimmet, P., Shaw, J. (2005). The metabolic syndrome – a new worldwide definition. *Lancet,* 366: 1059 - 1062.

Brunner, E. J., Marmot, M. G., Nanchahal, K., Shiplay, M. J., Stansfeld, S. A., Juneja, M., Alberti, K. G. (1997). Social inequality in coronary risk: central obesity and the metabolic syndrome: evidence from the Whitehall II Study. *Diabetologia,* 40:1341 - 1349.

Dallongeville, J., Cottel, D., Ferrieres, J., Arveiler, D., Bingham, A., Ruidavets, J. B., Haas, B., Ducimetiere, P., Amouyel, P. (2005). Household income is associated with the risk of metabolic syndrome in a sex-specific manner. *Diabetes Care,* 28: 409 - 415.

Everson, S. A., Maty, S. C., Lynch, J. W., Kaplan, G. A. (2002). Epidemiologic evidence for the relation between socioeconomic status and depression, obesity, and diabetes. *J. psychosom. Res.,* 53: 891 - 895.

Ford, E. S., Giles, W. H., Dietz, W. H. (2002). Prevalence of the metabolic syndrome among US adults: findings from the third National Health and Nutritional Examination Survey. *JAMA,* 287: 356 - 369.

Freiberg, M. S., Cabral, H. J., Heeren, T. C., Vasan, R. S., Ellison, R. C. (2004). Alcohol consumption and the prevalence of the metabolic syndrome in the U.S. *Diabetes* Care, 27: 2954 - 2959.

Groop, L. (2000). Genetics of the metabolic syndrome. *Br. J. nutr.,* 83 suppl. 1: S39-S48.

Gupta, R., Deedwania, P. C., Gupta, A., Rastogi, S., Panwar, R. B., Kothari, K. (2004). Prevalence of metabolic syndrome in Indian urban population. *Int. J. Cardiol.,* 97: 257 - 261.

Hao, Z., Konta, T., Takasaki, S., Abiko, H., Ishikawa, M., Takahashi, T. et al. (2007). The association between microalbuminuria and metabolic syndrome in the general population in Japan: the Takahata study. *Internal Medicine,* 46:341 - 346.

Hydrie, M. Z., Shera, A. S., Fawwad, A., Basit, A., Hussain, A. (2009). Prevalence of metabolic syndrome in urban Pakistan (Karachi): comparison of newly proposed International Diabetes Federation and modified Adult Treatment Panel III criteria. *Metabolic Syndrome Related Disorder,* 7: 119 - 124.

Katulanda, P., Ranasinghe, P., Jayawardana, R., Sheriff, R., Matthews, D. R. (2012). Metabolic syndrome among Sri Lankan adults: prevalence, patterns and correlates. *Diabetol. Metab. Syndr.,* 31: 24.

Lohman, T. G., Roche, A. F., Martorell. R. 1988. *Anthropometric Standardization Reference Manual*, Champaign, Illinois: Human Kinetics Books.

Mukhopadhyay, B., Sarkar, S. (2018). Lifestyle Correlates of Metabolic Syndrome among a Tribal Population Inhabiting Sikkim, India. In: *Anthropology in North East India*. Editor: Sarthak Sengupta. Gyan Publishing House, New Delhi. 261 - 274.

Park, S. Y., Park, Y. K., Cho, K. H., Choi, H. J., Han, J. H., Han, K. D. et al. (2015). Normal range albuminuria and metabolic syndrome in

South Korea: the 2011-2012 Korean National Health and Nutrition Examination Survey. *PloS One,* 10(5): e0125615. doi:10.1371/journal.pone.0125615.

Park, Y. W., Zhu, S., Palaniappan, L., Heshka, S., Carnethon, M. R., Heymsfield, S. B. (2003). The metabolic syndrome: Prevalence and association risk factor findings in the US population form the Third National Health and Nutrition Examination survey, 1988-1994. *Arch. Intern. Med.,* 163: 427 - 436.

Pickering, T. G. (2003). What will replace the mercury sphygmomanometer? *Blood Pressure Monitoring,* 8:23 - 25.

Ravikiran, M., Bhansali, A., Ravikumar, P., Bhansali, S., Dutta, P., Thakur, J. S. et al. (2010). Prevalence and risk factors of metabolic syndrome among Asian Indians: a community survey. *Diabetes Res. Clin. Pract.,* 89: 181 - 188.

Reaven, G. M. (1988). Banting Lecture 1988: Role of insulin resistance in human disease. *Diabetes,* 37:1595 - 1607.

Sarkar, S., Das, M., Mukhopadhyay, B., Chakraborty, C. S., Majumder, P. P. 2005. Prevalence of metabolic syndrome in two tribal populations of sub-Himalayan region of India: Ethnic and rural-urban difference. *Am. J. Hum. Biol.,* 17:814 - 817.

Sarkar, S., Mukhopadhyay, B. (2008). Age trends in blood pressure and obesity among the urban Bhutias of Sikkim. In: Bose, K. (editor). *Health and Nutrition Problems of Indigenous Populations. Tribes and Tribals (Special Volume 2).* Kamla-Raj Enterprises. 59 - 66.

Sarkar, S. (2013). Abdomen circumference is the best obesity related predictor of hypertension and dyslipidaemia: a study among the urban sub-Himalayan tribe of Sikkim, India. *Journal of Diabetes,* 5(suppl. 1): 115 [Abstract].

Soewondo, P., Purnamasari, D., Oemardi, M., Waspadji, S., Soegondo, S. 2010. Prevalence of metabolic syndrome using NCEP/ATP III criteria in Jakarta, Indonesia: the Jakarta primary non-communicable disease risk factors surveillance (2006). *Acta Med. Indones.,* 42:199 - 203.

Solomons, N. W., Gross, R. (1995). Urban nutrition in developing countries. *Nutr. rev.*, 53:90 - 95.

Timar, O., Sestier, F., Levy, E. (2000). Metabolic syndrome X: a review. *Can. J. Cardiol.,* 16: 779 - 789.

Torjensen, P. A., Birkeland, K. I., Anderssen, S. A., Hjermann, I., Holme, I., Urdal, P. (1997). Lifestyle changes may reverse development of the insulin resistance syndrome. The Oslo Diet and exercise Study: a randomized trial. *Diabetes care,* 20:26 - 31.

Vaughan, C., Schoo, A., Janus, E. D., Philot, B., Davis-Lameloise, N. et al. (2009). The association of levels of physical activity with metabolic syndrome in rural Australian adults. *BMC Public Health,* 9: 273.

Wardle, J., Waller, J., Jarvis, M. J. (2002). Sex differences in the association of socioeconomic status with obesity. *Am. J. pub. Health,* 92: 1299 - 1304.

Xi, B., He, D., Hu, Y., Zhou, D. (2013). Prevalence of metabolic syndrome and its influencing factors among the Chinese adults: the China Health and Nutrition Survey in 2009. *Preventive Medicine,* 57: 867 - 871.

Zimmet, P., Alberti, K. G., Shaw, J. (2001). Global and societal implications of the diabetes epidemic. *Nature,* 414: 782 - 787.

In: Obesity and Syndrome X
Editors: M. Das and K. Bose
ISBN: 978-1-53614-669-1

Chapter 5

Bisexual Differences in the Association of Adiposity Measures with the Risk of Hypertension among the Tribes of Gujarat, India

Gautam K. Kshatriya*
Department of Anthropology,
University of Delhi, Delhi, India

Introduction

Obesity is a global epidemic health issue which is leading to several health problems like hypertension, diabetes, cardiovascular diseases (CVDs) and metabolic abnormalities (WHO, 2000; Amin, Fatima, Islam & Gilani, 2015). Increased urbanization and modernization has led to sedentary lifestyle belonging to all the age groups living in urban as well as rural parts of India (Yusuf, Reddy, Ôunpuu & Anand, 2001, WHO, 2008, Bansal et al., 2012, Kshatriya & Acharya, 2016). It has been reported that

* Professor. Corresponding Author Email: g26_51@yahoo.co.in.

change in dietary and physical activity patterns are often the result of environmental and societal changes associated with development and lack of supportive policies in health, agriculture, transport, urban planning, food processing and education (WHO, 2016). According to 'A Global Brief on Hypertension' (WHO, 2013), about one million people around the world are affected by hypertension which causes strokes, heart attacks, kidney failure and other fatal conditions. Globally, complications out of increased blood pressure accounts for 9.4 million deaths every year (WHO, 2009; Lim et al., 2012). Furthermore, undetected high blood pressure has dangerous consequences which often lead to life-threatening complications (WHO, 2013).

It may be added here that hypertension is directly responsible for 57% of all stroke deaths and 24% of all coronary heart disease deaths in India (Anchalaet al., 2014). Studies revealed that prevalence of hypertension in urban India is about 29-45% in males and 25-38% in females (Gupta et al., 2003; Gupta & Gupta, 2009). Obesity has long been established as an important and independent risk factor for the development and complication of hypertension (Misra, 2000; Hossain, Kawar & El Nahas, 2007; Redónet al., 2008; Park et al., 2013; WHO, 2013; 2016; Moraes, Lacerda, Moreno, Horta & Carvalho, 2014; Rizwan et al., 2014; Hall, Do Carmo, Da Silva, Wang & Hall, 2015; Jiang, Lu, Zong, Ruan & Lin, 2016; Kshatriya & Acharya, 2016). Body Mass Index (BMI), Waist Circumference (WC), Waist-to-height ratio (WHtR) and Waist-hip ratio (WHR) are simple and valid anthropometric measures for the assessment of obesity and risk of hypertension (Mello et al., 2011; Rodea- Montero, Evia-Viscarra & Apolinar-Jiménez, 2014; Zhang et al., 2017). WC has stronger positive association with elevated blood pressure (Yalcin, Sahin & Yalcin, 2005). Nyamdorjet al. (2008) found the association of the development of hypertension with BMI as strong as that with central obesity indicators in Mauritian Indian and Mauritian Creole. Body composition measures such as visceral fat (VF) and percent body fat (PBF) are also considered to be significant indicators of body fat distribution in association with hypertension risk found in populations with different ethnicities worldwide (Despréset al., 2000; Gupta 2004; Lam, Koh, Chen, Wong & Fallows, 2015; Pereira et al., 2015). Asian Indians have higher abdominal body fat storage even at a lower BMI, and are susceptible to a higher risk of CVDs and metabolic syndrome (Chandalia, Abate, Garg, Stray-Gundersen & Grundy, 1999; Raji, Seely, Arky & Simonson, 2001, Raji et al., 2004; Forouhi, 2005; Bhat et al., 2005; Misra & Shrivastava 2013). Also, abdominal obesity leads to elevated blood pressure and insulin resistance (Poirier et al., 2005). Obese individuals with accumulated visceral fat have an increased risk for hypertension, type 2 diabetes mellitus and other cardiovascular events (Bidulescuet al., 2013) and variation in fat distribution mediates cardiometabolic risk factors (Neelandet al., 2012).

Several studies have reported the prevalence of hypertension in adults (Gupta & Mehrishi, 1997; Gupta, 2004; Thankappanet al., 2005; Kauret al., 2007; Kaur et al., 2012; Rizwanet al., 2014; Panda et al., 2017) and children in urban areas of India (Mohan et al., 2003; Singh, 2007; Durrani & Fatima, 2011; Shetty, Shetty, Sasidharan & Shenoy, 2013; Singh et al., 2013; Kumar et al., 2017). Studies (Gerber, Schwartz, Schnall & Pickering, 1995; Dua & Kapoor, 2000) have shown sex differences in association of adiposity measures with blood pressure in urban populations. WHR, WHtR and conicity index (CI) are found to be higher in females due to the gynoidal pattern of fat distribution (Mungreiphyet al., 2012). It has been found that males are more prone to abdominal fat deposition in comparison to females, which is responsible for higher central adiposity in them (Despreset al., 2000). Sex-wise studies on hypertension have highlighted that systolic blood pressure (SBP) levels increases with advancing age (Reddy, 1998; Raina, Chander, Prasher & Raina, 2016) and the increase has been reported to be more prominent in females than males (Dua, Bhuker, Sharma, Dhall & Kapoor, 2014; Raina et al., 2016).

Obesity and its association with elevated blood pressure has been reported among tribal populations of India (NNMB, 2009; Kapoor, Saluja, Verma & Kapoor, 2012; Kshatriya & Acharya, 2016). Meshram et al. (2012) found that the risk of hypertension was significantly higher among overweight/obese tribal men and women as compared to normal individuals. Similarly, Kapoor et al. (2012) reported a positive correlation of BMI and mid upper arm circumference (MUAC) and a negative correlation of PBF with risk of hypertension among tribal communities from different regions of India. Similar studies among tribes across varied ecological settings within India have observed association of hypertension with anthropometric indices (Babu, Kusuma & Naidu, 1996; Kusuma, Babu & Naidu, 2002; Mukhopadhyay & Mukhopadhyay, 2001; Kerketta, Bulliyya, Babu, Mohapatra & Nayak, 2009; Maken & Verte, 2016). The nomadic tribal groups of Rajasthan have shown an increased hypertensive tendency at elevated abdominal and visceral fat adiposity as well (Sachdev, 2011). BMI and abdominal adiposity showed positive correlation with hypertension in tribal population of India (Kshatriya, 2014). However, to the best of our knowledge there is hardly any study on the association of adiposity measures with blood pressure among the tribal population groups of India. Therefore, the present study is an attempt to investigate the bisexual variations in the association of adiposity measures with the risk of hypertension among the three tribal populations namely Dhodia, Kukna and Choudhuri of Gujarat, India for a better understanding of correlates of hypertension among these socially and economically deprived populations.

MATERIALS AND METHODS

Ethical Statement

Prior ethical clearance to conduct the research was obtained from the Institutional Review Committee, Department of Anthropology, University of Delhi. Informed written consent from each participant was obtained prior to the actual commencement of the study.

Area and People

The present study was conducted among three tribes namely Dhodia, Kukna and Choudhuri from Valsad and Surat districts of Gujarat, during August-September 2013 (Figure 1).

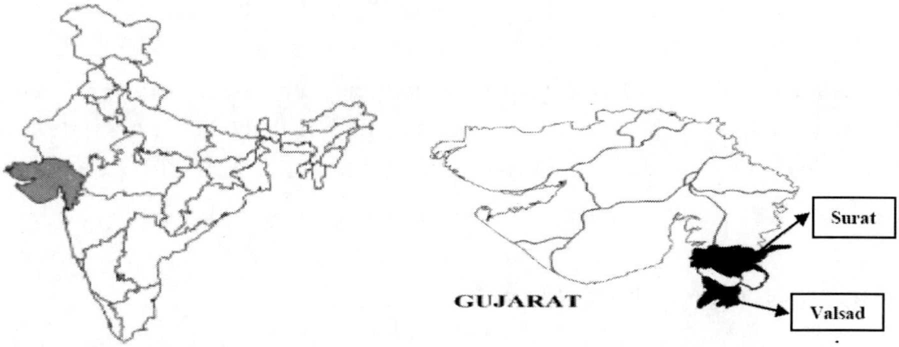

Source: https://www.mapsofindia.com/maps/gujarat/.

Figure 1. Geographical location of the selected districts in Gujarat.

The tribes of Gujarat are agriculturalists and have a sedentary life. They are also involved in other occupations such as government jobs, cattle rearing and manual labour. All the studied tribes have access to basic amenities such as water, electricity, education and healthcare. Ways of modern entertainments such as television, radio and music systems, mobile phones are making their way into the life of these tribal communities replacing the traditional community activities such as folk singing, narrations and dancing. Prevalence of alcohol consumption was low in the tribes of Gujarat.

Sampling Method and Sample Size

A total of 30 villages from two districts namely Valsad and Surat of Gujarat were chosen on the basis of the residence in acculturated areas of development (areas where development activities have reached). These areas have comparatively closed access to "urban centers." House listing was prepared for these selected villages. Subsequently, the age and sex composition of adult men and women was prepared for the studied three tribes from the house listing. A sample size of 120 adult men and 120 adult women from each of the three tribes was selected using simple random sampling. As a result, the study comprised of a total of 721 participants out of which 360 were men and 361 were women aged 20-60 years.

Exclusion criteria: People with any type of growth and developmental disorders, severe health issues in the past year, and the existence of any secondary cause of hypertension were not included in the current study. People who were hesitant about being part of the study were also excluded.

Data Collection and Measurements

Two trained anthropologists guided by the principal investigator constituted the field research team for data collection. To avoid any measurement of entry biases, one person was assigned the responsibility of taking all the measurements while the other used to enter data into the datasheet. Same set of instruments were used throughout for recording the measurements.

A structured format was used to collect demographic information such as name, age, sex, name of tribe from each of the participants.

Standard techniques were followed while taking all the anthropometric measurements (Lohman, Roche & Martorell, 1988). The standing height was measured to the nearest of 0.1 cm using a movable anthropometer. Skinfold thicknesses at four sites (biceps, triceps, sub-scapular and supra-iliac) were estimated using the Holtain's skinfold thickness calliper and sum of four skinfolds (SF_4) was measured.

Percent body fat (PBF) and visceral fat (VF) were estimated by bioelectrical impedance analysis (BIA) using Omron Karada Scan Body Composition Monitor (Omron Health Care Co., Kyoto, Japan), which is a hand-held impedance analyser. Each participant's particulars such as height, age and sex were recorded into the instrument after which the participant was instructed to stand on the platform with their feet placed on the scales present at the platform, the hand-held monitor was then held by them which scanned the body and gave recording of the impedance and body fat percentage calculation. The participants were encouraged to remove their shoes and heavy clothing before taking measurements. Weight was also recorded to the nearest 0.1kg with the help of this instrument.

Mid upper arm circumference (MUA), minimum waist circumference (MWC) and maximum hip circumference (MHC) were recorded using non-expandable measuring tape. Waist hip ratio (WHR) and waist height ratio (WHtR) were also estimated.

Blood pressure was measured following American Heart Association (AHA) guidelines (Liz, 2005). The systolic and diastolic blood pressure was measured using a standard mercury sphygmomanometer on the left upper arm of the participants in the sitting position. A minimum 15-minute rest before the measurement and a 5-minute interval between two consecutive measurements were ensured. The average of two readings was recorded.

Individual Classification

High body mass index (BMI) has been treated as a strong indicator of obesity and hypertension in various populations. Furthermore, the "obesity paradox" has been reported which indicated that low BMI was associated with hypertension (Hainer & Aldhoon-Hainerová, 2013). Therefore, we considered both low and high BMI statuses as predictors of hypertension risks. According to the World Health Organization (WHO) guidelines for Asian populations, individuals with BMI <18.5 kg/m^2 were considered as underweight; $\geq$18.5 kg/m^2 but <23 kg/m^{2}as normal; $\geq$23 kg/m^2 but <27.5 kg/m^2 as overweight and $\geq$27.5 kg/m^2 as obese (WHO, 1998; Kesavachandran, Bihari & Mathur, 2012). In the present study, we have combined the overweight and obese categories as the proportion for each of the two was found to be very low.

Several studies have demonstrated that WHtR is more closely associated with central obesity, encompassing the adjustment to various statures (Hsieh, Yoshinaga, Muto, Sakurai & Kosaka, 2000; Lin et al., 2002; Sayeed et al., 2003) and overcoming the negative correlation of height to metabolic syndromes (Henriksson, Kindblas, Agren, Nilsson-Ehle & Rastam, 2001). The mean height of Indian tribes is less than the mean height of the general Indian population (Gautam & Adak, 2006). Therefore, WHtR can be an ideal obesity measure and a strong indicator of health (Ashwell & Hsieh, 2005) in Indian tribal populations. In the present study, WHtR was classified in to two categories: (1) <0.50 as normal (Peng et al., 2013); and (2) ≥0.50 as at risk for both males and females. MWC and WHR have also been associated with central obesity and cut-offs also vary sex-wise because of the differences in the deposition of fat in males and females. In case of minimum waist circumference (MWC), males with <90cm and females with <80cm were considered as normal, while males with ≥90cm and females with ≥80 cm were considered as at-risk category (Alberti, Zimmet & Shaw, 2006; WHO, 2011). WHR was classified into two categories: 1) males with <0.90 and females with <0.85 as normal, and (2) males with ≥0.90 and females with ≥0.85 as at-risk category (WHO, 2011).

The 7th Joint National Committee on Prevention, Detection, Evaluation, and Treatment of High Blood Pressure cut off have been used for classifying the participants as normal, prehypertensive and hypertensive (Chobanianet al., 2003). Participants with SBP <120mm Hg and DBP <80mm Hg were recorded as normal, while those with SBP between 120 and 139 mm Hg or DBP between 80 and 89 mm Hg were classified as prehypertensive. Participants with blood pressure ≥140/90 mm Hg were considered hypertensive (James, 2014).

Statistical Analysis

Data entry was done in Microsoft Excel 2007, and further analyses were carried out using SPSS version 16.0 for Windows (SPSS Inc.,

Chicago, Illinois, USA). Descriptive statistics, such as mean and standard deviation (SD), were estimated for the selected anthropometric, body composition and physiometric variables. Student's t-test was performed to estimate the level of significance between the two sexes. Pearson's correlation coefficient was estimated for anthropometric, body composition measures and blood pressure. Furthermore, linear regression for total population as well as for males and females separately was used by taking SBP and DBP as dependent variables and MWC, MUAC, WHR, WHtR, BMI, SF_4, PBF and VF as independent variables. Data were cross tabulated by adiposity variables and sex, and analysed by using three-dimensional contingency chi-square test.

RESULTS

Table 1 describes the characteristics of the studied tribal populations of Gujarat. The mean values of height, weight, minimum waist circumference (MWC), mid upper arm circumference (MUAC), visceral fat (VF), waist hip ratio (WHR) and waist height ratio (WHtR) were observed to be higher in males as compared to females. The mean difference between males and females were found to be statistically significant.

Mean values of diastolic blood pressure (DBP), percent body fat (PBF) and sum of four skinfolds (SF_4) were found to be higher among females than males. Variables like PBF, DBP and SF_4 were found to be statistically significant between the two sexes.

Table 2 shows the partial correlation between adiposity variables (MWC, MUAC, BMI, WHR, WHtR, PBF, VF and SF_4) and physiometric variables (SBP and DBP) among the selected tribal groups of Gujarat. Findings indicate a significant positive correlation of all the adiposity measures with the physiometric variables.

Table 3 presents the linear regression analysis of physiometric measures with anthropometric and body composition measures as independent variables for the tribes of Gujarat. It can be seen that SBP and DBP have a significant positive impact on MWC (β-0.42, adj. R^2-0.08; β-0.61; adj. R^2-0.06) and PBF (β-0.14, adj. R^2-0.04; β- 0.16; adj. R^2-0.07) among the selected populations of Gujarat.

Table 4 shows sex-wise linear regression analysis for anthropometric and body composition measures with SBP and DBP as the dependent variables. It can be seen that among females, SBP has a significant positive impact on MWC (β-0.42; adj. R^2-0.11) and PBF (β-0.21; adj. R^2-0.09) while, DBP was found to have significant positive effect on MWC (β - 0.59; adj. R^2-0.08), PBF (β-0.16; adj. R^2-0.07) and VF (β- 0.38; adj. R^2-0.09). However, in case of males, SBP and DBP had significant positive impact only on MWC (β-0.38; adj. R^2-0.10; β- 0.68; adj. R^2-0.18).

Table 1. Characteristics of the studied tribal populations of Gujarat (n= 721)

Variables	Male (n=360)	Female (n=361)	T
	Mean ± S.D.	Mean ± S.D.	
Age (year)	40.8 ± 12.39	40.3 ± 11.61	0.61
Height (cm)	162.3 ± 6.48	150.4 ± 5.02	27.60***
Weight (kg)	53.4 ± 9.54	44.9 ± 7.47	13.33***
MWC (cm)	78.9 ± 10.48	67.2 ± 8.15	16.67***
MUAC (cm)	25.9 ± 2.69	22.6 ± 2.42	17.16***
SBP (mm Hg)	127.7 ± 20.57	126.8 ± 19.80	0.59
DBP (mm Hg)	78.2 ± 11.57	80.8 ± 12.44	-2.92**
PBF	22.3 ± 6.08	29.9 ± 6.03	-16.70***
BMI (kg/m^2)	20.2 ± 3.16	19.8 ± 3.15	1.72
VF	5.3 ± 3.89	3.4 ± 2.39	8.23***
WHR	0.9 ± .07	0.8 ± .06	29.89***
WHtR	0.5 ± .64	0.5 ± .06	8.61***
SF_4(mm)	31.7 ± 14.45	45.6 ± 21.05	-10.33***

***p<0.001, **p<0.0l.

Abbreviations: MWC- minimum waist circumference, MUAC- mid-upper arm circumference, SBP- systolic blood pressure, DBP- diastolic blood pressure, PBF- percent body fat, BMI- Body fat mass, VF- Visceral fat, WHR- waist hip ratio, WHtR- waist height ratio, SF_4- Sum of four skinfold thicknesses.

Table 2. Correlation of adiposity measures with physiometric variables (SBP and DBP) in the tribal populations of Gujarat (n= 721)

	MWC	MUAC	SBP	DBP	PBF	BMI	VF	WHR	WHtR	SF_4
MWC		.802**	.288**	.246**	.101**	.669**	.733**	.837**	.935**	.277**
MUAC			.177**	.170**	-.059	.658**	.659**	.630**	.705**	.286**
SBP				.709**	.212**	.217**	.226**	.178**	.313**	.149**
DBP					.267**	.290**	.260**	.074*	.274**	.230**
PBF						.384**	.271**	-.164**	.309**	.476**
BMI							.866**	.348**	.721**	.548**
VF								.526**	.737**	.341**
WHR									.740**	-.066
WHtR										.407**
SF_4										

** Correlation is significant at the 0.01 level (2-tailed).

* Correlation is significant at the 0.05 level (2-tailed).

Abbreviations: MWC- minimum waist circumference, MUAC- mid-upper arm circumference, SBP- systolic blood pressure, DBP- diastolic blood pressure, PBF- percent body fat, BMI- Body fat mass, VF- Visceral fat, WHR- waist hip ratio, WHtR- waist height ratio, SF_4- Sum of four skinfold thicknesses.

Table 3. Linear regression analysis of SBP and DBP with anthropometric and body composition measures among the tribes of Gujarat (n= 721)

Variables	SBP			DBP		
	β	T	Adj.R^2	β	T	Adj.R^2
MWC	0.421	2.737**	0.081	0.605	3.982***	0.059
MUAC	-0.046	-0.675	0.030	-0.076	-1.102	0.028
PBF	0.143	2.765**	0.044	0.163	3.177**	0.070
BMI	-0.182	-1.909	0.046	0.007	0.071	0.083
VF	0.066	0.806	0.050	0.054	0.666	0.066
WHR	-0.211	-2.369	0.030	-0.311	-3.535	0.004
WHtR	0.161	1.185	0.097	-0.105	-0.783	0.074
SF_4	-0.020	-0.400	0.021	0.012	0.243	0.052

***p<0.001, **p<0.0l.

Abbreviations: MWC- minimum waist circumference, MUAC- mid-upper arm circumference, SBP- systolic blood pressure, DBP- diastolic blood pressure, PBF- percent body fat, BMI- Body fat mass, VF- Visceral fat, WHR- waist hip ratio, WHtR- waist height ratio, SF_4- Sum of four skinfold thicknesses.

Table 4. Sex-wise linear regression analysis for anthropometric and body composition measures (n= 721)

Variables	Females (n= 361)						Males (n=360)					
	SBP			DBP			SBP			DBP		
	B	T	$AdjR^2$	β	T	$adjR^2$	β	T	$adjR^2$	β-	T	$adjR^2$
MWC	0.418	1.973*	0.107	0.594	2.767 **	0.083	0.375	2.015*	0.102	0.679	3.847 ***	0.179
MUAC	-0.059	-.548	0.029	-0.073	-.674	0.040	-0.027	-.333	0.043	0.043	.561	0.113
PBF	0.205	2.845 **	0.090	0.145	1.984*	0.072	0.048	.784	0.033	0.071	1.209	0.047
BMI	-0.226	-1.295	0.047	-0.155	-.878	0.067	-0.207	-1.547	0.041	-0.014	-.112	0.112
VF	0.151	1.036	0.069	0.379	2.564 **	0.094	0.102	.832	0.043	0.034	.292	0.102
WHR	-0.084	-.979	0.049	0.003	.038	0.028	-0.132	-1.185	0.062	-0.177	-1.671	0.080
WHtR	-0.029	-.134	0.109	-0.521	-2.384*	0.069	0.133	.652	0.095	-0.188	-.977	0.144
SF_4	-0.053	-.752	0.015	-0.032	-.455	0.021	0.024	.337	0.049	0.006	.081	0.085

***p<0.001, **p<0.0l, *p<0.05.

Abbreviations: MWC- minimum waist circumference, MUAC- mid-upper arm circumference, SBP- systolic blood pressure, DBP- diastolic blood pressure, PBF- percent body fat, BMI- Body fat mass, VF- Visceral fat, WHR- waist hip ratio, WHtR- waist height ratio, SF_4- Sum of four skinfold thicknesses.

Further, a mutually independent hypothesis and a number of partially independent hypotheses were tested for various categories of blood pressure (normal, PHTN and HTN), normal and at risk anthropometric variables and sex using three-dimensional chi-square analysis. In partially independent hypothesis, we tested: (a) sex as independent of blood pressure and normal and at risk anthropometric variables, (b) blood pressure as independent of sex, and normal and at risk anthropometric variables, and (c) normal and at risk anthropometric variables as independent of sex and blood pressure.

Tables 5, 6, 7 and 8 present the distribution of normal and at-risk categories of MWC, WHR, WHtR, BMI, and blood pressure by sex among the selected tribal groups of Gujarat. Our initial analysis showed that normal and at risk anthropometric variables, by sex and blood pressure were not mutually independent, which led us to test for partial independence. In partial independence, three of the one variable was tested as independent of the other two. It was found that except for BMI, all the chi-square tests for partial independence were statistically significant at p<0.05. Thus, it can be inferred that adiposity measures and risk of hypertension by sex are strongly associated.

Table 5. Distribution of normal and risk categories of MWC and blood pressure among the males and females of the selected tribal groups of Gujarat in three-dimensional contingency table and test for mutual independence (n=721)

	At risk (MWC)			Normal (MWC)			Total
	Normal	PHTN	HTN	Normal	PHTN	HTN	
Females (n=361)	2 (0.6%)	11 (3.0%)	15 (4.2%)	116 (32.1%)	142 (39.3%)	75 (20.8%)	361 (100%)
Males (n=360)	8 (2.2%)	18 (5.0%)	30 (8.3%)	124 (34.4%)	112 (31.1%)	68 (18.9%)	360 (100%)

Chi-square: 319.15; df: 7; p<0.05.

Table 6. Distribution of normal and risk categories of WHR and blood pressure among the males and females of the selected tribal groups of Gujarat in three-dimensional contingency table and test for mutual independence (n=721)

	At risk (WHR)			Normal (WHR)			Total
	Normal	PHTN	HTN	Normal	PHTN	HTN	
Females (n=361)	18 (5.0%)	31 (8.6%)	33 (9.1%)	100 (27.7%)	122 (33.8%)	57 (15.8%)	361 (100%)
Males (n=360)	110 (30.6%)	114 (31.7%)	90 (25.0%)	22 (6.1%)	16 (4.4%)	8 (2.2%)	360 (100%)

Chi-square: 319.15; df: 7; $p<0.05$.

Table 7. Distribution of normal and risk levels of WHtR and blood pressure among the males and females of the selected tribal groups of Gujarat in three-dimensional contingency table and test for mutual independence (n=721)

	At risk (WHtR)			Normal (WHtR)			Total
	Normal	PHTN	HTN	Normal	PHTN	HTN	
Females (n=361)	5 (1.4%)	25 (6.9%)	34 (9.4%)	113 (31.3%)	128 (35.5%)	56 (15.5%)	361 (100%)
Males (n=360)	29 (8.1%)	45 (12.5%)	61 (16.9%)	103 (28.6%)	85 (23.6%)	37 (10.3%)	360 (100%)

Chi-square: 114.94; df: 7; $p<0.05$.

Table 8. Distribution of BMI categories and blood pressure levels among the males and females of the selected tribal groups of Gujarat in three-dimensional contingency table and test for mutual independence (n=718)

	Underweight			Normal			Overweight			Total
	Normal	PHTN	HTN	Normal	PHTN	HTN	Normal	PHTN	HTN	
Females (n=361)	60 (16.6%)	60 (16.6%)	25 (6.9%)	49 (13.6%)	71 (19.7%)	41 (11.4%)	9 (2.5%)	22 (6.1%)	24 (6.6%)	361 (100%)
Males (n=357)	59 (16.5%)	35 (9.8%)	28 (7.8%)	59 (16.5%)	73 (20.4%)	37 (10.4%)	13 (3.6%)	20 (5.6%)	33 (9.2%)	357 (100%)

Chi-square: 52.16; df: 12; $p<0.05$.

DISCUSSION

The findings of the studied tribal communities of Gujarat showed that there are significant sex differences in several anthropometric measurements and blood pressure among the tribal populations. In addition, these groups also showed the risk of hypertension along with the burden of malnutrition (underweight and overweight). It may be noted here that obesity co-exists with underweight in India and hence, the country suffers from a double burden of malnutrition (Popkins, 2002; Kshatriya & Acharya, 2016). The development of obesity involves the amalgamation of numerous social, behavioural, cultural, physiological, metabolic and genetic factors (National Research Council [NRC], 1989; WHO, 2016). WHO (2011) reported the estimated prevalence for hypertension among the Indian National population as 32.5%, which was found to be higher than the estimated prevalence of 22.5% among tribal populations. Increasing trend of hypertension among tribal populations was also observed in various studies (NNMB, 2009; Naidu, Nayak & Sadi, 2016; Rizwan et al., 2014; Kshatriya & Acharya, 2016). Kshatriya & Acharya (2016) reported that hypertension was observed to be higher among females as compared to males in tribal populations of India. Only few studies (Deshmukh, Gupta, Dongre & Bharambe, 2006; Chockalingamet al., 2005; Ghosh, 2007; Guptaet al.,2007; Kapoor et al., 2012; Singh et al., 2013) have been carried out on the factors determining hypertension risk among Indian people. However, to the best of our knowledge this is the first attempt to find out the bisexual differences in the association of adiposity variables with blood pressure among the tribal populations of Gujarat.

Men in the studied tribal groups had significantly higher mean height, weight, MWC, MUAC, VF, WHR and WHtR, while mean values of DBP, PBF and SF_4 were significantly higher among females, indicating sexual differences in adiposity measures. Various studies have shown that adiposity measures play a significant role in predicting hypertension risk among males and females (Yalcin, 2005; Ghosh, Mukhopadhyay & Barik, 2016; Kandpal, Sachdeva & Saraswathy, 2016; Kshatriya & Acharya,

2016). Pal et al. (2014) found that rural Bengalee females had significantly higher PBF and fat mass while males had central adiposity resulting in higher mean values of anthropometric measures such as MWC, WHR and WHtR. Significant sex differences were also observed in numerous studies conducted on urban population groups residing in India (Sanjeev, Indech, Jit & Johnston, 1991; Bhadra, Mukhopadhyay & Bose, 2002; Deshmukh et al., 2006). However, few studies (Kapoor, Kapoor & Durnin, 1999; Misraet al., 2001; Mungreiphy & Kapoor, 2010; Bansal et al., 2012) have reported higher percentage of females to be overweight than males and have higher mean for WHR, WHtR and BMI due to relatively more gynoidal pattern of fat distribution. Furthermore, significant positive correlations between adiposity measures (MWC, MUAC, PBF, BMI, VF, WHR, WHtR, SF_4) and physiometric variables (SBP and DBP) were also obtained. A strong positive correlation between BMI, WHR, MWC, WHtR and SBP and DBP was observed in many studies as well (Deshmukh et al., 2006; Gupta et al., 2007; Chakraborty, Bose & Bisai, 2009; Pal, De, Sengupta, Maity & Dhara, 2014).

The regression analysis indicates that SBP and DBP have a significant positive impact on MWC and PBF among the selected population groups. Sex-wise regression analysis indicated that among females SBP had a significant positive impact on MWC and PBF, while DBP had a significant impact on MWC, PBF and VF; while in case of males, SBP and DBP had significant positive impact only on MWC, which could be because men are prone to abdominal fat deposition in comparison to women (Deprés, 2000; Mungreiphyet al., 2012). Similar results have also been reported in a few studies earlier (Ghosh et al., 2016; Kandpalet al., 2016; Kshatriya & Acharya, 2016).

It was also attempted in the present study to find out the association of normal and risk categories of adiposity markers such as MWC, WHR, WHtR and BMI with blood pressure levels (normal, PHTN and HTN) among both the sexes of selected tribal groups using three-dimensional contingency chi-square analysis. A mutually independent hypothesis along with various partially independent hypotheses were tested to investigate the association of adiposity measures with risk of hypertension by sex.

Bisexual differences were found to be statistically significant for MWC, WHR and WHtR and various categories of blood pressure. Mutual dependence was also reported between sex, anthropometric measures and blood pressure. Kshatriya & Acharya (2016) in their study reported that tribal women above 40 years of age are at a greater risk of suffering from undernutrition because of the social and gender disparities faced by them leading to chronic health conditions. Low BMI and undernutrition was reported to be a risk factor for CVD (Pal et al., 2014; Kshatriya & Acharya, 2016). An increased visceral fat mass is responsible for greater blood pressure due to activation of several mechanisms such as leptin resistance, insulin resistance and inflammation (Sniderman, Bhopal, Prabhakaran, Sarrafzadegan & Tchermof, 2007). Tainget al. (2016) also found MWC and WHtR to be strongly associated with blood pressure than BMI. People belonging to Asian ethnicities have a high total body fat and a greater amount of abdominal and visceral fat at a given BMI in comparison to other ethnic groups (Lear et al., 2007; Misra & Shrivastava, 2013). Therefore, anthropometric measures (MWC, WHR and WHtR) which take into consideration central fat distribution may be more helpful in determining the adverse health conditions in various communities in India.

Differences in blood pressure between various ethnic groups have been observed in India and various studies suggest that numerous factors are associated with SBP and DBP in rural as well as urban population. Higher SBP and DBP are associated with malnutrition, inaccessible health services, alcohol consumptions and smoking in rural groups (Reddy, Rao & Reddy,2002; Hazarika, Narain, Biswas, Kalita & Mahanta, 2004; Kusuma & Das, 2008; Kshatriya & Acharya, 2016), whereas sedentary lifestyle, unhealthy food habits, stress are being associated with high blood pressure levels in urban areas (Mungreiphy & Kapoor, 2010; Ibrahim & Damasceno, 2012; WHO, 2013). The tribal groups practicing farming have been reported for elevated risk of hypertension than those occupied in other occupations probably because of the unsatisfactory yield of crops leading to greater economic crisis and stress (Wasnik & Jawarkar, 2016).

Finally, the sex-wise differences and association of adiposity markers with hypertension observed in the current study will be helpful in extending these results to other tribal population groups for developing effective intervention strategies.

CONCLUSION

The findings of the present study show an increasing prevalence of prehypertension and hypertension among both the sexes in tribal areas at an alarming rate. The sex-wise differences and association of adiposity markers with hypertension in the current study would be helpful in designing better health care delivery systems in the areas of tribal concentration.

ACKNOWLEDGMENTS

The help rendered by Prof. Satwanti Kapoor, University of Delhi and Dr. Arnab Ghosh, Visva Bharati, Santi Niketan in formulation of the research problem is greatly appreciated. We express our gratitude to Subhendu Kumar Acharya, Miss Hemlata and Mr. Gajanan for participating in data collection. We sincerely acknowledge the support and co-operation of the participants of the selected villages. This study was funded to GKK by the Indian Council of Medical Research (ICMR), Government of India, bearing project reference number 5/4/8-2/2010 NCD-II. The author reports no conflicts of interest.

REFERENCES

Alberti, K. G. M. M., Zimmet, P., & Shaw, J. (2006). Metabolic syndrome—a new world-wide definition. A consensus statement from the international diabetes federation. *Diabetic Medicine*, *23*(5), 469-480.

Amin, F., Fatima, S. S., Islam, N., & Gilani, A. H. (2015). Prevalence of obesity and overweight, its clinical markers and associated factors in a high risk South-Asian population. *BMC Obesity*, *2*(1), 16.

Anchala, R., Kannuri, N. K., Pant, H., Khan, H., Franco, O. H., Di Angelantonio, E., & Prabhakaran, D. (2014). Hypertension in India: a systematic review and meta-analysis of prevalence, awareness, and control of hypertension. *Journal of Hypertension*, *32*(6), 1170.

Ashwell, M., & Hsieh, S. D. (2005). Six reasons why the waist-to-height ratio is a rapid and effective global indicator for health risks of obesity and how its use could simplify the international public health message on obesity. *International Journal of Food Sciences and Nutrition*, *56*(5), 303-307.

Babu, B. V., Kusuma, Y. S., & Naidu, J. M. (1996). Distribution of blood pressure and influence of subcutaneous fat on systolic and diastolic levels in a tribal population. *Journal of the Indian Medical Association*, *94*(8), 289-91.

Bansal, S. K., Goel, D., Saxena, V., Kandpal, S. D., Gray, W. K., & Walker, R. W. (2012). The prevalence of hypertension and hypertension risk factors in a rural Indian community: A prospective door-to-door study. *Journal of Cardiovascular Disease Research*, *3*(2), 117-123.

Bhadra, M., Mukhopadhyay, A., & Bose, K. (2002). Adiposity, central body fat distribution and blood pressure among young Bengalee adults of Kolkata, India: sexual dimorphism. *Journal of Physiological Anthropology and Applied Human Science*, *21*(6), 273-276.

Bhat, D. S., Yajnik, C. S., Sayyad, M. G., Raut, K. N., Lubree, H. G., Rege, S. S., ... & Kurpad, A. V. (2005). Body fat measurement in Indian men: comparison of three methods based on a two-compartment model. *International Journal of Obesity*, *29*(7), 842-848.

Bidulescu, A., Liu, J., Hickson, D. A., Hairston, K. G., Fox, E. R., Arnett, D. K., ... & Gibbons, G. H. (2013). Gender differences in the association of visceral and subcutaneous adiposity with adiponectin in African Americans: the Jackson Heart Study. *BMC Cardiovascular*

Disorders, *13*(1), 9. [accessed 2017 Aug 13]. https://www.ncbi.nlm.nih.gov/pmc/articles/PMC3586352/.

Chakraborty, R., Bose, K., & Bisai, S. (2009). Body mass index and blood pressure among adult Bengalee male slum dwellers of Kolkata, India. *Journal of Public Health*, *17*(5), 301.

Chandalia, M., Abate, N., Garg, A., Stray-Gundersen, J., & Grundy, S. M. (1999). Relationship between generalized and upper body obesity to insulin resistance in Asian Indian men. *The Journal of Clinical Endocrinology & Metabolism*, *84*(7), 2329-2335.

Chobanian, A. V., Bakris, G. L., Black, H. R., Cushman, W. C., Green, L. A., Izzo Jr, J. L., ... & Roccella, E. J. (2003). The seventh report of the joint national committee on prevention, detection, evaluation, and treatment of high blood pressure: the JNC 7 report. *Jama*, *289*(19), 2560-2571.

Chockalingam, A., Ganesan, N., Venkatesan, S., Gnanavelu, G., Subramaniam, T., Jaganathan, V., ... & Rafeeq, K. (2005). Patterns and predictors of prehypertension among "healthy" urban adults in India. *Angiology*, *56*(5), 557-563.

de Moraes, A. C. F., Lacerda, M. B., Moreno, L. A., Horta, B. L., & Carvalho, H. B. (2014). Prevalence of high blood pressure in 122,053 adolescents: a systematic review and meta-regression. *Medicine*, *93*(27).

Deshmukh, P. R., Gupta, S. S., Dongre, A. R., & Bharambe, M. S. (2006). Relationship of anthropometric indicators with blood pressure levels in rural Wardha. *Indian Journal of Medical Research*, *123*(5), 657.

Després, J. P., Couillard, C., Gagnon, J., Bergeron, J., Leon, A. S., Rao, D. C., ... & Bouchard, C. (2000). Race, visceral adipose tissue, plasma lipids, and lipoprotein lipase activity in men and women. *Arteriosclerosis, thrombosis, and vascular biology*, *20*(8), 1932-1938.

Dua, S., Bhuker, M., Sharma, P., Dhall, M., & Kapoor, S. (2014). Body mass index relates to blood pressure among adults. *North American journal of medical sciences*, *6*(2), 89.

Durrani, A. M., & Fatima, W. (2011). Determinants of blood pressure distribution in school children. *The European Journal of Public Health*, *22*(3), 369-373.

Forouhi, N. G. (2005). Ethnicity and the metabolic syndrome. In: Byrne, C. D., Wild, S. H. (Eds.), *The Metabolic Syndrome*. London: John Wiley and Sons.

Gautam, R. K., Adak, D. K. (2006). Nutrition and Genetic Variation among Central Indian tribes. In: *Proceedings of national symposium on Tribal Health*; Oct 19-20; Jaipur. Delhi: Regional Medical Research Centre for Tribals, Indian Council of Medical Research, National Family and Health Survey.

Gerber, L. M., Schwartz, J. E., Schnall, P. L., & Pickering, T. G. (1995). Body fat and fat distribution in relation to sex differences in blood pressure. *American journal of human biology*, *7*(2), 173-182.

Ghosh, A. (2007). Factor analysis of risk variables associated with metabolic syndrome in Asian Indian adolescents. *American Journal of Human Biology*, *19*(1), 34-40.

Ghosh, R. K., Bandyopadhyay, D., Hajra, A., Biswas, M., & Gupta, A. (2016). Cardiovascular outcomes of sodium-glucose cotransporter 2 inhibitors: a comprehensive review of clinical and preclinical studies. *International journal of cardiology*, *212*, 29-36.

Ghosh, S., Mukhopadhyay, S., & Barik, A. (2016). Sex differences in the risk profile of hypertension: a cross-sectional study. *BMJ open*, *6*(7), e010085.

Gupta, R., & Gupta, V. P. (2009). Hypertension epidemiology in India: lessons from Jaipur heart watch. *Current science*, 349-355.

Gupta, R., & Mehrishi, S. (1997). Waist-hip ratio and blood pressure correlation in an urban Indian population. *Journal of the Indian Medical Association*, *95*(7), 412-415.

Gupta, R., Rastogi, P., Sarna, M., Gupta, V. P., Sharma, S. K., & Kothari, K. (2007). Bodymass index, waist-size, waist-hip ratio and cardiovascular risk factors in urban subjects. *Japi*, *55*, 621-627.

Gupta, R., Sharma, A. K., Gupta, V. P., Bhatnagar, S., Rastogi, S., & Deedwania, P. C. (2003). Increased variance in blood pressure distribution and changing hypertension prevalence in an urban Indian population. *Journal of human hypertension*, *17*(8), 535-540.

Gupta, R. (2004). Trends in hypertension epidemiology in India. *Journal of human hypertension*, *18*(2), 73-78.

Hainer, V., & Aldhoon-Hainerová, I. (2013). Obesity paradox does exist. *Diabetes care*, *36*(Supplement 2), S276-S281.

Hall, J. E., do Carmo, J. M., da Silva, A. A., Wang, Z., & Hall, M. E. (2015). Obesity-induced hypertension: interaction of neurohumoral and renal mechanisms. *Circulation research*, *116*(6), 991.

Hazarika, N. C., Narain, K., Biswas, D., Kalita, H. C., & Mahanta, J. (2004). Hypertension in the native rural population of Assam. *Natl Med J India*, *17*(6), 300-4.

Henriksson, K. M., Lindblad, U., Ågren, B., Nilsson-Ehle, P., & Råstam, L. (2001). Associations between body height, body composition and cholesterol levels in middle-aged men. The coronary risk factor study in southern Sweden (CRISS). *European journal of epidemiology*, *17*(6), 521-526.

Hossain, P., Kawar, B., & El Nahas, M. (2007). Obesity and diabetes in the developing world—a growing challenge. *New England journal of medicine*, *356*(3), 213-215.

Hsieh, S. D., Yoshinaga, H., Muto, T., Sakurai, Y., & Kosaka, K. (2000). Health risks among Japanese men with moderate body mass index. *International journal of obesity*, *24*(3), 358.

Ibrahim, M. M., & Damasceno, A. (2012). Hypertension in developing countries. *The Lancet*, *380*(9841), 611-619.

James, P. A., Oparil, S., Carter, B. L., Cushman, W. C., Dennison-Himmelfarb, C., Handler, J., ... & Smith, S. C. (2014). 2014 evidence-based guideline for the management of high blood pressure in adults: report from the panel members appointed to the Eighth Joint National Committee (JNC 8). *Jama*, *311*(5), 507-520.

Jiang, S. Z., Lu, W., Zong, X. F., Ruan, H. Y., & Liu, Y. (2016). Obesity and hypertension. *Experimental and Therapeutic Medicine*, *12*(4), 2395-2399.

Kandpal, V., Sachdeva, M. P., & Saraswathy, K. N. (2016). An assessment study of CVD related risk factors in a tribal population of India. *BMC Public Health*, 16*(1), 434.*

Kapoor, A. K., Saluja, K., Verma, D., & Kapoor, S. (2012). Predictors of Hypertension among Adult Tribal Males of India. *International Journal of Tropical Disease Health, 2*(4), 241-256.

Kapoor, S. (2000). Blood pressure, waist to hip ratio and body mass index among affluent Punjabi girls of Delhi. *Acta Medica Auxologica*, *32*(3), 153-158.

Kapoor, S., Kapoor, A. K., & Durnin, J. V. G. A. (1999). Variation in body composition. In Bhatnagar, D. P., Verma, S. K., & Mokha, R. (Eds.), *Human Growth – A Multidisciplinary Approach* (pp. 12-21). Patiala: Exercise Science Publication Society.

Kaur, P., Rao, S. R., Radhakrishnan, E., Rajasekar, D., & Gupte, M. D. (2012). Prevalence, awareness, treatment, control and risk factors for hypertension in a rural population in South India. *International Journal of Public Health, 57*(1), 87-94.

Kaur, P., Rao, T. V., Sankarasubbaiyan, S., Narayanan, A. M., Ezhil, R., Rao, S. R., & Gupte, M. D. (2007). Prevalence and distribution of cardiovascular risk factors in an urban industrial population in south India: a cross sectional study. *Journal of Association of Physicians of India, 55*, 771-776.

Kerketta, A. S., Bulliyya, G., Babu, B. V., Mohapatra, S. S., & Nayak, R. N. (2009). Health status of the elderly population among four primitive tribes of Orissa India: a clinico-epidemiological study. *ZeitschriftfürGerontologie und Geriatrie, 42*(1), 53-59.

Kesavachandran, C. N., Bihari, V., & Mathur, N. (2012). The normal range of body mass index with high body fat percentage among male residents of Lucknow city in north India. *Indian Journal of Medical Research, 135*(1), 72–77.

Kshatriya, G. (2014). Changing perspectives of tribal health in the context of increasing lifestyle diseases in India. *Journal of Environmental and Social Science, 1*(1), 1-7.

Kshatriya, G. K., & Acharya, S. K. (2016). Gender Disparities in the Prevalence of Undernutrition and the Higher Risk among the Young Women of Indian Tribes. *PloS one*, *11*(7), e0158308.

Kshatriya, G. K., & Acharya, S. K. (2016). Triple Burden of Obesity, Undernutrition, and Cardiovascular Disease Risk among Indian Tribes. *PloS one*, *11*(1), e0147934.

Kumar, P., Kumar, D., Ranjan, A., Singh, C. M., Pandey, S., & Agarwal, N. (2017). Prevalence of Hypertension and its Risk Factors Among School Going Adolescents of Patna, India. *Journal of Clinical Diagnostic Research, 11*(1), 1-4.

Kusuma, Y. S., Babu, B. V., & Naidu J. M. (2002). Blood pressure levels among a few cross-cultural populations of Visakhapatnam district, Andhra Pradesh, India. *Annals of Human Biology, 29*(5), 502-512.

Kusuma, Y. S., & Das, P. K. (2008). Hypertension in Odisha, India: A cross-sectional study among some tribal, rural and urban populations. *Public Health,* 122*(10), 1120-1123.*

Lam, B. C. C., Koh, G. C. H., Chen, C., Wong, M. T. K., & Fallows, S. J. (2015). Comparison of body mass index (BMI), body adiposity index (BAI), waist circumference (WC), waist-to-hip ratio (WHR) and waist-to-height ratio (WHtR) as predictors of cardiovascular disease risk factors in an adult population in Singapore. *PLoS One, 10*(4).

Lear, S. A., Humphries, K. H., Kohli, S., Chockalingam, A., Frohlich, J. J., & Birmingham, C. L. (2007). Visceral adipose tissue accumulation differs according to ethnic background: results of the Multicultural Community Health Assessment Trial (M-CHAT). *American Journal of Clinical Nutrition, 86*(2), 353-359.

Lim, S. S., Vos, T., Flaxman, A. D., Danaei, G., Shibuya, K., Adair-Rohani, H., ... & Aryee, M. (2012). A comparative risk assessment of burden of disease and injury attributable to 67 risk factors and risk factor clusters in 21 regions, 1990–2010: a systematic analysis for the Global Burden of Disease Study 2010. *The Lancet*, *380*(9859), 2224-2260.

Lin, W. Y., Lee, L. T., Chen, C. Y., Lo, H., Hsia, H. H., Liu, I. L., ... & Huang, K. C. (2002). Optimal cut-off values for obesity: using simple anthropometric indices to predict cardiovascular risk factors in Taiwan. *International Journal of Obesity & Related Metabolic Disorders, 26*(9).

Lohman, T. G., Roche, A. F., & Martorell, R. (1988). *Anthropometric Standardization Reference Manual*. Chicago: Human Kinetics Books.

Maken, T., Varte, L. R. (2016). Anthropometric and Body Composition Differences among Rural and Urban Ao Naga Tribes: Correlation between Hypertension, Haemoglobin and Obesity. *International Journal of Biological and Medical Research, 7*(4), 5715-5721.

Map of India. [Accessed on Sept 4th, 2017]. Available on: https://www.mapsofindia.com/maps/gujarat/.

Mello, R. B., Moreira, L. B., Gus, M., Wiehe, M., Fuchs, F. D., & Fuchs, S. C. (2011). Central obesity is a risk factor for hypertension independent of body mass index in elderly individuals: Results of a Population-Based study [Abstract]. *Circulation*, 124, *A12691.*

Meshram, I. I., Arlappa, N., Balkrishna, N., Rao, K. M., Laxmaiah, A., & Brahmam, G. N. V. (2012). Prevalence of hypertension, its correlates and awareness among adult tribal population of Kerala state, India. *Journal of Postgraduate Medicine, 58*(4), 255.

Misra, A., Pandey, R. M., Devi, J. R., Sharma, R., Vikram, N. K., & Khanna, N. (2001). High prevalence of diabetes, obesity and dyslipidaemia in urban slum population in northern India. *International Journal of Obesity, 25*(11), 1722.

Misra, A., & Shrivastava, U. (2013). Obesity and dyslipidemia in South Asians. *Nutrients, 5*(7), 2708-2733.

Misra, A. (2000). Risk factors for atherosclerosis in young individuals. *Journal of Cardiovascular Risk, 7*(3), 215-229.

Mohan, B., Kumar, N., Aslam, N., Rangbulla, A., Kumbkarni, S., Sood, N. K., & Wander, G. S. (2003). Prevalence of sustained hypertension and obesity in urban and rural school going children in Ludhiana. *Indian Heart Journal, 56*(4), 310-314.

Mukhopadhyay, B., Mukhopadhyay, S. (2001). Blood pressure and its biocultural correlates among the Lepchas of Sikkim, India: A micro level epidemiological study. *Collegium Antropologicum, 25*(1), 97-110.

Mungreiphy, N. K., Dhall, M., Tyagi, R., Saluja, K., Kumar, A., Tungdim, M. G., ... & Kapoor, A. K. (2012). Ethnicity, obesity and health pattern among Indian population. *Journal of Natural Science, Biology and Medicine,* 3(1), 52-59.

Mungreiphy, N. K., & Kapoor, S. (2010). Socioeconomic changes as covariates of overweight and obesity among Tangkhul Naga tribal women of Manipur, North-East India. *Journal of Biosocial Science,* 42*(3), 289-305.*

Naidu, S. A., Nayak, M. S., & Sadi, N. (2016). Prevalence of hypertension among reproductive age group tribal women in Visakhapatnam district, Andhra Pradesh, India. *International Journal of Research in Medical Sciences*, *4*(4), 1224-1228.

Neeland, I. J., Turer, A. T., Ayers, C. R., Powell-Wiley, T. M., Vega, G. L., Farzaneh-Far, R., ... & de Lemos, J. A. (2012). Dysfunctional adiposity and the risk of prediabetes and type 2 diabetes in obese adults. *JAMA*, *308*(11), 1150-1159.

National Nutrition Monitoring Bureau. (2009). *Diet and nutritional status of tribal population and prevalence of hypertension among adults—Report on second repeat survey* [NNMB Technical Report No. 25]. Hyderabad: National Institute of Nutrition.

National Research Council. (1989). *Diet and health: implications for reducing chronic disease risk*. Washington: National Academies Press.

Nyamdorj, R., Qiao, Q., Söderberg, S., Pitkäniemi, J., Zimmet, P., Shaw, J., ... & Chitson, P. (2008). Comparison of body mass index with waist circumference, waist-to-hip ratio, and waist-to-stature ratio as a predictor of hypertension incidence in Mauritius. *Journal of Hypertension*, *26*(5), 866-870.

Pal, A., De, S., Sengupta, P., Maity, P., & Dhara, P. C. (2014). Relationship of body compositional and nutritional parameters with blood pressure in adults. *Journal of Human Nutrition and Dietetics*, *27*(5), 489-500.

Panda, P. S., Jain, K. K., Soni, G. P., Gupta, S. A., Dixit, S., & Kumar, J. (2017). Prevalence of hypertension and its association with anthropometric parameters in adult population of Raipur city, Chhattisgarh, India. *International Journal of Research in Medical Sciences*, *5*(5), 2120-2125.

Park, S. H., Park, J. H., Song, P. S., Kim, D. K., Kim, K. H., Seol, S. H., ... & Park, J. (2013). Sarcopenic obesity as an independent risk factor of hypertension. *Journal of the American Society of Hypertension*, *7*(6), 420-425.

Peng, Y. G., Li, Y., Guo, M., Tian, Y., Li, X., Li, S. H., ... & Zhao, L. C. (2013). The optimal cut-off value of waist-to-height ratio for detecting severe central obesity and low body weight adult Chinese population. *Zhonghuaxinxue guan bingzazhi,* 41*(7), 607-610.*

Pereira, P. F., Serrano, H. M. S., Carvalho, G. Q., Ribeiro, S. M. R., Peluzio, M. D. C. G., Franceschini, S. D. C. C., & Priore, S. E. (2015). Measurements of body fat distribution: assessment of collinearity with body mass, adiposity and height in female adolescents. *Revista Paulista de Pediatria* (English Edition), 33(1), 63-71.

Poirier, P., Lemieux, I., Mauriège, P., Dewailly, E., Blanchet, C., Bergeron, J., & Després, J. P. (2005). Impact of waist circumference on the relationship between blood pressure and insulin. *Hypertension*, *45*(3), 363-367.

Popkin, B. M. (2002). The shift in stages of the nutrition transition in the developing world differs from past experiences!. *Public health nutrition*, *5*(1A), 205-214.

Raina, S. K., Chander, V., Prasher, C. L., & Raina, S. (2016). Prevalence of hypertension in a tribal land locked population at high altitude. *Scientifica, 2016.*

Raji, A., Gerhard-Herman, M. D., Warren, M., Silverman, S. G., Raptopoulos, V., Mantzoros, C. S., & Simonson, D. C. (2004). Insulin resistance and vascular dysfunction in nondiabetic Asian Indians. *The Journal of Clinical Endocrinology & Metabolism*, *89*(8), 3965-3972.

Raji, A., Seely, E. W., Arky, R. A., & Simonson, D. C. (2001). Body fat distribution and insulin resistance in healthy Asian Indians and

Caucasians. *The Journal of Clinical Endocrinology & Metabolism, 86*(11), 5366-5371.

Reddy, B. N. (1998). Blood pressure and adiposity: A comparative study of socioeconomically diverse groups of Andhra Pradesh, India. *American Journal of Human Biology*, *10*(1), 5-21.

Reddy, K. K., Rao, A. P., & Reddy, T. P. (2002). Socioeconomic status and the prevalence of coronary heart disease risk factors. *Asia Pacific journal of clinical nutrition*, *11*(2), 98-103.

Redón, J., Cea-Calvo, L., Moreno, B., Monereo, S., Gil-Guillén, V., Lozano, J. V., ... & investigators of the PREV-ICTUS Study. (2008). Independent impact of obesity and fat distribution in hypertension prevalence and control in the elderly. *Journal of hypertension*, *26*(9), 1757-1764.

Rizwan, S. A., Kumar, R., Singh, A. K., Kusuma, Y. S., Yadav, K., & Pandav, C. S. (2014). Prevalence of hypertension in Indian tribes: a systematic review and meta-analysis of observational studies. *PLoS one*, *9*(5), e95896.

Rodea-Montero, E. R., Evia-Viscarra, M. L., & Apolinar-Jiménez, E. (2014). Waist-to-height ratio is a better anthropometric index than waist circumference and BMI in predicting metabolic syndrome among obese Mexican adolescents. *International Journal of Endocrinology, 2014*.

Sachdev, B. (2011). Prevalence of hypertension and associated risk factors among Nomad Tribe groups (Screening of Hypertension, Adiposities and ABO Blood Group among Select Nomad Tribes of Rajasthan, India). *Antrocom Online Journal of Anthropology, 7*(2), 181-189.

Sanjeev, Indech, G. D., Jit, I., & Johnston, F. E. (1991). Skinfold thicknesses, body circumferences and their relationship to age, sex, and socioeconomic status in adults from northwest India. *American Jorunal of Human Biology, 3*(5), 469–477.

Sayeed, M. A., Mahtab, H., Latif, Z. A., Khanam, P. A., Ahsan, K. A., Banu, A., & Azad, K. A. (2003). Waist-to-height ratio is a better obesity index than body mass index and waist-to-hip ratio for predicting diabetes, hypertension and lipidemia. *Bangladesh Medical Research Council Bulletin*, *29*(1), 1-10.

Shetty, S., Shetty, S. S., Sasidharan, S., & Shenoy, V. (2013). Prevalence of pre-hypertension and hypertension in asymptomatic urban school going children of Mangalore and its correlation with BMI. *Journal of Dental and Medical Sciences*, *9*(1), 76-79.

Singh, N., Parihar, R. K., Saini, G., Mohan, S. K., Sharma, N., & Razaq, M. (2013). Prevalence of metabolic syndrome in adolescents aged 10-18 years in Jammu, J. and K. *Indian Journal of Endocrinology and Metabolism*, *17*(1), 133.

Singh, R., Bhansali, A., Sialy, R., & Aggarwal, A. (2007). Prevalence of metabolic syndrome in adolescents from a north Indian population. *Diabetic Medicine*, *24*(2), 195-199.

Sniderman, A. D., Bhopal, R., Prabhakaran, D., Sarrafzadegan, N., & Tchernof, A. (2007). Why might South Asians be so susceptible to central obesity and its atherogenic consequences? The adipose tissue overflow hypothesis. *International Journal of Epidemiology*, *36*(1), 220-225.

Taing, K. Y., Farkouh, M. E., Moineddin, R., Tu, J. V., & Jha, P. (2016). Age and sex-specific associations of anthropometric measures of adiposity with blood pressure and hypertension in India: a cross-sectional study. *BMC Cardiovascular Disorders*, *16*(1), 247.

Thankappan, K. R., Sivasankaran, S., Sarma, P. S., Mini, G. K., Khader, S. A., Padmanabhan, P., & Vasan, R. S. (2005). Prevalence-correlates-awareness-treatment and control of hypertension in kumarakom, kerala: baseline results of a community-based intervention program. *Indian Heart Journal*, *58*(1), 28-33.

Wasnik, V. R., & Jawarkar, A. K. (2016). Prevalence of prehypertension and hypertension in rural area of Amravati District of Maharashtra, India. *International Journal of Research in Medical Sciences*, *4*(2), 549-555.

World Health Organization. (1998). *Obesity, preventing and managing the global epidemic* [Report of a WHO consultation on obesity]. Geneva: World Health Organization.

World Health Organization. (2000). *Obesity: preventing and managing the global epidemic*. Geneva: World Health Organization.

World Health Organization. (2008). *Global Strategy on Diet, Physical Activity and Health.* Accessed from http://www.who.int/dietphysical activity/factsheet_inactivity/en/.

World Health Organization. (2008). *Waist circumference and waist-hip-ratio* [Report of WHO expert consultation]. Geneva: World Health Organization.

World Health Organization. (2009). *Global health risks: mortality and burden of disease attributable to selected major risks*. Geneva: World Health Organization.

World Health Organization. (2011). *Waist circumference and waist-hip ratio* [Report of a WHO expert consultation]. Geneva, Switzerland: World Health Organization.

World Health Organization. (2013). *A global brief on hypertension: silent killer, global public health crisis: World Health Day 2013*. Geneva: World Health Organization.

World Health Organization. (2016). *Obesity and overweight.* Accessed from http://www.who.int/mediacentre/factsheets/fs311/en/.

Yalcin, B. M., Sahin, E. M., & Yalcin, E. (2005). Which anthropometric measurements is most closely related to elevated blood pressure?. *Family practice*, *22*(5), 541-547.

Yusuf, S., Reddy, S., Ôunpuu, S., & Anand, S. (2001). Global burden of cardiovascular diseases. *Circulation*, *104*(23), 2855-2864.

Zhang, Q., Mahapatra, T., Huang, F., Tang, W., Guo, Y., Tang, S., ... & Zhang, J. (2017). Association between Anthropometric Measures and Indicators for Hypertension Control among Kazakh-Chinese Hypertension Patients in Xinjiang, China: Results from a Cross-sectional Study. *PloS one*, *12*(1), e0170959.

PART II: ANALYTICAL ASPECT

In: Obesity and Syndrome X
Editors: M. Das and K. Bose
ISBN: 978-1-53614-669-1

Chapter 6

OBESITY AS AN IMPORTANT PREDICTOR OF HYPERTENSION AMONG RAJSHAHI UNIVERSITY STUDENTS IN BANGLADESH: A CROSS-SECTIONAL STUDY

Md. Golam Hossain[1,*], Sadekur Rahman[1], Suhaili Mohd[2], Saw Aik[2], Rashidul Alam Mahumud[3,†], Premananda Bharati[4,‡] and Pete E. Lestrel[5,#]

[1]Health Research Group, Department of Statistics, University of Rajshahi, Rajshahi, Bangladesh
[2]National Orthopaedic Centre of Excellence for Research and Learning (NOCERAL), Department of Orthopaedic Surgery, Faculty of Medicine, University of Malaya, Kuala Lumpur, Malayasia
[3]Health Economics and Financing Research Group, Centre for Equity and Health System, International Centre for Diarrhoeal Disease Research, Bangladesh, Dhaka, Bangladesh

---

[*] Corresponding Author Email: hossain95@yahoo.com.
[†] Senior Research Officer.
[‡] Professor Emeritus.
[#]Formerly, Associate Professor

[4]Biological Anthropology Unit, Indian Statistical Institute, Kolkata, India
[5]Sections of Orthodontics and Oral Biology, School of Dentistry, University of California at Los Angeles, CA, US

Abbreviations

BP:	Blood Pressure;
SBP:	Systolic Blood Pressure;
DBP:	Diastolic Blood Pressure;
BPC:	Blood Pressure Category;
WHO:	World Health Organization;
BMI:	Body Mass Index;
mmHg:	Millimeter of Mercury;
SPSS:	Statistical Package for Social Science;
IBM:	*International Business Machines*;
AOR:	Adjusted Odds Ratio;
SE:	Standard Error;
CI:	Confidence Interval;
R:	Reference category.

Introduction

Hypertension or raised blood pressure is one of the important components of metabolic syndrome (Grundy et al., 2004). It is one of the major risk factors for cardiovascular diseases and affects one billion people in worldwide, leading to heart attacks and strokes (WHO, 2013). It is considered a major global public-health challenge because of its high frequency and has concomitant risks of cardiovascular and kidney diseases (Oyewole and Oritogun, 2012). The incidence and prevalence of hypertension continues to increase around the world (Chen and Lipscombe 2008; Karen et al., 2008). Globally, cardiovascular diseases account for approximately 17 million deaths a year, nearly one third of the reported total deaths (WHO, 2008). Of these, complications of hypertension account for 9.4 million deaths worldwide every year (Lim et al., 2012). Hypertension is one of the leading reported causes of death in Bangladesh and approximately 17,000 or 2.28% of total deaths is due to hypertensive problem as reported by World Health Organization (WHO) in 2014 (WHO, 2014).

The prevalence of pre-hypertension and hypertension in different countries, particularly among university students was reported for Saudi Arabian females at 13.5% (Koura et al., 2012), West Bank 27.1% (male 38% and female 11.2%) (Tayem et al., 2012), Malaysia 42.9% (Lee et al., 2010), and Kuwait 39.5% (Al-Majed and Sadek, 2012). Among medical students, 67% presented with pre-hypertension and hypertension (Kulkarni et al., 2011) in India, 12.8% in Chile (Palomo et al., 2006) and 6.9% to 24.9% in Portugal (Dores et al., 2010). Once hypertension is identified, the patients should be regularly checked for their blood pressure (BP), in order to monitor and maintain the blood pressure under control (Black and Hawks, 2005). Gender, age, parental history of hypertension, and behavioral factors, like body mass index(BMI), sleep duration, smoking status have all been identified as the risk factors in hypertension (Tadesse and Alemu, 2014).

Many studies have been carried out on hypertension among university students in Western countries (Tayem et al., 2012; Simào et al., 2008; Hujova 2013; Soliman et al., 2014). While in Bangladesh researchers have investigated the association between hypertension and socio-economic and demographic factors among patients and in the general population (Rahman et al., 2015; Yinon et al., 2013). University students need to be considered a valuable asset for any nation; thus, special attention should be paid to them because of their potential influence on their families and their contribution to the nation's workforce in the future. Thus, it is important to determine the prevalence of hypertension and pre-hypertension among university students and to investigate the relationship between high blood pressure and socio demographic factors such as gender, residence, smoking, parents' history of hypertension, body mass index, religion, number of family members, parents' education, family income, sleeping duration and physical activities, in order to determine possible corrective measures.

Therefore, the aim of this study was to investigate the prevalence and associated factors of hypertension among university students in Bangladesh.

METHODS

Data

The cross-sectional study sample consisted of 911 (727 males and 184 females) university students. Data were collected from Rajshahi University, Bangladesh. Students were interviewed from January to June 2014. The age range of the subject's was 18-27 years old at the time of measurement. Rajshahi University was selected because it is the second largest university in Bangladesh, having a student population of nearly 25,000 students at any particular time. These students come from different parts of the country. Data were collected using a semi-structured pre- and post-tested questionnaire containing pre-coded and open-ended questions. Body height was measured as the distance from the top of the head in the midsagittal plane to the floor and body weight was taken while wearing thin clothing using an electronic weighing machine [Digital Display Height and Weight Tester (sgsport.en.alibaba.com)]. Body mass index was calculated as the ratio of weight in kilograms divided by the square of height in meters. i.e., $BMI = weight (kg)/(height(m))^2$. BMI was categorized into four groups as follows: underweight, $BMI \leq 18.5$; normal weight, $18.5 < BMI < 25$; overweight, $25 \leq BMI < 30$; and obese, $BMI \geq 30$ (Hossain et al., 2012).

Outcome Variable

Blood pressure (BP) was considered as an outcome variable. Systolic blood pressure (SBP) and diastolic blood pressure (DBP) were taken from each subject three times in the sitting position using mercury sphygmomanometers (Pickering et al., 2005), and the average value was taken for the analysis. Each subject was allowed to rest 5 minutes between measurements, and without having any drinks or smoking. The sample was classified into four classes according the range of blood pressure (BP); (i) Hypotension (SBP $<$ 90mmHg or DBP $<$ 60mmHg), (ii) Normal ($90 \leq$ SBP $<$ 120mmHg and $60 \leq$ DBP $<$ 80mmHg), (iii) Pre-hypertension ($120 \leq$ SBP $<$ 140 or $80 \leq$ DBP $<$ 90 mmHg), and (iv) Hypertension (SBP $\geq$ 140 mmHg or DBP $\geq$ 90mmHg) (Tadesse and Alemu, 2014).

Independent Variables

In this study, we attempted to establish the relationship between hypertension and some of the selected risk factors. The possible predictors for hypertension of university students were selected based on the published studies of university students in other countries (Tayem et al., 2012; Simào et al., 2008; Hujova, 2013; Soliman et al., 2014). Gender was classified as male (code 1) and female (code 2), permanent residence, was classified into two groups; rural (code 1) and urban (code 2), cigarette smoking behavior was divided into two groups; non smoker (no, code 0) and smoker (yes, code 1). Fathers' and mothers' education, were classified into four levels; uneducated (code 0), primary education (code 1), secondary education (code 2) and high education (code 3). Fathers' occupation was classified into three groups; agriculture (code 1), service (code 2) and business (code 3). Mothers' occupation was categorized into two groups; housewife (code 1) and non housewife (code 2). On the basis of the parents' history of hypertension the sample was categorized into two groups; parents' with hypertension, yes (code 1) and no (code 0). Body size was classified into three groups; underweight (code 1), normal (code 2) and overweight or obese (code 3), the subjects' religion was divided into two groups; Non-Muslim (code 0) and Muslim (code 1), family members were set up as $\leq$4 persons (code 1), 5-7 persons (code 2) and $\geq$8 persons (code 3). Parents' family income was divided into three groups; monthly income $<$ Taka 10000 (code 1), 10000-20000 Taka (code 2) and $\geq$Taka 20000 (code 3). Sleeping hours a night of the subjects was classified into two classes; $<$7 hours (code 1) and $\geq$7 hours (code 2), and finally, physical activity with 45 minutes a day on at least five days a week, was divided into two groups; no (code 0) and yes (code 1).

Sample Size Determination and Sampling

Since our target population is known (approximately 25000; male 20000 and female 5000), thus the significant sample size for this study would be calculated on the basis of population size, and the following formula was used for determining the sample size: $n = \frac{N}{1 + Nd^2}$ where, n = required sample size, N = population size (in here 25000), d = marginal error (we used, d = 0.032), lastly, a 95% confidence level was utilized (Rana et al., 2015). The formula provided the minimal sample size of 900 for this study. However, a total of 930 selected students were asked by one of our coauthors, using a standard questionnaire, to report their socio-demographic characteristics. Nineteen (female 12 and male 7) students who did not agree to provide their information were excluded from the current analysis. Consequently, 911 students were included in this study.

The population was considered heterogeneous, divided into two different groups (male and female). However, they were considered homogeneous within the groups. A two-stage stratified random sampling technique with a proportional allocation was used for selecting the samples from Rajshahi University. The proportional allocation technique indicated that 727 males and 184 female students would be needed for this study.

Statistical Analysis

The prevalence of each category of BP was determined using by frequency distributions. The Chi-square test was utilized to find the association between the categories of BP and some of the selected socio-economic, demographic, anthropometric and behavioral factors. Finally, multinomial logistic regression analysis was used to find the effect of socio-economic, demographic and behavioral factors on pre-hypertension and hypertension of university students. Data were analyzed using the Statistical Package for Social Sciences (SPSS, IBM version 20). A value of $p < 0.05$ was regarded as statistically significant in the analysis.

RESULTS

Background Information

A total of 911 university students were interviewed and examined. Among them 727 (79.8%) students were male and 184 (20.2%) were female. The age of the subjects varied from 18 to 27 years, with a mean age of 22.27 ± 1.86 years. The present study demonstrated that the prevalence of pre-hypertension and hypertension among university students were 42.50% and 25.60% respectively, while the prevalence of hypotension among university students was very low (1.50%) (Figure 1). Students with hypotension were excluded from further statistical analysis.

Three categories; normal, pre-hypertension and hypertension were considered in the further statistical analysis.

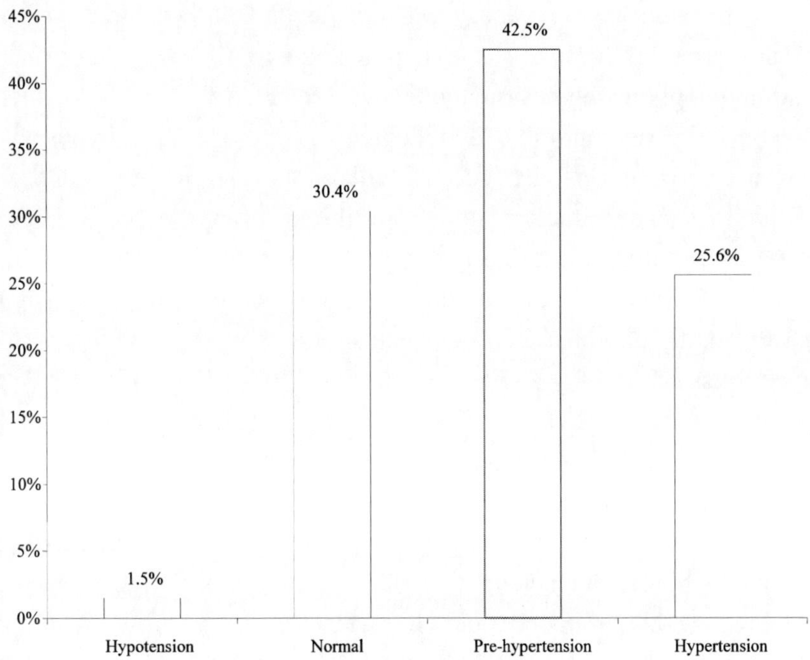

Figure 1. Prevalence of hypotension, normal, pre-hypertensive and hypertension of Rajshahi University students.

Association between Hypertension and Other Selected Variables

The Chi-square test (χ^2-test) was used to find the association between the blood pressure categories (BPC) and various socio-economic, demographic, anthropometric and behavioral factors among the university students in Bangladesh. In this study, gender $p < 0.001$), residence ($p < 0.05$), cigarette smoking behavior ($p < 0.05$), body mass index ($p < 0.001$, parents' education level ($p < 0.05$), fathers' occupation BPC ($p < 0.01$), family income ($p < 0.05$), sleeping duration a night ($p < 0.05$) and physical activity ($p < 0.01$) were significantly associated factors of university students' BPC.

Factors Influencing Hypertension in University Students

Blood pressure (BP) category was our dependent variable, and it was three categories (i) normal (ii) hypertension and (iii) hypertension, the multinomial logistic regression model was selected to find the effect of socio-economic, demographic and behavior factors on pre-hypertension and hypertension, normal BP was considered as reference case. Only the significant associated factors got from the χ^2-test were considered as independent variable of multinomial logistic model (Table 2).

The coefficients and adjusted odds ratio (AOR) of multinomial logistic regression model demonstrated that male students were more likely to get pre-hypertension [AOR = 5.80, 95% CI, 3.67-9.16; $p < 0.01$] and hypertension [AOR = 26.90, 95% CI, 11.41-63.45; $p < 0.01$] than female students. Students slept less than 7 hours a night who was more porn to get pre-hypertension [AOR = 0.65, 95% CI, 0.46-0.92; $p < 0.05$] and hypertension [AOR = 0.67, 95% CI, 0.45-0.95; $p < 0.05$] compared with who slept ≥7 hours. Over-weight or obese students had higher chance in developing pre-hypertension and hypertension than those who were underweight [AOR = 0.15, 95% CI, 0.06-0.41; $p < 0.01$] and [AOR = 0.03, 95% CI, 0.01-0.11; $p < 0.01$], and those of normal weight [AOR = 0.45,

Table 1. Association of blood pressure and socio-economic, demographic and behavior factors of university students

Variables, N (%)	Normal, N (%)	Pre-hypertension, N (%)	Hypertension, N (%)	χ^2-value	p-value
Gender					
Male, 717 (79.9)	152(21.2)	339(47.3)	226(31.5)	164.91	0.001
Female, 180 (20.1)	125(69.4)	48(26.7)	7(3.9)		
Residence					
Rural, 733(81.7)	211(28.8)	326(44.5)	196(26.7)	8.24	0.016
Urban, 164(18.3)	66(40.2)	61(37.2)	37(22.6)		
Cigarette Smoking behavior					
No, 761(84.8)	249(32.7)	324(42.6)	188(24.7)	8.99	0.011
Yes, 136(15.2)	28(20.6)	63(46.3)	45(33.1)		
Father hypertension					
No, 620(69.1)	191(30.8)	264 (42.6)	165(26.6)	0.47	0.715
Yes, 277(30.9)	86(31.0)	123(44.4)	68(24.5)		
Mother hypertension					
No, 619(69.0)	204(33.0)	262(42.3)	153(24.7)	4.31	0.116
Yes, 278(31.0)	73(26.3)	125(45.0)	80(28.8)		
Body mass index					
Under-weight, 120 (13.4)	73(60.8)	36(30.0)	11(9.2)	82.89	0.001
Normal, 709(79.0)	197(27.8)	325(45.8)	187(26.4)		
Over-weight or obese, 68(7.6)	7(10.3)	26(38.2)	35(51.5)		
Religion					
Non-Muslim, 79(8.8)	26(32.9)	32(40.5)	21(26.6)	0.27	0.875
Muslim, 818(91.2)	251(30.7)	355(43.4)	212(25.9)		
Household size					
≤4, 261(29.1)	82(31.4)	108(41.4)	71(27.2)	0.82	0.936
(5-7), 495(55.2)	150(30.3)	220(44.4)	125(25.3)		
≥8, 141(15.7)	45(31.9)	59(41.8)	37(26.2)		
Fathers' education					

Table 1. (Continued)

Variables, N (%)	Normal, N (%)	Pre-hypertension, N (%)	Hypertension, N (%)	χ^2-value	p-value
No education, 282(31.4)	99(35.1)	112(39.1)	71(25.2)	16.25	0.012
Primary, 138(15.4)	27(19.6)	63(45.7)	48(34.8)		
Secondary, 209(23.3)	74(35.4)	90(43.1)	45(34.8)		
Higher, 268(29.9)	77(28.7)	122(45.5)	69(25.7)		
Mothers' education					
No education, 87(9.7)	38(43.7)	30(34.5)	19(21.8)	24.96	0.001
Primary, 178(19.8)	39(21.9)	73(41.0)	66(37.1)		
Secondary, 356(39.7)	121(34.0)	159(44.7)	76(21.3)		
Higher, 276(30.8)	79(28.6)	125(45.3)	72(26.1)		
Fathers' occupation					
Farmer, 419(46.7)	108 (25.8)	198(47.3)	113(27.0)	15.30	0.004
Service, 245(27.3)	79(32.2)	94(38.4)	72(29.4)		
Business, 233(26.0)	90(38.6)	95(40.8)	48(20.6)		
Mothers' occupation					
Housewife, 835(93.1)	252(30.2)	367(44.0)	216(25.9)	3.81	0.149
Others, 62(6.9)	25(40.3)	20(32.3)	17(27.4)		
Family income					
≤Taka 10000, 447(49.8)	121(27.1)	200(44.7)	126(28.2)	9.07	0.049
Taka 10001-20000 Taka, 160(17.8)	63(39.4)	63(39.4)	34(21.2)		
≥20001 Taka, 290(32.4))	93(32.1)	124(42.8)	73(25.2)		
Sleeping hour					
≥7 Hours, 451(50.3)	155(34.4)	184(40.8)	112(24.8)	5.18	0.045
<7 Hours, 446(49.7)	122(27.4)	203(45.5)	121(27.1)		
Physical activity					
No, 798 (88.9)	233(29.2)	344(43.1)	221(27.7)	14.86	0.001
Yes, 99(11.1)	44(44.4)	43(43.4)	12(12.1)		
Extra salt intake					
No, 481(53,6)	136(28.3)	216(44.9)	129(26.8)	3.31	0.191
Yes, 416(46.4)	141(33.9)	171(41.1)	104(25.0)		

Table 2. Effect of socio-economic, demographic and behavior factors on university students' hypertension

	Variable	Category	AOR	95%CI for AOR			Variable	Category	AOR	95%CI for AOR	
				Lower	Upper					Lower	Upper
Pre-hypertension	Gender	Male	5.80**	3.67	9.16	Hypertension	Gender	Male	26.90**	11.41	63.45
		Female^R	.	.	.			Female^R	.	.	.
	Father's education	No education	0.92	0.53	1.61		Father's education	No education	0.89	0.45	1.74
		Primary	1.11	0.53	2.33			Primary	0.98	0.43	2.26
		Secondary	0.66	0.40	1.07			Secondary	0.63	0.34	1.15
		Higher^R	.	.	.			Higher^R	.	.	.
	Mother's education	No education	0.60	0.32	1.16		Mother's education	No education	0.79	0.36	1.76
		Primary	0.59	0.29	1.21			Primary	1.08	0.49	2.43
		Secondary	0.54	0.33	0.89			Secondary	0.46	0.25	0.83
		Higher^R	.	.	.			Higher^R	.	.	.
	Residence	Rural	1.05	0.64	1.73		Residence	Rural	1.02	0.56	1.89
		Urban^R	.	.	.			Urban^R	.	.	.
	Cigarette smoking behavior	Yes	1.12	0.66	1.89		Cigarette smoking behavior	Yes	1.18	0.67	2.13
		No^R	.	.	.			No^R	.	.	.
	Father's occupation	Farmer	1.35	0.83	2.09		Father's occupation	Farmer	1.21	0.68	2.12
		Service	0.94	0.55	1.58			Service	1.43	0.76	2.70
		Business^R	.	.	.			Business^R	.	.	.
	Monthly family income (Taka)	≤10000	0.87	0.55	1.36		Monthly family income (Taka)	≤10000	1.02	0.59	1.75
		10001-20000	0.72	0.43	1.20			10001-20000	0.70	0.37	1.30
		>20000^R	.	.	.			>20000^R	.	.	.
	Sleeping time (hour)	≥7	0.65*	0.46	0.92		Sleeping time (hour)	≥7	0.67*	0.45	0.95
		<7^R	.	.	.			<7^R	.	.	.
	BMI category	Underweight	0.15**	0.06	0.41		BMI category	Underweight	0.03**	0.01	0.11
		Normal	0.45*	0.18	0.90			Normal	0.19**	0.07	0.47
		Overweight/obese^R	.	.	.			Overweight/obese^R	.	.	.
	Physical activities	No	1.14	0.68	1.91		Physical activities	No	2.38*	1.12	5.04
		Yes^R	.	.	.			Yes^R	.	.	.

N.B.: AOR, Adjusted Odds Ratio; **, 1% level of significance; *, 5% level of significance; R, Reference case.

95% CI, 0.18-0.90; $p < 0.05$] and [AOR = 0.19, 95% CI, 0.07-0.47; $p < 0.05$] students, respectively. Students performed a certain level of physical activity with 45 minutes a day on at least five days a week who was less likely to get hypertension [AOR = 2.38, 95% CI, 1.12-5.04; $p < 0.01$] than their counterparts (Table 2).

DISCUSSION

This study was aimed at assessing the prevalence and associated factors of pre-hypertension and hypertension among university students in Bangladesh. A total of 911 students from 7 residence halls at Rajshahi University were recruited using a simple random sampling strategy. The study duration was conducted from January to June, 2014. The cross-sectional study identified pre-hypertension and hypertension as a significant health problem among these university students aged 18-27 years. The present study demonstra-ted that more than one-third and near to one-fourth of the students were pre-hypertensive and hypertensive respectively of the students was pre-hypertensive. University students are young adults who are more likely to be in a pre-hypertension mode rather than displaying full hypertension. The category of pre-hypertension was created to alert people to their risk of developing high blood pressure (HBP) so they could make the necessary lifestyle changes that may avoid the development of hypertension. If the students could be induced to change to their lifestyle and food habits this may help in avoiding the development of high blood pressure and therefore avoiding hypertension in their life in the future.

Hypertension among university students in Bangladesh was identified as lower than in other developing countries such as the university students in Gambia (38.0%) (Van der Sande et al., 2000), Tunisia (35.1%) (Hajer et al., 2012) and Ethiopia (28.3%) (Awoke et al., 2012). However, the hypertension of Bangladeshi university students was higher than in some other countries such as in Nigeria (19.3%) (Isezuo et al., 2011), Kuwait (7%) (Al-Majed and Sadek, 2012) and Saudi Arabia (9.3%) (Ibrahim et al.,

2014). The present study demonstrated that male students were more likely to get hypertension compared to female students, and our results agree with the findings of studies in Kuwait (Al-Majed and Sadek, 2012), Tunisia (Awoke et al., 2012), Hungary (Katona et al., 2011), Qatar (Bener et al., 2004) and USA (Everett and Zajaacova, 2015). In this study, we observed that the prevalence of risk factors such as overweight or obese and cigarette smoking behavior among male students was higher than that of female students, while more number of female students (19.4%) performed physical activities than male (8.9%), these were the important reasons for gender differentiation in hypertension. Same causes were found in one of the USA studies, they also found young men were less likely to be aware of their hypertensive status compared to young women (Everett and Zajaacova, 2015).

It is also important to note that overweight or obese students were at higher risk of getting hypertension compared to underweight and normal weight students. This finding supports previous reports from Tunisia, Portugal, and sub-Saharan African countries (Tadesse and Alemu, 2014). A study conducted in sub-Saharan countries showed that blood pressure was associated with BMI (Tasfaye et al., 2007). A study in Tunisia also demonstrated this relationship between BMI and hypertension (Hajer at al., 2012). Physical activities can reduce body fat, and it is suggested as a significant lifestyle modification that may help in the prevention of hypertension. It was noted that only 11.1% Rajshahi university students performed physical activity with 45 minutes a day on at least five days a week, also observed that university students who performed physical activates was less likely to get hypertension. Same result had been found in other studies (Diaz and Shimbo, 2013; Kokkinos et al., 2009). It was found that habitual short sleep duration at night was an important risk cause for hypertension (Calhoun and Harding, 2010). This study also demonstrated that students who slept less than 7 hours at night had a higher probability of getting hypertension than their counterparts. It is thought that over time, a lack of sleep can damage human body's ability to regulate stress hormones, leading to hypertension, sleep can helps to control human blood pressure and helps nervous system remain healthy. The duration of sleep at night seven to eight hours may play a role in the treatment and prevented of high blood pressure.

Limitation of the Study

Only students staying in the residence halls of Rajshahi University were involved in this study; therefore, the present data cannot reflect the prevalence of hypertension among university students in Bangladesh as a whole. This study should not be limited to only university students but must involve other young adults of the same age range, especially those who may have dropped out from school/college and are working. During the study, some students were not willing to freely give information about BP, while others agreed but gave incorrect information especially regarding their parents' income and social status, so these students had to be excluded. This study was conducted as preliminary work to investigate the prevalence of pre-hypertension and hypertension and its association with selected anthropometric measures, socio-demographic and behavior factors. However, it was not possible to look at other important factors that may also be directly related to hypertension, such as diabetes mellitus, alcohol consumption (Tadesse and Alemu, 2014), environmental factors (Simào et al., 2008), and sedentary lifestyle (Tayem et al., 2012). Clearly, more studies of this type are required.

Conclusion

The purpose of this study was to investigate the prevalence and associated factors of pre-hypertension and hypertension among Rajshahi University students in Bangladesh. The study showed that gender, residence, cigarette smoking behavior, BMI, parents' education, fathers' occupation, family income, duration of sleep a night and physical activities were significantly associated with categories of blood pressure among university students. Multinomial logistic regression exhibited that male students, less than 7 hours sleep in night and overweight or obese students were more likely to become pre-hypertensive and hypertension compared to their counterparts. It is also observed that a student did not perform a certain level of physical activity at least 45 minutes in a day (at least 5 days in a week) who was more likely to get hypertension than his/her counterpart.

The findings of this study have policy implications as well as leading to recommendations that would be helpful to health authorities and policy makers to lead to substantial improvements in the area of hypertension and public health. It would especially assist the government and other policy makers to take the proper initiatives to promote the awareness among young adults about the dangers of becoming hypertensive in Bangladesh and to begin to take steps to attempt to reduce the prevalence of hypertension. Government and non-government organization need to have awareness and provide the necessary counseling regarding the risks of overweight and obesity among university students. Physical activates is a most important predictors of hypertension, and it can help to reduce the body fat. The health authorities of Bangladesh government and university authorities should take initiative to ensure that all university students must perform exercise at least 45 minutes for at least 5 days in a week.

Additional Points

Availability of Data and Materials

Primary data was used in this study and data was collected from university students in Bangladesh. Many variables were collected from subjects. The dataset will be used for other propose, we do not wish to share our data.

Ethical Approval

This study obtained the permission from the authority of the University of Rajshahi, and the research has been approved by the ethical committee of the i*nstitute of Biological Science (IBSC), Rajshahi University, Bangladesh.*

Consent

Written consent was taken from each participant after a detailed oral explanation about the study. We got consent from all subjects for publishing their data.

Disclosure

There was no grant, technical or corporate support for this research project.

Conflicts of Interest

All authors declared that there were no conflicts of interests in relation to this study.

Authors' Contributions

Golam Hossain and Sadekur Rahman designed the study, wrote the proposal, collected the data, analyzed the data and wrote the manuscript. Suhaili Mohd, Rashidul Alam Mahumud and Pete E. Lestrel approved the proposal and revised the manuscript.

ACKNOWLEDGMENTS

We appreciate the authority of Students' Residence Hall, University of Rajshahi, Bangladesh for giving permission to take data from students.

REFERENCES

Al-Majed HT, Sadek AA. 2012. Pre-hypertension and hypertension in college students in Kuwait: a neglected issue. *J Family Community Med.* 19:105-112.

Aounallah-Skhiri H, El Ati J, Traissac P, Ben Romdhane H, Eymard-Duvernay S, Delpeuch F, Achour N, Maire B. 2012. Blood pressure and associated factors in a North African adolescent population. A national cross-sectional study in Tunisia. *BMC Public Health.* 12:98. doi: 10.1186/1471-2458-12-98.

Awoke A, Awoke T, Alemu S, Megabiaw B. 2012. Prevalence and associated factors of hypertension among adults in Gondar, Northwest Ethiopia: a community based cross-sectional study. *BMC Cardiovasc Disord.* 12:113. doi: 10.1186/1471-2261-12-113.

Bener A, Al-Suwaidi J, Al-Jaber K, Al-Marri S, Dagash MH, Elbagi IE. 2004. The prevalence of hypertension and its associated risk factors in a newly developed country. *Saudi Med J.* 25: 918-922.

Black JM, Hawks JH. 2005. *Medical-surgical nursing: Clinical management for positive outcomes.* (7thed.). St. Louis, Mo: Elsevier Saunders.

Calhoun DA, Harding SM. 2010. Sleep and Hypertension. *Chest.* 138:434–443.

Chen Y, Factor-Litvak P, Howe GR, Parvez F, Ahsan H. 2006. Nutritional influence on risk of high blood pressure in Bangladesh: A population-based cross-sectional study. *Am J Clin Nutr.* 84:1224-1232.

Diaz KM, Shimbo D. 2013. Physical activity and the prevention of hypertension. *Curr Hypertens Rep.* 15: 659-668. doi: 10.1007/s11906-013-0386-8.

Dores H, Santos P, Salvador F, Maia J, Paixão L, Pereira R, Gonçalves N, Leitão A, Fonseca C, Ceia F. 2010. Blood pressure in young adults. *Rev Port Cardiol*. 29:1495-1508.

Everett B, Zajacova A. 2015. Gender differences in hypertension and awareness among young adults. *Biodemography Soc Biol.* 61: 1-17. doi:10.1080/19485565.2014.929488.

Grundy SM, Brewer HB Jr, Cleeman JI, Smith SC Jr, Lenfant C; National Heart, Lung, and Blood Institute; American Heart Association. 2004. Definition of metabolic syndrome: report of the National Heart, Lung, and Blood Institute/American Heart Association conference on scientific issues related to definition. *Arterioscler Thromb Vasc Biol.* 24:e13-8.

Hossain MG, Bharati P, Aik S, Lestrel PE, Abeer A, Kamarul T. 2012. Body mass index of married Bangladeshi women: Trends and association with socio-demographic factors. *J Biosoc Sci.* 44: 385-399.

Hujová Z. 2013. The prevalence of obesity and hypertension among first-year students at Trnava University in Slovakia. *Int. J. Med. Med. Sci.* 5:361-367.

Ibrahim NK, Mahnashi M, Al-Dhaheri A, Al-Zahrani B, Al-Wadie E, Aljabri M, Al-Shanketi R, Al-Shehri R, Al-Sayes FM, Bashawri J. 2014. Risk factors of coronary heart disease among medical students in King Abdul-Aziz University, Jeddah, Saudi Arabia. *BMC Public Health.* doi: 10.1186/1471-2458-14-411.

Isezuo SA, Sabir AA, Ohwovorilole AE, Fasanmade OA. 2011. Prevalence, associated factors and relationship between pre-hypertension and hypertension: a study of two ethnic African populations in Northern Nigeria. *J Hum Hypertens.* 25: 224-230.

Karen Tu, Zhongliang Chen, Lorraine L Lipscombe. 2008. Prevalence and incidence of hypertension from 1995 to 2005: a population-based study. *CMAJ*. 178: 1429–1435.

Katona E, Zrínyi M, Komonyi E, Lengyel S, Paragh G, Zatik J, Fülesdi B, Páll D. 2011. Factors influencing adolescent blood pressure: the Debrecen hypertension study. *Kidney Blood Press Res.* 34:188-195.

Kokkinos PF, Giannelou A, Manolis A, Pittaras A. 2009. Physical activity in the prevention and management of high blood pressure. *Hellenic J Cardiol.* 50: 52-59.

Koura MR, Al-Dabal BK, Rasheed P, Al-Sowielem LS, Makki SM. 2012. Prehypertension among young adult females in Dammam, Saudi Arabia. *East Mediterr Health J.* 18:728-734.

Kulkarni MM, Hemagiri K, Malavika, Patil RS. 2011. Pre-hypertension and associated factors among medical students of SSIMS &RC, Davangere-a cross-sectional study. *J Indian Med Assoc.* 109:733-736.

Lee P, Ong T, Muna S, Syed Alwi S, Kamarudin K. 2010. University students have high cardiovascular risk? A pilot study from University Malaysia Sarawak (UNIMAS). *Malaysian* Family *Physician,* vol. 5, no. 1, pp. 41-43, 2010. *Malays Fam Physician.* 5:41-43.

Lim SS, Vos T, Flaxman AD, Danaei G, Shibuya K, Adair-Rohani H, Amann M, Anderson HR, Andrews KG, Aryee M, Atkinson C, Bacchus LJ, Bahalim AN, Balakrishnan K, Balmes J, Barker-Collo S, Baxter A, Bell ML, Blore JD, Blyth F, Bonner C, Borges G, Bourne R, Boussinesq M, Brauer M, Brooks P, Bruce NG, Brunekreef B, Bryan-Hancock C, Bucello C, Buchbinder R, Bull F, Burnett RT, Byers TE, Calabria B, Carapetis J, Carnahan E, Chafe Z, Charlson F, Chen H, Chen JS, Cheng AT, Child JC, Cohen A, Colson KE, Cowie BC, Darby S, Darling S, Davis A, Degenhardt L, Dentener F, Des Jarlais DC, Devries K, Dherani M, Ding EL, Dorsey ER, Driscoll T, Edmond K, Ali SE, Engell RE, Erwin PJ, Fahimi S, Falder G, Farzadfar F, Ferrari A, Finucane MM, Flaxman S, Fowkes FG, Freedman G, Freeman MK, Gakidou E, Ghosh S, Giovannucci E, Gmel G, Graham K, Grainger R, Grant B, Gunnell D, Gutierrez HR, Hall W, Hoek HW, Hogan A, Hosgood HD 3rd, Hoy D, Hu H, Hubbell BJ, Hutchings SJ, Ibeanusi SE, Jacklyn GL, Jasrasaria R, Jonas JB, Kan H, Kanis JA, Kassebaum N, Kawakami N, Khang YH, Khatibzadeh S, Khoo JP, Kok C, Laden F, Lalloo R, Lan Q, Lathlean T, Leasher JL, Leigh J, Li

Y, Lin JK, Lipshultz SE, London S, Lozano R, Lu Y, Mak J, Malekzadeh R, Mallinger L, Marcenes W, March L, Marks R, Martin R, McGale P, McGrath J, Mehta S, Mensah GA, Merriman TR, Micha R, Michaud C, Mishra V, Mohd Hanafiah K, Mokdad AA, Morawska L, Mozaffarian D, Murphy T, Naghavi M, Neal B, Nelson PK, Nolla JM, Norman R, Olives C, Omer SB, Orchard J, Osborne R, Ostro B, Page A, Pandey KD, Parry CD, Passmore E, Patra J, Pearce N, Pelizzari PM, Petzold M, Phillips MR, Pope D, Pope CA 3rd, Powles J, Rao M, Razavi H, Rehfuess EA, Rehm JT, Ritz B, Rivara FP, Roberts T, Robinson C, Rodriguez-Portales JA, Romieu I, Room R, Rosenfeld LC, Roy A, Rushton L, Salomon JA, Sampson U, Sanchez-Riera L, Sanman E, Sapkota A, Seedat S, Shi P, Shield K, Shivakoti R, Singh GM, Sleet DA, Smith E, Smith KR, Stapelberg NJ, Steenland K, Stöckl H, Stovner LJ, Straif K, Straney L, Thurston GD, Tran JH, Van Dingenen R, van Donkelaar A, Veerman JL, Vijayakumar L, Weintraub R, Weissman MM, White RA, Whiteford H, Wiersma ST, Wilkinson JD, Williams HC, Williams W, Wilson N, Woolf AD, Yip P, Zielinski JM, Lopez AD, Murray CJ, Ezzati M, AlMazroa MA, Memish ZA. 2012. A comparative risk assessment of burden of disease and injury attributable to 67 risk factors and risk factor clusters in 21 regions, 1990-2010: a systematic analysis for the Global Burden of Disease Study 2010. *The Lancet.* 380: 2224-2260.

Oyewole OO, Oritogun KS. 2012. Pre-hypertension and hypertension in adolescence: how much does it occur in a Nigerian community. *West Afr J Med.* 31:71-75.

Palomo IF, Torres GI, Alarcón MA, Maragaño PJ, Leiva E, Mujica V. 2006. High prevalence of classic cardiovascular risk factors in a population of university students from south central Chile. *Rev Esp Cardiol.* 59:1099-105.

Pickering TG, Hall JE, Appel LJ, Falkner BE, Graves J, Hill MN, Jones DW, Kurtz T, Sheps SG, Roccella EJ. Recommendations for blood pressure measurement in humans and experimental animals: part 1: blood pressure measurement in humans: a statement for professionals from the Subcommitteeof Professional and Public Education of the

American Heart Association Council on High Blood Pressure Research. *Circulation.* 111:697-716.

Rahman MM, Gilmour S, Akter S, Abe SK, Saito E, Shibuya K. 2015. Prevalence and control of hypertension in Bangladesh: a multilevel analysis of a nationwide population-based survey. *J Hypertens.* 33:465-472.

Rana M, Sayem A, Karim R, Islam N, Islam R, Zaman TK, Hossain G. 2015. Assessment of knowledge regarding tuberculosis among non-medical university students in Bangladesh: a cross sectional study. *BMC Public Health.* 15:716, DOI 10.1186/s12889-015-2071-0.

Simão M, Hayashida M, dos Santos CB, Cesarino EJ, Nogueira MS. 2008. Hypertension among undergraduate students from Lubango, Angola. *Rev Lat Am Enfermagem.* 16:672-678.

Soliman M, El-Salamony O, El-Khashab K, El-Sherbiny NA, Safaa Khamis S. 2014. Study of hypertension among Fayoum University students. *In J Public Health Res.* 2:15-19.

Tadesse T, Alemu H. 2014. Hypertension and associated factors among university students in Gondar, Ethiopia: a cross-sectional study. *BMC Public Health.* 14:937. Doi:10.1186/1471-2458-14-937.

Tayem YI, Yaseen NA, Khader WT, Abu Rajab LO, Ramahi AB, Saleh MH. 2012. Prevalence and risk factors of obesity and hypertension among students at a central university in the West Bank. *Libyan J Med.* doi: 10.3402/ljm.v7i0.19222.

Tesfaye F, Nawi NG, Van Minh H, Byass P, Berhane Y, Bonita R, Wall S. 2007. Association between body mass index and blood pressure across three populations in Africa and Asia. *J Hum Hypertens.* 21:28-37.

van der Sande MA, Milligan PJ, Nyan OA, Rowley JT, Banya WA, Ceesay SM, Dolmans WM, Thien T, McAdam KP, Walraven GE. 2000. Blood pressure patterns and cardiovascular risk factors in rural and urban Gambial communities. *J Hum Hypertens.* 14:489-496.

World Health Organization (WHO). *A global brief on hypertension,* 2013.

World Health Statistics. *World Health Organization (WHO) Report* 2014.

World Health Organization (WHO). *Causes of Death* [online database]. Geneva. *WHO.* http://www.who.int/healthinfo/global_burden_disease/cod_2008_sources_methods.pdf.

Yinon L, Chen Y, Parvez F, Bangalore S, Islam T, Ahmed A, Rakibuz-Zaman M, Hasan R, Sarwar G, Ahsan H. 2013. A prospective study of variability in systolic blood pressure and mortality in a rural Bangladeshi population cohort. *Prev Med.* 57:807-812.

In: Obesity and Syndrome X
Editors: M. Das and K. Bose ISBN: 978-1-53614-669-1

Chapter 7

INCREASING INCIDENCE OF MACROSOMIA: THE IMPACT OF MATERNAL SOMATIC AND BEHAVIORAL PARAMETERS ON NEWBORN WEIGHT STATUS

Sylvia Kirchengast*, PhD
Department of Anthropology, University of Vienna, Vienna, Austria

INTRODUCTION

The prevalence of obesity and the so called "syndrome x" has increased drastically worldwide during the last 20 years. Consequently, many authors already warn of global epidemics (Ford & Mokard 2008, Rheeder 2006). 10 years ago, the number of obese people on earth exceeded the number of people suffering from starvation and malnutrition for the first time in the long history of *Homo sapiens* (FAO 2008). Currently more than 1.9 billion adults, 18 years and older, are overweight

* Corresponding Author Email: sylvia.kirchengast@univie.ac.at.

and more than 600 million are obese (WHO 2016). Obesity is commonly defined, as a level of adiposity that is sufficiently excessive to damage health, demonstrated by an increased risk of metabolic and cardiovascular diseases, such as diabetes, hypertension, stroke and some forms of cancer (Danaei et al. 2009). The clustering of metabolic symptoms, in particular insulin resistance, dyslipidemia (with hypertriglyceridaemia and low levels of high density lipoprotein cholesterol) and cardiovascular symptoms such as hypertension are called "syndrome x", which is significantly related to obesity (Reaven 1988, Dwyer et al. 2002). The most severe expression of syndrome x is found in combination with central obesity and is often referred as the metabolic syndrome. To determine obesity commonly the body mass index (BMI) based on body weight and height (kilograms per square meter) is used. (WHO 1995). The World Health Organization (WHO) defines overweight as a BMI above 25.00kg/m^2, while a BMI above 30.00kg/m^2 is an indicator of obesity. A BMI above 40.00kg/m^2 is seen as morbidly obese (WHO 1995). These cut offs are defined for adults. Obesity however, is not only a problem of the adult population, currently overweight or obesity affects one in ten children or adolescents worldwide (WHO 2016). In Europe, one in five children can be classified as overweight or obese (WHO 2016). Since sub adult individuals are still growing, and the growth patterns differ according to sex, the use of BMI cutoffs for determining obesity is problematic among sub adults. Therefore, BMI percentiles for each separate sex and age class are widely used for the determination of overweight and obesity among children and adolescents (Wang & Wang 2000).

The strong association between obesity and the risk of several chronic diseases such as heart disease, stroke, hypertension, but also pancreatitis, osteoarthritis and cancer makes the high rates of obesity among children as well as adults to a major concern of public health (Kulie et al. 2011, WHO 2016). This is especially true of the association between obesity and insulin resistance. Insulin resistance or type II diabetes is one of the most serious metabolic diseases with disastrous long term consequences such as blindness, nephropathy or the amputation of the lower extremities. The past president of the American Diabetes association, Francine Kaufman pointed out exceptionally strong interaction between obesity and type II diabetes and introduced the term "diabesity" (Kaufmann 2005). There is no doubt that obesity and insulin resistance but also syndrome x represent a global health crisis that threatens the economies worldwide (Hu 2011). Consequently the prevention of obesity as well as syndrome x is the major goal of public health strategies. In order to develop strategies to reduce the risk of developing obesity and syndrome x, it is necessary to analyze the potential risk factors. During the last decade several potential risk factors of syndrome x have been identified. It is well documented, that beside genetic factors life style patterns such as hyper alimentation and physical inactivity have a significant impact on the development of obesity and syndrome x. The life style factors promoting syndrome x can be seen in a close context with westernized life style patterns and modernization (Fall 2001, Harell et al. 2015).

OBESITY, SYNDROME X AND NEWBORN SIZE

Recently there is growing interest in the association between newborn size and the risk of obesity, and syndrome x in later life (Ramadhani et al. 2006). Newborn size, mainly expressed by birth weight, reflects intrauterine growth patterns, which are determined by genetic factors but also intrauterine environment. Obesity and insulin resistance during later life are more common among small for gestational age newborns (SGA) but also among large for gestational age newborn (LGA) (Ramadhani et al. 2006, Hermann et al. 2010, Wang et al. 2009, Bamberg et al. 2013, Yu et al. 2015).

During the 1980s and the early 1990s the British epidemiologists Barker and Hales proposed the concept that environmental stress factors such as malnutrition in utero, might influence the development of obesity and syndrome x later on in life (Barker & Clark 1997; Barker 1999). According to Barkers so called thrifty phenotype hypothesis fetal undernutrition and therefore fetal programming are the causative factors a of later life metabolic diseases (Barker 1999, Robert & Woods 2014). In utero nutritional deficiencies lead to small for gestational age newborns who respond to their low level of nutritional intake in early life through alterations in growth and metabolism which increase the risk of obesity and syndrome x in later life (Barker 1999). According to Barker and Hales hypothesis small for gestational age newborns have metabolically thrifty mechanisms for fat storage and glucose sparing with reduced rates of glucose oxidation in insulin-sensitive target tissues (Barker 1999). Consequently, low birth weight, which has been defined as a birth weight below 2500g regardless of gestational age, is on the one hand one of the strongest single risk factors for early neonatal mortality and morbidity (Mahumud et al. 2017). On the other hand low birth weight is also an important risk factor for developing obesity and syndrome x in later life. This association is of special concern because according to the World Health Organization (WHO) the prevalence of low birth weight is 15.5% globally and 96.5% of low birth weight infants are born in developing countries (Mahumud et al. 2017).

Macrosomia

As pointed out above birth weight as a predictor of health in later life showed a u-shaped curve with both low birth weight as well as high birth weight associated with increased risks. High birth weight or large for gestational age newborn is commonly called macrosomia, which defined a birth weight above 4000g or 4500g (Dennedy & Dunne 2013). The American College of Obstetricians and Gynecologists supports the use of a 4500g cutoff, irrespective of gestational age because a birth weight of more than 4500g increases the risk of adverse maternal and perinatal outcome (ACOG 2000). Unfortunately for the definition of macrosomia the cut offs of 4000g and 4500g are still used simultaneously. Another definition of macrosomia is a birth weight greater than 90% for gestational age after correcting for neonatal sex and ethnicity. Ye et al. (2015) plead for a population specific definition of macrosomia and suggested a cut-off of 4500g for African and Latin American newborn but a cut off of 4000g for

Asian populations. Based on these, definitions macrosomia affects 1 to 10% of pregnancies worldwide. As to be expected the prevalence of macrosomia (birth weight above 4000g) widely from a low of 0.5% in India to a high of 14.9% in Algeria (Koyanagi et al., 2013). In Western countries macrosomia (> 4000g) is encountered in up to 10% of deliveries (Campbell 2014). In the United States approximately 7% of newborn had birth weight above 4000g, 1% had birth weight higher than 4,500g, and 0.1% had birth weight higher than 5000g (Dennedy & Dunne 2013).

Using the definition of fetal macrosomia as a neonate with a birth weight above 4.5 kg the prevalence of macrosomia ranges from 1.3 – 1.5% of all births in developed countries. Only few neonates are extremely large. According to the Guinness world record the heaviest infant born to a healthy mother, weighing 10.2kg was born in Italy in 1955. Few other infants weighing more than 6kg are recorded such as a newborn weighing 7kg from Cambria, UK in 1992, and an infant weighing 7.6kg in Bahia Brazil in 2005. In 2007, a newborn weighing 6.6kg was born in Cancun Mexico. In China, an infant weighing 6.2kg was born 2006 and in 2008, a Chinese baby weighing 5.5kg was delivered. The largest baby ever recorded in Bangladesh was born in 2008 weighing 6kg (Sultana et al. 2007). Without any doubt such extraordinary heavy newborn are extremely rare. What we can observe however are changes in mean birth weight. A secular trend in birth weight was observable in some countries from the mid to the late 20th century (Bralic et al. 2006; Oken 2013, Begic et al. 2016, Chegeni et al. 2016). In Moscow, Russia, for instance, the mean birth weight of boys increased from 3450g in 1987 to 3500g in 2002, among girl mean birth weight increased from 3360g to 3450g (Treyak et al. 2005). In Sweden, the mean weight at birth increased from 3596g to 3631g during the period 1992 and 2002 (Surkan et al. 2005). Furthermore, the prevalence of macrosome newborns (> 4500g) increased from 3.7% to 4.6% during this period (Surkan et al. 2005).

According to popular press and public perceptions birth weight seems to increase steadily during the last decades, but this is not true. Recent data indicate that in developed countries the mean birth weight has begun to decline. In the United States the incidence of low weight newborn (<

2500g) increased, while the prevalence of newborn weighing more than 5000g decreased. (Oken 2013). Similar trends are observed for France and Australia (Oken 2013). In Austria the prevalence of macrosome newborn (> 4500g) decreased from 7.1% in 2006 to 6.4% in 2016. (Statistik Austria 2017) These trends may be due to changes in population mixture but mainly due to changes in obstetric practice. Induction of labor, but also increased monitoring of diabetic and prediabetic women during pregnancy account for this decrease in macrosome newborn.

This reduction of macrosomia is of special importance because macrosomia increases maternal as well as newborn morbidity and mortality. Higher stillbirth rates but also higher fetal mortality rates are associated with a birth weight above 4250g in non-diabetic mothers and with a birth weight above 4000g among diabetic mothers (Mondestin et al. 2002, Najafian & Cheraghi 2012). Furthermore, macrosomia increases birth complication in particular the risk of shoulder dystocia and trauma to the birth canal, bladder, perineum and anal sphincter (Campbell 2014). This is especially true of birth weights higher than 4500 g and particularly among birth weight, which exceeds 5000 g. Consequently, fetal macrosomia is associated with increased risks for emergency Cesarean section (CS) and instrumental delivery (Campbell 2014). For the newborn macrosomia associated complications, include beside increased mortality, brachial plexus or facial nerve injuries, fractures of the humerus or clavicle and birth asphyxia (Campbell 2014)

Consequently, macrosomia is clearly associated with birth complications and maternal as well as newborn morbidity and mortality (Najafian & Cheraghi 2012, Campbell 2014). Additionally, many studies have shown that macrosomia is a risk factor or obesity and syndrome x in later life (Yu et al. 2008, Hermann et al. 2010). Therefore, the analysis of potential risk factors of macrosomia is essential.

Factors strongly associated with fetal macrosomia include genetics, ethnic factors, duration of gestation, presence of gestational diabetes, and maternal diabetes mellitus types I and II (Li et al. 2014, Kamana et al. 2015). It is well documented, that maternal diabetes- pregestational as well as gestational diabetes - is one of the strongest risk factors associated with macrosomia (Hammoud et al. 2013). Furthermore, maternal prepregnancy weight status affects birthweight (Pölzlberger et al. 2017). Obese women but also women experiencing excessive gestational weight gain are more likely to give birth to larger infants (Kirchengast & Hartmann 2018). Additionally some studies plead for an association between macrosomia and multiparity as well as older maternal age (Li et al. 2015). An important fetal factor is sex. Male infants are heavier than female ones at any gestational age and the prevalence of macrosomia is higher among male newborns.

As mentioned above beside the perinatal complications, macrosomia represents an important risk factor of syndrome x and obesity in later life (Herrmann 2010). Therefore, the analysis of potential risk factor of macrosomia despite of maternal diabetes is of special importance. In the present study, the impact of fetal sex but also maternal prepregnancy weight status and maternal behavior on newborn size was tested among more than 10 000 term births in Vienna, Austria.

MATERIAL AND METHODS

Data Set

This retrospective study is based on a data set of 10231 singleton births, which took place at the University Clinic of Gynecology and Obstetrics in Vienna, Austria between 1995 and 2000. Although, a total of 18425 births were collected, only 10231 met the strict inclusion and exclusion criteria. Following inclusion criterions have been defined:

1. Births between the 38th and 41th week of gestation, because only term births should be included in analyses to make maternal pregnancy weight gain and newborn anthropometric data more comparable.

2. Only pregnant women ageing between 18 and 45 years were enrolled in the present study whose first prenatal check took place during the eighth week of gestation.
3. All prenatal check-ups of the mother-child passport were completed.
4. Delivery of a single infant without congenital malformations
5. No registered maternal diseases before and during pregnancy i.e., no hypertension (BP < 150/90 mmHg), no preeclampsia, no protein or glucose in the urine, no pregnancy related immunization.

Additionally the following exclusion criteria have been defined:

1. Early Teenage pregnancy i.e., maternal age below sixteen years.
2. Coincident medical diseases such as diabetes mellitus or nephropathy.
3. Drug or alcohol abuse.
4. Twin birth or IVF.

Gestational age was calculated in terms of the number of weeks from the beginning of the last menstrual bleeding to the date of delivery (= duration of amenorrhoea). All subjects originated from Austrian or central Europe.

Maternal Parameters

All 10231 women enrolled in the present study aged between 17 and 49 years (mean = 25.3 yrs SD = 5.7). The following maternal somatometric parameters were determined at the first prenatal visit: Stature height was measured to the nearest 0.5cm and prepregnancy weight (PPW), was measured to the nearest 0.1kg on a balance beam scale. Additionally maternal weight at the end of pregnancy (EPW) was measured before birth. The weight gain during pregnancy (PWG) was calculated by subtraction of pre-pregnancy weight from body weight at the end of pregnancy. Maternal weight status before pregnancy was described by means of the body mass index (BMI) (kg/m^2). Weight status was classified according to the recommendations of the WHO (1995).

< 18.50 = underweight
18.50 - 24.99 = normal weight
25.00 - 29.99 = overweight
30.00 - 39.99 = obese
> 40.00 = morbid obese

Newborn Parameters

Birth weight, birth length, head circumference, diameter fronto-occipitalis and acromial circumference were taken directly from newborn immediately after birth. Newborn weight status was defined as follows: low < 2500g, normal 2500 - 3999g, high 4000 - 4500g and macrosome > 4500g (Dennedy & Dunne 2013). Furthermore, the one- and the five minute APGAR scores (Casey et al. 2001) for the evaluation of the newborn were determined.

Mode of Delivery

Spontaneous vaginal birth and caesarean section were recorded. Caesarean sections requested by the mother without any medical indication were not carried out at this hospital.

Statistical Analyses

Statistical analyses were performed by means of SPSS for Windows program Version 22.0. After calculating descriptive statistics (means, SDs), group differences were tested regarding their statistical significance using Duncan analyses. Furthermore, χ^2 analyses and odds ratios were computed. Multiple regression analyses were performed to test the impact of maternal prepegnancy BMI, stature height, gestational weight gain on birth weight. Additionally binary logistic regressions were computed in order to test the association between maternal parameters and newborn weight status. Normal birthweight was coded as 1, high birth weight and macrosomia were coded as 2.

RESULTS

Sample Description

Altogether 10231 newborns have been enrolled in the present study. The number of male newborn (n = 5249; 51.3%) surpassed the number of female ones (n = 4991; 48.7%). The majority of mothers (73.3%) corresponded to the WHO definition of normalweight.8.9% of the mothers were classified as underweight because their prepregnancy body mass index was below 18.50 kg/m^2. 14.2% of the mothers were classified as overweight (BMI 25.00 to 29.99kg/m^2) and only 3.6% corresponded to the definition of obesity i.e., a prepregnancy BMI above 30.00 kg/m^2. Only 0.3% of the mothers were classified as morbidly obese (BMI > 40.00 kg/m^2). The mean weight gestational gain was 12.9kg (SD = 5.5) ranging from 2 to 38 kg. The majority of mothers were nonsmokers before pregnancy (64.2%) and during pregnancy (72.0%). 22.8% of the mothers were classified as heavy smokers (> 10 cigarettes per day) before pregnancy and 7.6% of the mothers were still heavy smokers (>10 cigarettes per day) during pregnancy.

The Prevalence of High Birth Weight and Macrosomia

As to be expected the majority of newborn (90.3%) corresponded to the definition of normal weight (2500 - 3999g). 1.8% of the newborn were classified as low weight (< 2500g). 7.3% corresponded to the definition of high birthweight (4000 - 4499g) and only 0.8% corresponded to the definition of macrosomia (> 4500g). Male and female newborn differed significantly in weight status ($p < 0.0001$). The prevalence of high birthweight and macrosomia was significantly higher among male newborn. 9.5% of the male newborn showed a birth weight between 4000 and 4500g, 0.7% were heavier than 4500g. Among female newborn the prevalence of high birth weight was only 4.9% and only 0.2% of the female newborn were classified as macrosome.

As demonstrated in Table 1, high weight newborn and macrosome newborn were not only heavier than their normal weight and low weight counterparts, they were also significantly longer and exhibited significantly larger head dimensions and significantly higher acromial circumferences. Concerning vital parameters, however it turned out the one minute and five minute appear scores of high weight and macrosome newborn were only slightly decreased in comparison to their normal weight counterparts.

The Impact of Maternal Parameters on Newborn Weight Status

Newborn weight status was significantly associated with various somatic but also behavioral parameters of the mothers. As demonstrated in Table 1 the mothers of high weight or macrosome newborn were significantly older, taller and heavier than the mothers of normal weight or low weight newborns. Furthermore, they exhibited significantly larger pelvic dimensions and experienced a significantly higher gestational weight gain ($p < 0.0001$). Maternal prepregnancy overweight and obesity increased the risk of giving birth to high weight and macrosome newborn significantly. While the prevalence of high weight and macrosome newborn was below 5% among underweight mothers and 6.9% among normal weight mothers, 12.3% of overweight women, 13.9% of obese women and 33.4% of morbidly obese women gave birth to high weight or macrosome offspring. Smoking before and during pregnancy reduced the risk to give birth to a macrosome newborn.

Table 1. Maternal and newborn characteristics according to newborn weight status

n	Birth weight categories				
	< 2500g	2500 - 3999g	4000 - 4500g	> 4500g	.
	185	9241	746	59	Sig
	mean (Sd)	mean (Sd)	mean (Sd)	mean (Sd)	p-value
Maternal characteristics					
Maternal age (yrs)	25.4 (6.2)	25.2 (5.6)	26.3 (5.4)	28.0 (5.8)	< 0.0001
Stature height (cm)	161.1 (6.8)	163.0 (6.4)	165.6 (6.7)	166.7 (6.3)	< 0.0001
Prepregnancy weight (kg)	55.2 (9.5)	59.1 (9.9)	64.8 (11.8)	69.6 (11.9)	< 0.0001
End of pregnancy weight (kg)	65.0 (11.1)	72.4 (11.7)	81.3 (13.6)	95.9 (13.6)	< 0.0001
Prepregnancy BMI (kg/kh^2)	21.22 (3.15)	22.18 (3.47)	23.59 (4.21)	25.05 (4.61)	< 0.0001
Gestational weight gain (kg)	10.4 (5.3)	12.8 (5.4)	14.9 (5.6)	15.6 (5.2)	< 0.0001
Distantia spinarum (cm)	24.3 (2.0)	24.9 (2.0)	25.5 (2.1)	25.8 (1.6)	< 0.0001
Distantia cristarum (cm)	27.5 (2.0)	28.0 (2.1)	28.8 (2.0)	29.4 (1.7)	< 0.0001
Newborn characteristics					
Birth length (cm)	45.6 (1.9)	49.7 (1.7)	52.3 (1.5)	53.6 (1.6)	< 0.0001
acromial circumference (cm)	32.7 (1.4)	36.6 (2.1)	40.1 (1.9)	42.5 (2.2)	< 0.0001
Head circumference (cm)	32.0 (1.2)	34.3 (1.3)	35.9 (1.2)	36.8 (1.1)	< 0.0001
Diameter fronto-occipitalis	10.6 (0.7)	11.2 (0.7)	11.7 (0.7)	12.0 (0.7)	< 0.0001
Apgar 1 minute	8.0 (1.9)	8.6 (1.2)	8.4 (1.4)	8.2 (1.5)	< 0.0001
Apgar 5 minute	9.4 (1.4)	9.8 (0.7)	9.7 (0.8)	9.7 (0.6)	< 0.0001

These findings were corroborated by the results of the multiple and the binary logistic regression analyses (see Tables 2 and 3). Maternal age, stature height, prepregnancy weight status and gestational weight gain were significantly positively associated with birth weight and macrosomia. Nicotine consumption before and during pregnancy were significantly negatively associated with birth weight however only insignificantly negatively with macrosomia.

Table 2. Impact of maternal characteristics on newborn size. Multiple regression analyses

	R^2	B	Sig	95% CI
Dependent variable. Newborn weight				
Maternal age	0.28	4.59	< 0.001	2.42 – 6.77
Stature height		12.77	< 0.001	10.91 – 14.62
Prepregnancy BMI		25.37	< 0.001	22.19 -- 28.54
Gestational weight gain		17.38	< 0.001	15.14 – 19.62
Newborn sex		- 126.4	< 0.001	-150.15 - -102.61
Prepregnancy nicotine consumption		- 2.96	< 0.001	- 4.57 - - 1.34
Nicotine consumption during pregnancy		- 8.53	< 0.001	- 11.07 - - 5.99

Table 3. Impact of maternal characteristics on macrosomia. Multiple regression analyses

	Exp (B)	Sig	95% CI
Dependent variable: newborn weight status			
Maternal age	1.07	0.034	1.01 – 1.14
Stature height	1.09	0.003	1.03 – 1.16
Prepregnancy BMI	1.18	0.001	1.102 – 1.27
Gestational weight gain	1.11	0.001	1.04 – 1.18
Newborn sex	0.54	0.130	0.24 – 1.20
Prepregnancy nicotine consumption	0.99	0.646	0.94 – 1.04
Nicotine consumption during pregnancy	0.95	0.267	0.86 – 1.04

Newborn Weight Status and Delivery Mode

Delivery mode differed significantly according to newborn weight status (Chi-square = 24.8; $p < 0.0001$). Caesarean section rate of the whole sample was 21.5%. The lowest cesarean section rate was found among normal weight newborn (21.1%) the highest rate among low weight newborn (37.0%). High weight newborn (4000 - 4399g) and macrosome newborn (> 4500g) showed a CS rate of 23.0% and 23.6% respectively. High birth weight (OR = 1.12 CI 0.93 - 1.32) and macrosomia (OR = 1.16, CI 0.62 - 2.15) increased slightly the risk to give birth via caesarean section in comparison to normal weight newborn.

DISCUSSION

Macrosomia is clearly an important risk factor of obesity and syndrome x during childhood and adult life (Yu et al. 2008, Wang et al. 2009, Hermann et al. 2010). Large for gestational age infants show distinctly different growth patterns from normal weight newborns during childhood. They experience higher weight gains and show significantly higher body mass indices than their normal weight counterparts (Yu et al. 2008, Bocca-Tjeertes et al. 2014). These high rates of obesity increase the risk of metabolic disorders from early childhood onwards (Bocca-Tjeertens et al. 2014). Therefore, the analysis of factors promoting macrosomia is of special importance. In the present study, the impact of fetal sex but also maternal somatometric factors as well as maternal behavioral factors on birth weight was analyzed. In detail a large sample of term births taking place in Vienna Austria were enrolled in the present analysis. Only 1.8% of the newborn were classified as low weight or small for gestational age (< 2500g). This is much lower than the general prevalence of small for gestational age newborn in Austria (Statistik Austria 2016). Between 2007 and 2016 the rate of small for gestational age newborns ranges between 6.4 and 7.2%. This discrepancy is due to the fact, that exclusively term births have been included into the present study. The prevalence of high birth weight newborn (4000 - 4499g) was 7.3%. This rate is in accordance with macrosomia rates (> 4000g) in other high- income countries (Campbell 2014). Only 0.8% of the newborn were heavier than 4500g. This low incidence of macrosomic newborn is comparable to that of the United States where about 1% of the newborn exhibit a birth weight above 4500g (Dennedy & Dunne 2013.) In the present study, fetal sex had a significant impact on macrosomia. The birth weight of 9.5% of the male newborn was between 4000 and 4500g, while only 4.9% of newborn girls were weighing between 4000 and 4500g and only 0.2% exhibited a birth weight above 4500g. These significant sex differences are in accordance with the results of several other studies. Male newborns typically weigh more than female newborns, in detail male newborns are generally approximately 150 - 200 g heavier than female newborn of the same gestational age near term

(Kirchengast 2014). Furthermore, male newborn are more likely to be macrosomic than female ones (Di Renzo et al. 2007).

As to be expected, macrosome newborn were not only heavier they also were longer and had larger heads. This fact may be the main reason that caesarean section rates were significantly higher among mothers of macrosome newborns. In the present study, more than 23.0% of newborn weighing above 4500g were delivered via Caesarean section. This finding is in accordance with the results of numerous previous studies, which yielded significantly increased caesarean section rates among mothers of macrosome newborns (Barber et al. 2011, Kirchengast & Hartmann 2017)

Concerning maternal parameters, prepregnancy weight status was significantly associated with birth weight. While less than 7% of normal weight mothers gave birth to a newborn heavier than 4000g, this was true of more than 12% of overweight mothers, nearly 14% of obese mothers and more than 33% of morbidly obese mothers (BMI > 40.00kg/m^2). Maternal obesity is general seen as a main risk factor of newborn macrosomia (lit.). Additionally mothers of high birth weight (4000 - 4499g) and macrosome newborns (> 4500g) are taller and experienced a higher gestational weight gain than mothers of low weight and normal weight newborns. These findings corroborate the results of several previous study (Clausen et al. 2005, Pölzlberger et al. 2017). Furthermore, the pelvic dimensions of mothers of high weight and macrosome newborns are larger than those of mothers of normal weight or low weight newborn. These increased pelvic dimensions may enable mothers of large fetuses to experience vaginal delivery despite of the large dimensions of the fetus.

Concerning maternal behavioral factors, the impact of nicotine consumption before and during pregnancy on newborn size was tested. Smoking before and during pregnancy increased the risk of giving birth to a small for gestational age newborn, but reduced the risk of giving birth to a macrosome one smoking however, should not be used to reduce the risk of macrosomia.

Macrosomia and associated obesity and syndrome x during later life are important issues of public health and obstetrics but these association patterns are also of interest from view point of evolutionary biology. Of course, it is not the task of evolutionary biology and/or evolutionary anthropology to develop new treatment strategies, but they may focus on the evolutionary basis of the prevalence of macrosomia on the one hand and the association between macrosomia and later life health issues on the hand. Evolution is the central paradigm in biological science and consequently Theodosius Dobzhansky stated "*Nothing in biology makes sense except in the light of evolution*" (Dobzhansky 1973). From this point of view, macrosomia and associated health risks in later life have to be considered, within the framework of human evolution.

The first hazard of an evolutionary analysis of macrosomia and associated health risks is that we have no information regarding newborn size and birth weight of our hominid ancestors. Only few fossil remains of hominid infants are known, for example the Neanderthal neonates from Mezmaiskaya 1 (Russia) and Le Moustier 2 (France) (Weaver et al. 2016). These rare skeletal remains allow us to reconstruct birth patterns among Neanderthals (Ponce de Leon et al. 2008), but we have no information regarding mean birth weights among different hominid species. The analysis of birth weight among our hominid ancestors is quite difficult. Wells (2009) used maternal height as predictor of birth weight and reconstructed birth weight trends from the Paleolithic onwards. According to Wells analyses birth weight declined from about 3500 to 3300 g during Paleolithic to about 2900 to 3000g during Neolithic times. Consequently, the transition from the Paleolithic hunter-gatherer subsistence to Neolithic agriculture was associated with a decrease of birth weight but also a deterioration of health. Nevertheless, we cannot assume that macrosomia was a common condition during Paleolithic times. The typical life style of our Paleolithic ancestors was characterized by a high level of physical activity because high levels in daily activity in search of food, water and sleeping sites were necessary. Diets consisted to a high degree of vegetable food, protein (50 to 80%) and a low fat content (Konner and Eaton 2010). It can be assumed, that typical non-communicable diseases such as hypertension, heart disease, cancer, diabetes or obesity have been rare or rather unknown during Paleolithic times (Lieberman 2003). The Neolithic transition changed the lifestyle of our ancestors drastically (Larson 1995).

The adoption of agriculture and animal husbandry allowed the production of a surplus of food and consequently population growth. Our ancestors developed semi-permanent settlements and gave up their mobile lifestyle. Dietary breadth declined dramatically and diet consisted of high carbohydrate crops such as rice, barley or wheat and tuber such as potatoes (Larsen 1995). Analyses of Neolithic skeletal remains indicate protein deficiencies and periodic food shortages. Furthermore, domestication of animals and plants changed the environments dramatically. The close proximity to domesticated animals exposed humans to a variety of new pathogens resulting in an increased frequency of infectious diseases (Armelagos et al. 1991). The use of feces as fertilizer and the construction of irrigation increased the contact with parasites. Many of these diseases had an important impact on early life. On the one hand, birth weight declined and this trend increased the risk of infectious diseases and increased infant mortality. On the other hand, maternal stature decreased during Neolithic transition and smaller birth size may be interpreted as an adaptation to this maternal somatic change (Wells 2009).

Birth weight increased again in recent times. The increase of macrosomia, which is evident for the last fifty years, can be interpreted as result of increasing affluence in developed but also developing countries. Rapid changes of our life style resulted in an obesogenic environment, which increased rates of obesity and type II diabetes but also gestational diabetes. Diabetes, first of all gestational diabetes are major risk factors for large for gestational age newborn (Kamana et al. 2015).

From an evolutionary viewpoint, increased rates of macrosomia in the second half of the 20th century may an indicator of a mismatch between recent life circumstances and the environment in which our ancestors evolved. Modernization as well as urbanization took place, eating habits and physical workload changed dramatically. Especially a rapid transition in nutritional habits and general lifestyle increases the risk to be obese and to suffer from type II diabetes (Popkin 2003). This is especially true of rising economies in Asia. In 1980 less than 1% of Chinese adults suffered from obesity and diabetes type II, in 2008 the prevalence had reached nearly 10% (WHO 2016). The prevalence of macrosomia (> 4000g) increased from 2.6% in the 1970s to 13.25 in the 1990s. Greatest increase occurred in urban areas. In Shanghai, the percentage of macrosomia increased by 50% from 1989 to 1999 (Yu et al. 2008).

Rapid modernization seems to enhance macrosomia rates. This is especially true of indigenous people experiencing rapid westernization. During the last 30 years, the incidence of macrosomia increased dramatically among indigenous populations in Canada. Among First Nations in Quebec and Ontario the a third of newborns is heavier than 4000g and a tenth is heavier than 4500g (Auger et al. 2013). Especially high rates of adult obesity and type II diabetes associated with westernization and modernization occur among Pacific Islanders (Jowitt 2014). The prevalence rates macrosomia (> 4500g) among Samoan mothers was 2.4%, while in developed countries less than 1% of the newborn are heavier than 4500g (Tsitas et al. 2015).

Macrosomia seems to be a problem of obesogenic environments, affluence and rapid modernization.

Conclusion

Macrosomia is strongly related to obesity and syndrome x in later life and have to be seen within the same context. Maternal obesity and high gestational weight gains enhance the risk of macrosomia independent of gestational diabetes. On the other hand macrosomia increases the risk of obesity and syndrome x.

References

American College of Obstetricians and Gynecologists ACOG. (2000). *Practice Bulletin Fetal Macrosomia.*

Armelagos, G. J., Goodman, A. H. & Jacobs, K. H. (1991). The origins of agriculture: Population growth during a period of declining health. *Popul. Environ*, *13*, 9-22.

Auger, N., Park, A. L., Zoungrana, H., Sing, M. F., Lo, E. & Luo, Z. G. (2013). Widening inequality in extreme macrosomia between indigenous and non-indigenous populations of Quebec, Canada. *Austral NZealand J Pub health*, *37*, 58-62.

Bamberg, C., Hinkson, L. & Henrich, W. (2013). Prenatal detection and consequences of fetal macrosomia. *Fetal Diagn Ther*, *33*, 143-148.

Barber, E. L., Lundsberg, L., Belanger, K., Pettiker, C. M., Funai, E. F. & Illuzzi, J. L. (2011). Contributing indications to the rising cesarean delivery rate. *Obstet Gynecol*, *118*, 29-38.

Barker, D. J. P. & Clark, P. M. (1997). Fetal undernutrition and disease in later life. *Rev Reprod*, *2*, 105-112.

Barker, D. J. P. (1999). Fetal origins of type 2 diabetes mellitus *Ann Int Med*, *130*, 322-324.

Begic, A., Halilovic, J. H., Mesalic, L. & Hialilovic, S. H. (2016). Secular trend of anthropometric parameters of newborns in municipalities of Tuzla Canton (1976-2007). *Med Glas*, *13*, 125-135.

Bocca-Tjeerttes, I. F. A., Kerstjens, J. M., Reijneveld, S. A., Veldman, K., Bos, A. F. & deWinter, A. F. (2014). Growth patterns of large for gestational age children up to four years. *Pediatrics*, *133*, 643-649.

Bralic, I., Rodin, U., Vrdoljak, J., Plavec, D. & Capkun, V. (2006). Secular birth weight trend changes in liveborn infants before, during and after the 1991-1995 homeland war in Croatia. *Croat Med J*, *47*, 305-312.

Campbell, S. (2014). Fetal macrosomia: a problem in need of a policy. *Ultrasound Obstet Gynecol*, *43*, 3–10.

Chegeni, M., Fotouhi, A., Emamian, M. H. & Mohammed, K. (2016). Secular trend of birth weight in a population of Iranian neonates during 1991 and 2011. *Int J Health Studies*, *2*, 14-18.

Clausen, T., Burski, T. K., Oyen, N., Godang, K., Bollerslev, J. & Henriksen, T. (2005). Maternal anthropometric and metabolic factors in the first half of pregnancy and risk of neonatal macrosomia in term pregnancies. A prospective study. *Eur J Endocrinol*, *153*, 887-894.

Danaei, G., Ding, E. L., Mozaffarian, D., Taylor, B., Rehm, J., Murray, C. J. & Ezzati, M. (2009). The preventable causes of death in the United States: comparative risk assessment of dietary, lifestyle and metabolic risk factors. *PLoS Med*, *6*, e1000058.

Dennedy, M. C. & Dunne, F. (2013). Macosomia: defining the problem worldwide. *The Lancet*, *381*, 435-436.

Di Renzo, G. C., Rosati, A., Sarti, R. D., Cruciani, L. & Cutuli, A. M. (2007). Does fetal sex affect pregnancy outcome? *Gender Medicine.*, *4*, 19–30.

Dobzhansky, T. (1973). Nothing in Biology makes sense except in the light of evolution. *The American Teacher*, *35*, 125-129.

Dwyer, T., Blizzard, L., Venn, A., Stankovich, J. M., Ponsonby, A. L. & Morley, R. (2002). Syndrome x in 8-y-old Australian children: stronger associations with current body fatness than with infant size or growth. *Int J Obes*, *26*, 1301-1309.

FAO. (2008). The state of food insecurity in the world 2008. *Food and Agriculture Organization of the United Nations.* Rome.

Fall CHD. (2001). Non-industrialized countries and affluence. *Brit Med Bull*, *60*, 33-50.

Ford, E. S. & Mokdad, A. H. (2008). Epidemiology of obesity in the Western hemisphere. *J Clin Endocrinol Metab*, *93*, S1-S8.

Hammoud, N. M., Visser, G. H. A., Peter, S. A. E., Graatsma, E. M., Pistorius, L. & de Valk, H. W. (2013). Fetal growth profiles of macrosomic and non-macrosomic infants of women with pregestational or gestational diabetes. *Ultrasound Obstet Gynecol*, *41*, 390-397.

Harell, M., Ussery, E., Green-Cramer, B., Ranjit, N. & Sharma, S. V. (2015). The influence of 2westernization" on nutrition and physical activity behaviors of adolescents in New Delhi, India: Are we exporting an epidemic of obesity? *J Appl Res Children Inform Policy Children Risk*, *6*, 1-22.

Hermann, G., Dallas, L. M., Haskell, S. E. & Roghair, R. D. (2010). Neonatal macrosomia is an independent risk factor for adult metabolic syndrome. *Neonatalogy*, *98*, 238-244.

Hu, F. B. (2011). Globalization of diabetes. *Diabetes Care*, *34*, 1249-1257.

Jowitt, L. M. (2014). Ethnicity and type 2 diabetes in Pacific Island adults in New Zealand. *Int J Diab Clin Res*, *1*, 1-5.

Kamana, K. C., Shakya, S. & Zhang, H. (2015). Gestational diabetes mellitus and macrosomia: a literature review. *Ann Nutr Metab*, *66*, 14-20.

Kaufmann, F. (2005). *Diabesity*. Bantam Books NewYork.

Kirchengast, S. (2014). Sexual dimorphism in newborn size and its relationship to newborn vital parameters. *Folia Anthropologica*, *13*, 37-45.

Kirchengast, S. & Hartmann, B. (2017). Maternal obesity increases the risk of primary as well as secondary caesarean section. *Ann Obes Dis*, *2*, 1017-1021.

Kirchengast, S. & Hartmann, B. (2018). Maternal prepregnancy nutritional status influences newborn size and mode of delivery. *AIMS Medical Science*, *5*, 53-66.

Konner, M. & Eaton, S. B. (2010). Paleolithic nutrition. *Nutr Clin Pract* 25:594-602.

Koyanagi, A., Zhang, J., Dagvadorj, A., Hirayama, F., Shibhuya Souza, J. P. & Gülmezoglu, A. M. (2013). Macrosomia in 23 developing countries: an analysis of a multi-country, facility-based, cross-sectional survey. *The Lancet*, *381*, 476-483.

Kulie, T., Slattengren, A., Redner, J., Counts, H., Ehglash, A. & Schrager, S. (2011). Obesity and women´s health: an evidence-based review. *J Am Board Fam Med*, *24*, 75-85.

Larsen, C. (1995). Biological changes in human populations with agriculture. *Ann Rev Anthropol*, *24*, 185-213.

Li, Y., Liu, Q. F., Zhang, D., Shen, Y., Ye, K., Lai, H. L., Wang, H. Q., Hu, C. L., Zhao, Q. H. & Li, L. (2015). Weight Gain in Pregnancy, Maternal Age and Gestational Age in Relation to Fetal Macrosomia. *Clin Nutr Res.*, *4*, 104–109.

Li, G., Kong, L., Li, Z., Zhang, L., Fan, L., Zou, L., Chen, Y., Ruan, Y., Wang, X. & Zhang, W. (2014). Prevalence of macrosomia and ist risk factors in China: a multicentre survey based on birth data involving

101723 singleton term infants. *Paediatric Perinatal Epidemiol*, *28*, 345-350.

Lieberman, L. S. (2003). Dietary, evolutionary and modernizing influences on the prevalence of type 2 diabetes. *Ann Rev Nutr*, *23*, 345-377.

Mahumud, R. A., Sultaa, M. & Sarker, A. R. (2017). Distribution and determinants of low birth weight in developing countries. *J Prev Med Pub Health*, *50*, 18-28.

Mondestin, A. M. J., Ananth, C. V., Smulian, J. C. & Vintzloes, A. M. (2002). Birth weight and fetal death in the United States: the effect of maternal diabetes during pregnancy. *Am J Obstet Gynecol*, *187*, 922-926.

Najafian, M. & Cheraghi, M. (2012). Occurrence of fetal macrosomia rate and its maternal and neonatal complications: a 5 year cohort study. *Obstet Gynecol* DOI: 10.5402/2012/353791.

Oken, E. (2013). Secular trends in birthweight. *Nestle Nutr Inst Workshop*, *71*, 103-114.

Pölzlberger, E., Hartmann, B., Hafner, E., Stümpflein, I. & Kirchengast, S. (2017). Maternal height and pre-pregnancy weight status are associated with foetal growth patterns and newborn size. *Jbiosoc Sci*, *49*, 392-407.

Ponce de León, M. S., Golovanova, L., Doronichev, V., Romanova, G., Akazawa, T., Kondo, O., Ishida, H. & Zollikofer, C. P. (2008). Neanderthal brain size at birth provides insights into the evolution of human life history. *Proc Natl Acad Sci*, *105*, 13764-8.

Popkin, B. M. (2003). The nutrition transition in the developing world. *Develop Policy Rev*, *21*, 581-597.

Ramadhani, M. K., Grobbee, D. E., Bots, M. L., Cabezas, M. C., Vos, L. E., Oren, A. & Uiterwaal, C. S. P. M. (2006). Lower birth weight predicts metabolic syndrome in young adults: The Atheriosclerosis risk in young adults (ARYA)-study. *Atheriosclerosis*, *184*, 21-27.

Reaven, G. M. (1988). Role of insulin resistance in human disease. *Diabetes*, *37*, 1595-1607.

Rheeder, P. (2006). Type 2 diabetes: the emerging epidemic. *SA Fam Pract*, *48*, 20.

Roberts, E. & Wood, P. (2014). Birth weight and adult health in historical perspective. Evidence from a NewZealand cohort 1907-1922. *Soc Sci Med*, *107*, 154-161.

Statistik, Austria. (2017). *Statistical Yearbook.* Vienna, Austria.

Sultana, S., Ferdous, S., Hossein, N. & Basak. (2007). Newborn baby having birth weight of 6kg. Is it heaviest birth weight ever recorded in Bangladesh? *Bangladesh J Child Health.*, *31*, 43-45.

Surkan, P. J., Hsieh, C. C., Johansson, A. L. V., Dickman, P. W. & Cnattingius, S. (2004). Reasons for increasing trends in large for gestational age births. *Obstet Gynecol*, *104*, 720-726.

Tretyak, A., Godina, E. & Zadorozhnaya, L. (2005). Secular trends of sizes at birth in Russian infants born between 1987 and 2002. *J Physiol Anthrop*, *24*, 404-406.

Tsitas, M., Schmid, B. C., Oehler, M. K. & Tempfer, C. B. (2015). Macrosomic and low birth weight neonates in Pacific Islanders from Samoa: a case–control study. *Arch Gynecol Obstet*, *292*, 1261-1266.

Wang, Y. & Wang, J. Q. (2000). Standard definitions of child overweight and obesity worldwide. *Brit Med J*, *321*, 1158.

Wang, Y., Gao, E., Wu, J., Zhou, J., Yang, Q., Walker, M. C., Mbikay, M., Sigal, R. J., Nair, R. C. & Wen, S. W. (2009). Fetal macrosomia and adolescence obesity: results from a longitudinal cohort study. *Int J Obes*, *33*, 923-928.

Weaver, T. D., Coqueugniot, H., Golovanova, L. V., Doronichev, V. B., Maureille, B. & Hublin, J. J. (2016). Neonatal postcrania from Mezmaiskaya, Russia, and Le Moustier, France, and the development of Neandertal body form. *PNAS*, *113*, 6472-6477.

Wells, J. C. K. (2009). What was human birth weight in the past? Simulations based on data on stature from the Paleolithic to the present. *J Life Sci*, *1*, 115-120.

WHO. (1995). Physical status the use and interpretation of anthropometry. *WHO technical Reports Series* 854, Geneva.

WHO. (2016). Global Report on Diabetes, *WHO*, Geneva.

Ye, J., Torloni, M. R., Ota, E., Jayaratne, K., Pileggi-Castro, C., Ortiz-Panozo, E., Lumbiganon, P., Morisaki, N., Laopaiboon, M., Mori, R.,

Tuncalp, Ö., Fang, F., Yu, H., Souza, J. P., Vogel, J. P. & Zhang, J. (2015). Searching for the definition of macrosomia through an outcome-based approach in low- and middle-income countries: a secondary analysis of the WHO global survey in Africa, Asia and Latin America. *BMC Pregnancy and Childbirth* DOI: 10.1186/s12884-015-0765-z.

Yu, Z., Sun, J. Q., Haas, J. D., Gu, Y., Li, Z. & Lin, X. (2008). Macrosomia is associated with high weight for height in children aged 1-3 years in Shanghai, China. *Int J Obes*, *32*, 55-60.

Yu, Z. B., Han, S. B., Zhu, G. Z., Zhu, C., Wang, X. J., Cao, X. G. & Guo, X. R. (2011). Birth weight and subsequent risk of obesity: a systematic review and meta-analysis. *Obes Rev*, *12*, 525-542.

In: Obesity and Syndrome X
Editors: M. Das and K. Bose
ISBN: 978-1-53614-669-1

Chapter 8

METABOLIC DISORDER AND TYPE-2 DIABETES ASSOCIATIONS WITH ANTHROPOMETRIC MEASURES AMONG ADULT ASIAN INDIANS

Sampriti Debnath[1], Nitish Mondal[2,*] and Jaydip Sen[1]
[1]Department of Anthropology, University of North Bengal, Darjeeling, West Bengal, India
[2]Department of Anthropology, Assam University, Diphu Campus, KarbiAnglong, Assam, India

INTRODUCTION

The concept of the metabolic disorder (MetD) has now been in existence for several years. The MetD also known as syndrome-X was first described by Gerald Reaven in 1988. It is mainly characterized by insulin resistance, hyperinsulinemia, hyperglycemia, dyslipidemia and arterial hypertension. The MetD is defined as glucose intolerance, impaired

[*] Corresponding Author Email: nitishanth@gmail.com.

glucose tolerance (IGT) or diabetes mellitus, or insulin resistance together with two or more other components {e.g., Raised arterial pressure, i.e., ≥140/90 mmHg; raised plasma triglyceride (≥ 150 mg/dl) and/or low HDL-C (<35 mg/dl in men and <39 mg/dl in women); central obesity, i.e., waist/hip ratio (WHR) >0.90 in men and >0.85 in women and/or body mass index (BMI) >30.00 kg/m^2, micro-albuminuria, i.e., urinary albumin excretion rate ≥ 20 μgm/minute or albumin/creatinine ratio ≥ 30 μgm/mg} (Parikh and Mohan 2012; Awasthi et al. 2017; Ricci et al. 2017). The MetD can also be defined in terms of the associations between obesity, insulin resistance (IR), hypertension and dyslipidemia (NCEP 2001; Grundy et al. 2004; Furukawa et al. 2017). Some other study groups have suggested several other definitions of MetD {For example, The European Group for Study of Insulin Resistance (EGIR); American Association of Clinical Endocrinologists (AACE) and International Diabetes Federation (IDF)} (Yankey et al. 2017) (Table 1). The main cause of increase in MetD is observed to be the increasing prevalence of obesity in populations worldwide (Grundy 2016; Saltiel and Olefsky 2017).

Type-2 diabetes mellitus (T2DM) comprises of different degrees of β-cell failure relative to varying degrees of insulin resistance (Cnop et al. 2005; Tripathi and Srivastava 2006). The T2DM, also known as non-insulin-dependent diabetes mellitus (NIDDM) is a chronic condition that affects the way of metabolizing glucose. In this condition the body either resists the effect of insulin on glucose or does not produce enough insulin that can metabolize glucose (Tripathi and Srivastava 2006) (Figure 1). The T2DM is described as the MetD of multiple aetiology which can be characterized by chronic hyperglycaemia with disturbances of carbohydrate, fat and protein metabolism resulting from the defects in insulin secretion, insulin action or both (Kharroubi and Darwish 2015; Heindel et al. 2017). In this case hepatic insulin resistance is the leading cause of the inability to suppress hepatic glucose production and peripheral glucose uptake impaired by peripheral insulin resistance. This combination gives rise to fasting and postprandial hyper-glycemia (Tripathi and Srivastava 2006). It is a long-term disorder that affects other health problems in individuals. The T2DM mainly occurs due to excess body adiposity or obesity but some studies also observed the effect of genetics and environment in it. Environmental factors also have significant effect on the predisposition of T2DM and excess adiposity. It also increases the risk of other major problems like Cardio-Vascular disease (CVD) and coronary heart disease (CHD) in population.

Table 1. Different criteria for Type-2 diabetes mellitus proposed by different organizations

Reference	Criteria for Type-2 Diabetes Mellitus (T2DM) or Non-Insulin Dependent Diabetes Mellitus (NIDDM)
WHO (1999)	Insulin resistance (glucose uptake in the euglycemic clamp below the lowest quartile for the general population) or impaired glucose regulation (impaired fasting glycemia, impaired glucose tolerance, or type-2 diabetes), with 2 or more of the following: 1) BP of 140/90 mm Hg or higher, 2) Triglyceride levels of 150 mg/dL (1.7 mmol/L) or higher and/or HDL-C levels less than 35 mg/dL (0.9 mmol/L) in men and less than39 mg/dL (1.0 mmol/L) in women, 3) Waist-hip ratio >0.90 in men and >0.85 in women and/or Body mass index (BMI, calculated as weight in kilograms divided by the square of height in meters) greater ≥30.00 kg/m^2) and microalbuminuria.
NCEP (2001)	Insulin resistance and the presence of 3 or more of the following components: 1) Fasting plasma glucose concentration greater than 110 mg/dL (6.1 mmol/L), 2) Triglyceride concentration of 150 mg/dL (1.69 mmol/L) or greater,3) HDL-C concentration less than 40 mg/dL (1.04 mmol/L) in men and less than 50 mg/dL (1.29 mmol/L) in women,4) BP of 130/85 mm Hg or greater and 5), waist circumference (WC) greater than 102 cm in men and 88 cm in women.
NCEPATP3 (2005)	Presence of any three or more of the following: 1) Blood glucose greater than 5.6 mmol/L (100 mg/dl) or drug treatment for elevated blood glucose; 2) HDL cholesterol < 1.0 mmol/L (40 mg/dl) in men, < 1.3 mmol/L (50 mg/dl) in women or drug treatment for low HDL-C; 3) Blood triglycerides > 1.7 mmol/L (150 mg/dl) or drug treatment for elevated triglycerides; 4) Waist > 102 cm (men) or > 88 cm (women); 5) Blood pressure > 130/85 mmHg or drug treatment for hypertension.
International Diabetes Federation (IDF) (2006)	Presence of three or more of the five risk factors established by the American Heart Association/National Heart, Lung, and Blood Institute (AHA/NHLBI): 1) Abdominal obesity (WC ≥90 cm in men and ≥80 cm in women), 2) Hypertriglyceridemia (triglycerides ≥150 mg/dL or use of medications to lower triglycerides), 3) Low HDL-C.

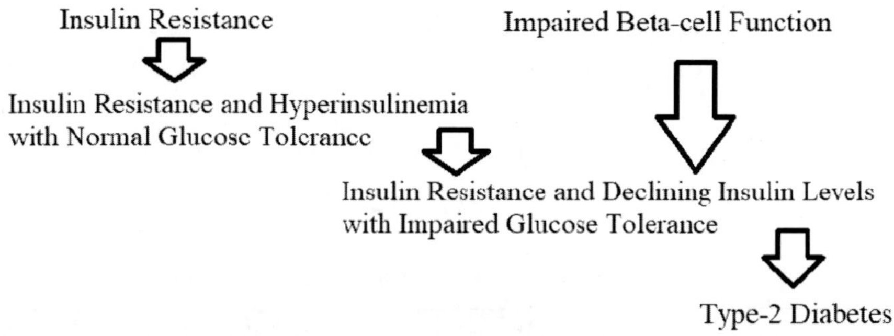

Figure 1. Development of type-2 diabetes mellitus.

RELATIONSHIP BETWEEN TYPE-2 DIABETES MELLITUS AND METABOLIC DISORDER

According to, National Cholesterol Education Program Adult Treatment Panel III (NCEP-ATP III), traits of the MetD include an increased waist circumference (WC), blood pressure elevation, low HDL cholesterol, high triglycerides and hyperglycemia (NCEP 2001; Grundy 2004; Nsiah et al. 2015) (Table 1). When at least 3 of the 5 traits are present and affected individuals are insulin resistant then the condition is considered as MetD. Several studies have reported that MetD is a common problem among the individuals with T2DM. The presence of T2DM increases the risk of MetD to a great extent (NCEP 2001; Wilson et al. 2005) (Table 1). Studies have reported that obese individuals with high BMI and MetDs were also predisposed with T2DM (Meigs et al. 2006; Kautzky-Willer et al. 2016). Obesity contributes to the premature mortality and morbidities associated with MetD (Furukawa et al. 2017; Saltiel and Olefsky 2017) including preventable non-communicable diseases in population (WHO 2000; WHO Expert Consultation 2004; Deaton 2017) (Figure 2). The prevalence of obesity has exploded during the past two decades so the occurrence of MetD. Among the several MetDs (e.g., T2DM, hypertension, dyslipidaemia and CHD) insulin resistance is one of the most prevalent problem occurring due to obesity in developing countries (Ruderman et al. 2013; Misra and Bhardwaj 2014; Pozza and

Isidori 2018). According to IDF (2013) report, global prevalence of T2DM in adults (20-79 years) was 8.3% (382 million people; 198 million men and 184 million women). The number is expected to rise beyond 592 million by 2035 with the global prevalence of 10.1%. In India, over 62 million individuals are diagnosed with T2DM and topped by 31.7 million in 2000 in the world with the highest number of people with T2DM followed by China (20.8 million) and United States (17.7 million) in second and third place, respectively (Joshi and Parikh 2007; Kumar et al. 2013).

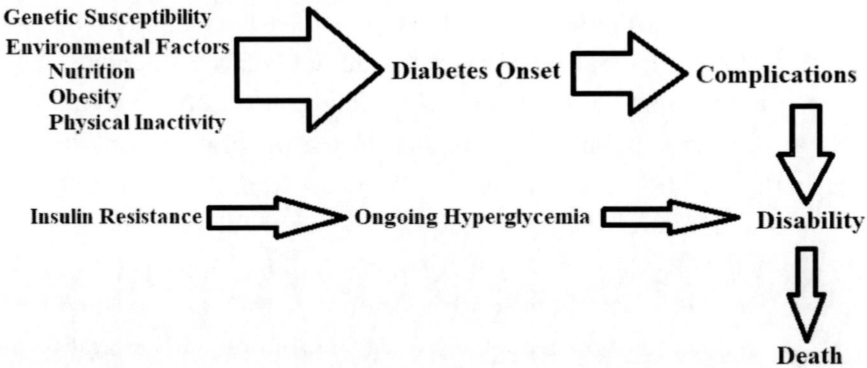

Source: American Diabetes Association (1998, 2003).

Figure 2. The continuum of type-2 diabetes mellitus.

In the developed countries obesity and MetD (e.g., insulin resistance and CVD) have reached epidemic proportions (Berghofer et al. 2008; van Vliet-Ostaptchouk et al. 2014). Among the United States adults, the prevalence of obesity (BMI $\geq$ 30.00 kg/m^2) has increased from 15% in the early 1970s to the most recent estimate of 34% in 2009–2010 (Freedman 2011; Ogden et al. 2012; van Vliet-Ostaptchouk et al. 2014). Developing countries like India are experiencing rapid demographic, epidemiological and economic transitions (Subramanian et al. 2007; Prasad et al. 2010; Kapil and Sachdev 2012; Popkin et al. 2012; Mondal et al. 2017; Phua et al. 2017). These transitions are the main contributing factors for rapid increase in sedentary lifestyles, less physical work outs leading to increased adiposity levels. According to the preliminary National Family Health Survey (NFHS)–4 data, obesity prevalence rates have rapidly increased across India in the past 10 years bringing the national average prevalence to 20% for both women (20.8%) and men (19.9%) (McMurry et al. 2017).

The NFHS-3 study in India reported that 13%of women and 9% of men are overweight or obese. The prevalence of obesity is more pronounced among those living in the urban areas as compared to the rural areas (Laxmaiah et al. 2007; Subramanian et al. 2007; Yang et al. 2009; Sen et al. 2013; Varadharajan et al. 2013; Mondal et al. 2015, 2017; Ajayi et al. 2016). The prevalence of insulin resistance or T2DM is a major global health problem based on the Diabetes atlas (International Diabetic Federation 2009). India having over 20 million diabetic patients have become diabetic capital of the world (Khandelwal et al. 2017). About 80% of T2DM is preventable by changing diet, increasing physical activity and improving the living environment. However, because of lack of effective prevention and control programs, the occurrence of diabetes is likely to continue rising worldwide (Chatterjee et al. 2017; Perreault 2018). Therefore, there is an urgent need to focus on the problem associated with T2DM to reduce the relative burden of morbidity and mortality in population.

Role of Anthropometry in Adiposity Assessment and Metabolic Disorders

Anthropometry is a widely used non-invasive, in-expensive and easy-to-use technique to assess nutritional status, adiposity and body composition in both epidemiological and clinical settings in populations. Anthropometric indicators have been widely used {e.g., BMI, WC and WHR} to assess the body composition, nutritional status and excess adiposity in both epidemiological and clinical investigations. It is evident that the Asian populations have shown the greater prevalence of morbidity and mortality at lower levels of body mass index (BMI= weight/height, kg/m^2) and smaller WC values in adults (WHO, 2000; WHO Expert

Consultation, 2004). Moreover, this BMI classification measures relative weight gain that has been directly related to health risks and morbidity patterns in different populations. BMI has been used extensively in most of the studies for evaluating excess adiposity patterns and overweight-obesity (Snehalatha et al. 2003; Mohan and Deepa 2007; Prasad et al. 2010; Sen et al. 2013; Sengupta et al. 2014; Girdhar et al. 2016). BMI relates weight to height and is the most widely used measure of body size and to estimate the prevalence of obesity within a population (WHO 1999; Khullar et al. 2014). BMI has been extensively used to assess body size but it does not account for the variation in body adiposity distribution and abdominal fat mass (WHO 1999; Wells and Fewtrell 2006). Excess abdominal adiposity is associated with greater risk of obesity and obesity-related morbidity (Visscher et al. 2002; Després 2017) (Figure 3). The associations of T2DM and standard epidemiological translations of BMI and WC have been observed in adults (Alberti et al. 2007; Hsu et al. 2015) (Table 2). In terms of clinical perspective, central obesity (approximated by WC or WHR) provides more information than general BMI (Vazquez et al. 2007). Thus, measurements of WC and WHR are viewed as alternatives to BMI, with both measures regularly used in the clinical and research settings. WC has been shown to be the best simple measure of both intra-abdominal fat-mass and total adiposity (Barreira et al. 2014; Ashwell and Gibson 2016). Several studies have observed that WC alone reflects abdominal adiposity (Mohan and Deepa 2007; Barreira et al. 2014; Ashwell and Gibson 2016).

Table 2. Co-morbidity risks associated with suggested BMI and WC in Asian adults (WHO 2000)

Classification	BMI (kg/m^2)	Risk of co-morbidity (WC)	
		<90 cm (in men)	≥90 cm (in men)
		<80 cm (in women)	≥80 cm (in women)
Underweight	<18.50	Low but increased risk of other clinical problems	Average
Normal range	18.50-22.99	Average	Increased
Overweight	≥23.00		
At Risk	23.00-24.99	Increased	Moderate
Obesity I	25.00-29.99	Moderate	Severe
Obesity II	30.00	Severe	Very Severe

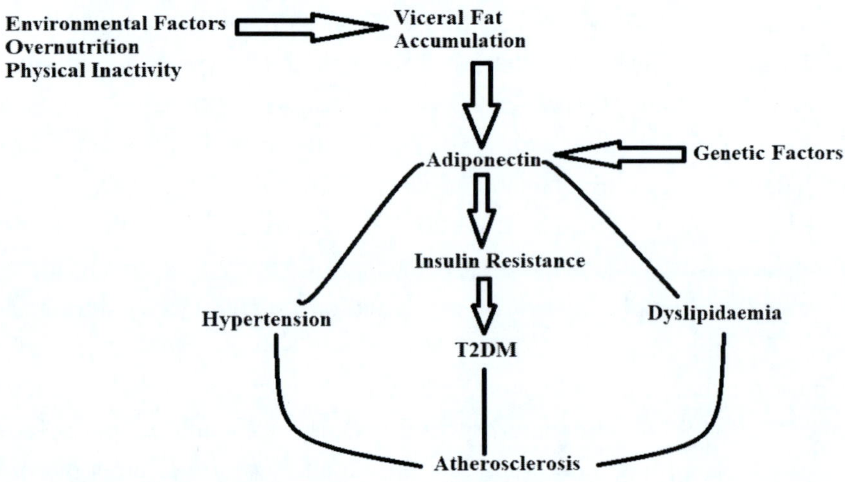

Figure 3. Factors affecting T2DM and Metabolic disorder.

In 1999, the WHO definition included a measure of obesity and defined obesity in terms of either BMI or WHR. WC in combination with BMI has been implemented in guidelines for the assessment and treatment of excess adiposity (obesity) related mortalities and morbidities (WHO 2000; Deurenberg-Yap et al. 2002; Mohan and Deepa 2007; Barreira et al. 2014; Ashwell and Gibson 2016). WHO (2000) has suggested co-morbidity risks associated with different levels of BMI with higher WC among Asian adults. Hence, WC has been advocated as a simple clinical alternative to BMI for detecting adults with possible health risks due to obesity (WHO 2000; WHO Expert Consultation 2004; Mohan and Deepa 2007; Pratyush et al. 2012; Barreira et al. 2014; Ashwell and Gibson 2016). Abdominal obesity which is a condition due to increased amount of intra-abdominal fat including visceral adipose tissue (WHO 2000; Sullivan et al. 2015) is a major cause of T2DM. WC and WHR are useful indicators of abdominal obesity. Increased WC and WHR among the Asian populations reflect increased visceral adipose tissue and increased risks of MetDs (Deurenberg-Yap et al. 2002; Prasad et al. 2010; Soares and Müller 2017). Several studies have observed a higher percentage of body-fat, increased prevalence of metabolic risk factors at lower BMI levels among various Asian populations (Deurenberg-Yap et al. 2002; WHO 2004; Misra and Khurana 2011; Soares and Müller 2017). Increased prevalence of abdominal obesity in Asians as compared with those in Caucasians has also been reported (Deurenberg-Yap et al. 2002; Wang et al. 2005; Mohan and Deepa 2007; Misra and Khurana 2011). Hence, abdominal obesity assessed using WC is considered to be more appropriate to predict MetDs than generalized adiposity assessed using BMI. Several studies have suggested that Asian individuals tend to have increased level of WC (Prasad et al. 2010) with excess body-fat accumulation, abdominal and truncal/regional adiposity and insulin resistance (Hung et al. 2017). Several recent studies have observed strong relationship between waist to height ratio and T2DM (Liu et al. 2016; Hardy et al. 2017; Nagar and Jain 2017; Uday et al. 2017). The conicity index (CI) [CI = WC (m) / 0.109 × √{Weight (kg)/ Height(m)}] which was developed as an indicator of obesity can also be used as an anthropometric indicator for T2DM. Body fat distribution and neck circumference (NC) have significant relationship with the occurrence of T2DM and obesity (Marques et al. 2015; Hingorjo et al. 2016; Papazafiropoulou et al. 2016; Wu et al. 2016; Marcadenti et al. 2017). Neck circumference (NC) was also observed to be associated with body adiposity and T2DM (Ghosh and Bandyopadhyay 2014; Marques et al. 2015; Papazafiropoulou et al. 2016; Wu et al. 2016; Marcadenti et al. 2017).

ASSOCIATION OF ADIPOSITY, TYPE-2 DIABETES MELLITUS AND ANTHROPOMETRIC MEASURES

According to WHO (1995, 2000), the health risks increase above the BMI cut-off $\geq$25.00 kg/m^2 that defined overweight in the current WHO classification (WHO 1995, 2000). According to WHO (2000), greater proportion of Asian people with lower BMI levels than the existing WHO cut-off ($\geq$25.00 kg/m^2) are at a high risk ofT2DM. Due to this variation

WHO (2000) has proposed a re-defined criteria of overweight (≥23.00 kg/m^2) and obesity (≥25.00 kg/m^2) among Asian populations as instances of co-morbidities and health risk factors occurred at the lower BMI (Table2). It is evident that the age-sex specific body-adiposity distribution pattern and increase in excess adiposity ethnically vary among populations (WHO 2000; WHO Expert Consultation 2004; Subramanian et al. 2007; Sen et al. 2013). The proportion of Asian populations with a high risk of T2DM are substantial at BMIs lower than the existing WHO cut-off for overweight (BMI≥25.00 kg/m^2) and obesity (BMI≥30.00 kg/m^2). The cut-offs for observed risk varied from 22.00 kg/m^2 to 25.00 kg/m^2 in different Asian populations and the high risk group this cut-off varied from 26.00 kg/m^2 to 31.00 kg/m^2. Although, the WHO Expert Consultation (2004) reported that the current BMI cut-off should be retained as the international classification. It has been recommended for the purpose of public health action. These cut-offs (23.00 kg/m^2, 27.50 kg/m^2, 32.50 kg/m^2 and 37.50 kg/m^2) and proposed methods could be considered and countries could make decisions for redefining obesity to take public health action (WHO Expert Consultation 2004). There are evidences of the association between high adiposity levels and the prevalence of T2DM in population (Yajnik 2004; Mohan and Deepa 2007; Mohan et al. 2007; Mondal and Sen 2014; Shrestha 2015; Jain et al. 2017)(Figure 3). The CI is another anthropometric index which is able to identify fat distribution and the risk of diseases therefore used as an indicator of obesity in populations (Roriz et al. 2016). The association between degree of excess adiposity, body-fat distribution and excess weight gain with subsequent incidence of T2DM, CHD and CVD has been examined in several prospective studies (Mohan et al. 2007; Mondal and Sen 2014; Shrestha 2015; Jain et al. 2017). The excess adiposity (e.g., BMI) is now a well-established independent risk factor for their development (Snehalatha et al. 2003; Yajnik 2004; Mohan and Deepa 2007; Mohan et al. 2007; Mondal and Sen 2014; Shrestha 2015; Jain et al. 2017).

Association of Adiposity, Type-II Diabetes Mellitus and Anthropometry in Asian Indians

The prevalence of obesity is considered to be the defined cluster of risk factors for non-communicable diseases (T2DM, CVD, dyslipidaemia and certain types of cancer). Most of the studies assessing the adiposity level have used BMI as an indicator. Several studies showed the need for a national level study based on obesity indices to determine the thresholds for obesity parameters for detecting high risk groups for metabolic abnormalities (Snehalatha et al. 2003; Nandimath et al. 2016). A study to identify obesity thresholds in rural Wardha, India (Deshmukh et al. 2006) showed the threshold for the obesity parameter (e.g., BMI) was same as compared to other studies in Asian Indians. Several recent studies have observed high prevalence of T2DM in Indian populations (Mahalakshmi et al. 2014; O'Keefe et al. 2016). There are geographical variations in obesity parameters and its associations with metabolic abnormalities (Ramachandran et al. 2001). Such regional variations have also been reported in the prevalence of T2DM with increasing BMI (Ramachandran et al. 2001; WHO Expert Consultation 2004). The risk of developing T2DM is high at relatively low BMI values in subjects originating from the South-east Asian populations when compared to the Caucasoids (Snehalatha et al. 2003; Yajnik 2004; Misra and Khurana 2011; Mondal and Sen 2014; Krugger et al. 2017). The BMI might not correspond to the same body-adiposity in different populations because of variations in body proportions, which can be the reason for lower BMI in Indians (WHO 2000; WHO Expert Consultation 2004). The relationship of T2DM and impaired glucose tolerance for BMI value of >22.00 kg/m^2 had been established in Asian Indian populations (Ramachandran et al. 2001; Snehalatha et al. 2003; Yajnik 2004; Mondal and Sen 2014; Jayawardana et al. 2017). It has also been reported that the South Asian populations have BMI cut-off values lower than the Western populations due to greater

Table 3. Indian studies done on type-2 diabetes mellitus (T2DM) or metabolic disorders (MetD) and anthropometry in adults

Population	Region/area	N	Measurements	Cut-off used for BMI or Type-2 Diabetes	Result	Cut-off proposed	Reference
Diabetic and non-diabetic individuals	Central India	100	BMI and Blood pressure	American Heart Association and US Center for Disease Control and Prevention	Anthropometric parameters were found to be high in diabetic subjects compared with non-diabetic subjects.	-	Meshram et al. 2013
Type-2 diabetics and non-diabetics of >30 years of age.	Karnataka, India	700	NC and BMI	WHO (1997) and Yang et al. (2010)	The NC in diabetics was significantly higher than in non-diabetics	-	Aswathappa et al. 2013
Asian Indian youth with type-2 diabetes mellitus and prediabetes	Chennai, India	114	BMI and WC	WHO Consultation group for Diabetes Mellitus (1999)	T2DM in Asian Indian youth and prediabetes subjects had higher BMI, WC and fasting insulin than NGT subjects	-	Mohan et al. 2013
Indian adults (aged: 20–90 years)	States and UT's of India	16,607	Weight, height, WC and BMI	WHO (2006)	29.5% had hypertriglyceridemia	-	Joshi et al. 2014
Overweight and obese people of semi-urban area of Assam	Assam, India	300	Weight, BMI and WC	WHO (2000, 2004)	Prevalence of T2DM and hypertension increases with increasing weight of the individuals	-	Mandal 2014
Healthy adults (20-30 years of age) of Amritsar	Punjab, India	200	BMI, WHR and WHtR	WHO (1995, 2000)	All the derived anthropometric indices were significantly increased in young healthy adults (20-30yrs of age) having positive family history of T2DM.	-	Khanna and Sharma 2015

Population	Region/area	N	Measurements	Cut-off used for BMI or Type-2 Diabetes	Result	Cut-off proposed	Reference
Indian population	India	875,711	BMI	-	7% adults with diabetes	-	Akhtar and Dhillon 2017
102 individuals	South India	102	BMI, WHR and WC	WHO (2004, 2008)	A strong association between obesity indices and diabetes was identified. BMI and WC could be used in clinical practice for suggesting life style modifications.	-	Awasthi et al. 2017
Urban slum	India		BMI, WC and WHR	-	Indian Diabetes Risk Score (IDRS)can be used as an effective tool for screening undiagnosed diabetes	-	Dudeja et al. 2017
Adult patients of type-2 diabetes	Surat, India	120	BMI, WC and WHR	WHO (1995), IDF (2006)	More than half (52.5%) of lean patients and 82.5% of IBW (Ideal Body Weight) patients had abnormal high WHR where as in obese group all patients (100%) were having abnormal WHR.	-	Gamit et al. 2017
Students aged 17–19 years	India	526	BMI	ADA (2005)	BMI and WC estimation can be done for early detection of pre-diabetes in adolescents	Cut-offs for WC for predicting pre-diabetes was found to be ≥82.5 cm for boys and ≥80.3 cm for girls.	Pandeya et al. 2017

level of mortality and morbidities in lower adiposity (WHO 2000; WHO Expert Consultation 2004; Hsu et al. 2015; Kruger et al. 2017). China being the largest developing country in the world is experiencing an epidemic of MetD (Lao et al. 2011; Li et al. 2016) and studies have observed high prevalence of MetD in both North and South China. This prevalence also varies due to diverse populations of different regions, cultural behaviours, lifestyle habits and the use of different diagnosis criteria (Zhao et al. 2011; Lao et al. 2014; Xiao et al. 2015).

Recent Developments in Anthopometry, Regional Adiposity andType-2 Diabetes Melitus

Several recent studies showed that there are many medical conditions e.g., obesity, hypertension, elevated cholesterol levels (combined hyperlipidemia) and other MetDs which are also related to regional adiposity levels and can potentially give rise to T2DM (Alberti et al. 2005; Olokoba et al. 2012). A majority of individuals suffering from T2DM are obese, with central visceral adiposity. Therefore, the deposition of excess adipose tissue plays a crucial role in the pathogenesis of T2DM (Olokoba et al. 2012). Increasing trend of obesity, abdominal obesity and MetD is particularly worrisome since Asian Indians develop T2DM and atherogenic dyslipidemia at lower levels of BMI and WC (Gupta et al. 2012; Bodicoat et al. 2014). Onset of dyslipidemia and MetD are early contributing factors to the onset of T2DM (Gulati and Misra 2017). Several studies have used anthropometry as indicator of T2DM in Indian population using different cut-offs for adiposity levels (Table 3). Studies have shown that the proportion of intra-abdominal visceral adipose tissue specifically truncal/abdominal subcutaneous adiposity is higher in South Asians mainly in those with T2DM (Raji et al. 2001; Anoop et al. 2016; Gulati and Misra 2017). Moreover, a number of recent studies have reported in South Asians that there is excess of deep subcutaneous and abdominal adipose tissue which has high metabolic activity and may cause insulin resistance and

CVD (Anand et al. 2011; Marinou et al. 2014). In a recent study by Anoop et al. (2016) it has been found out that increased adipose deposition in liver and pancreas in Asian Indians have potentials of predicting diabetes. Interestingly, the abdominal/regional subcutaneous adipocyte area is increased among South Asians (Anand et al. 2011). Further, Chandalia et al. (2007) observed that subcutaneous adipocyte size was inversely correlated to glucose disposal rate (the rate of glucose uptake from the blood by the peripheral tissues, such as skeletal muscle) in South Asians. This is also independent of intra-peritoneal body adiposity. Several researchers have reported that heightened insulin resistance in South Asians was observed to be more related to increased truncal subcutaneous fat and adipose tissue dysfunction than to excess intra-abdominal visceral adipose deposition (Chandalia et al. 2007; Anand et al. 2011; Gulati and Misra 2017). Studies have observed low physical activity and low-protein diets among South Asians than among white Caucasians (Bhatt et al. 2012). Another study by Eastwood et al. (2014) observed there are relationships between T2DM, CHD and thigh muscle area which is lower in South Asians. Anbalagan et al. (2013) observed that in South Indian population 39.5% of the patients had pre-sarcopenia (characterized by low muscle mass, without any decrease in muscle strength or physical performance) which was independently associated with diabetes. These associations between adipose tissues/regional adiposity levels and diabetes observed by recent studies suggests that anthropometry by which adiposity levels can be measured almost accurately with high precession can be used as a very important tool in future for detection and screening of T2DM in populations.

Genetic and Environment Factors Effecting Type-2 Diabetes Mellitus in Asian Indians

T2DMbeing a complex disease involves a wide-range of genetic, lifestyle and environmental factors. Several studies have observed significant associations of T2DM, genetics and environment (Staiger et al. 2009; Banoo et al. 2015; Kharroubi and Darwish 2015) (Figure 3). It is typically a multi-factorial disease involving multiple genes and various environmental factors with different extents. Moreover, it is not an autoimmune disorder (Banoo et al. 2015). In most of the individual or populations there are susceptible genes predisposing to NIDDM which have not been identified till now (Banoo et al. 2015). Heterogeneity of the genes responsible for the susceptibility to T2DM may be one of the reasons for this problem of identification (Banoo et al. 2015). The variations in T2DM are directly or indirectly affected by overall genetic background of the individual, family or populations which are further more complicated by the interaction with variable environmental conditions/factors (Staiger et al. 2009; Kharroubi and Darwish 2015). Although, there are problems of identification of the genes but several research studies have observed genetic susceptibility of T2DM. Studies have also reported more than 200 T2DM susceptible genes such as Insulin receptor, GLUT, Glycogen Synthase (Mahajan et al. 2014; Zhao et al. 2017). Association between genetic polymorphisms and T2DM have also been observed in the genes encoding the peroxisome proliferators activated receptor, Insulin Receptor Substrate, inward rectifying potassium channel, zinc transporter and calpain-10 (Ali 2013; Banoo et al. 2015). The mechanisms increasing susceptibility of these genetic loci to T2DM are not clear, but most of them are predicted to be altering the function/development/insulin secretion (Banoo et al. 2015). Studies have observed Caucasians are affected by T2DM by 1 to 2% but it is much higher in some ethnic groups e.g., Pima-Indians and Arabs among South Indians it approaches 50% (Banoo et al. 2015). The risk of diabetes increases with age and in most of the cases it has been diagnosed at the age of 40 years and above. It is becoming an epidemic in some countries due to increase in aging population.

Genetic predisposition is a major reason among Asian Indians also called as "*Asian Indian phenotype*" which contributes to the increased predisposition of T2DM among Asian Indians (Mohan et al. 2007; Vimaleswaran et al. 2016; Soares and Müller 2017). Despite having lower prevalence of obesity as defined by BMI, Asian Indians tend to have greater WC and WHR thus having a greater degree of central obesity. Other reasons of T2DM are fast food culture and sedentary lifestyle in Indian population due to the major epidemiological changes going on in the country (Deepa et al. 2017; Mastorci et al. 2017). Genetic factors play an important role in the development of T2DM and mutations in a single gene or a multi-factorial origin can act as the genetic cause of T2DM (Horikawa et al. 2000; Kharroubi and Darwish 2015).

EFFECT OF MIGRATION AND TYPE-2 DIABETES MELLITUS IN ASIAN INDIANS

Several studies worldwide on migrant Indians have shown that Asian Indians have an increased risk of developing T2DMand related metabolic abnormalities (e.g., MetDs) compared to other ethnic groups (Mohan et al. 2007; Soares and Müller2017). Genetic factors and environmental conditions are the main causes of these physiological conditions among Asian Indians. Migration is the movement of individual/population from one environment to another and it can bring several changes due to external or internal factors (e.g., social and cultural changes) among population. Studies have reported that migration from rural areas to urban slums in a metropolitan city in India have led to obesity, glucose intolerance and dyslipidaemia (Mohan et al. 2007). Several factors include genetic and pre-migration history (e.g., socioeconomic level, lifestyle habits, exposure to infections), as well as the quality of healthcare in the countries of destination controls the link between migration and prevalence of disease (Montesi et al. 2016; Girardi et al. 2017). Moreover, there are many factors (viz., urbanization, mechanization, changes in nutrition and lifestyle including physical inactivity, genetic environment/susceptibility interactions and stress) which expose the migrants to a higher risk of developing certain diseases after arrival in the host countries (Misra and Ganda 2007; Montesi et al. 2016; Girardi et al. 2017). Several conditions experienced by migrants moving from a poverty-ridden rural area in early life to an obesogenic urban environment in their later life increases the risk of obesity and T2DM among both inter- and intra-country migrants in developed and developing countries (Girardia et al. 2017). The adoption of sedentary lifestyles and availability and abundance of calorie-dense/low fibre foods is associated with increased risks of morbidity and mortality among the migrated populations. Several studies have investigated the link between migration and T2DM(Misra and Ganda 2007). Several studies have also reported that migration itself contribute to the increase in truncal/subcutaneous abdominal adiposity, which is also an observed phenomena in Asian Indians and South Asians (Raji et al. 2001; Girardiet al. 2017).

ASIAN ENIGMA IN REGIONAL ADIPOSITY, METABOLIC DISORDERS ANDTYPE-2 DIABETES MELLITUS

Several studies have observed that South Asian populations have 3%-5% of greater body-adiposity than Caucasians at any given BMI with low adipokine production, lower lean body mass. Ethnic/genetic, environment, demographic, cultural, lifestyle and socioeconomic factors are being considered as potential contributors to an early age-onset of obesity-linked CVD risk and MetDs (WHO Expert Consultation 2004; Prasad et al. 2010; Misra and Khurana 2011; Hudda et al. 2017). The WHO has revised the BMI cut-off for Asian Indians and suggested a BMI ≥25.00 kg/m^{2}to define obesity against the ≥30.00 kg/m^2 recommended for Europeans (WHO 2000) (Table 1). Asian Indians have the increased predispositions to T2DM (WHO 2000; WHO Expert Consultation 2004; Yajnik 2004; Ramachandran et al. 2014). This predisposition has been attributed to the Asian Indian Phenotype which is characterized by lesser than the generalized obesity as measured by BMI but greater than the central obesity with respect to the WC and WHR (WHO 2000; Prasad et al. 2010; Vimaleswaran et al. 2016; Little 2017). This is the cause of biochemical and hormonal changes including higher plasma insulin levels, greater insulin resistance, lower HDL cholesterol, higher triglyceride levels, increased small dense LDL cholesterol as well as small dense HDL cholesterol and C-reactive protein and leptin levels but decreased adiponectin levels (Lele et al. 2006; Manoria et al. 2010). Asian Indians have higher total abdominal and visceral adiposity for any given BMI (WHO Expert Consultation 2004; Raji et al. 2001) and for any given body adiposity they have increased insulin resistance (Soares and Müller 2017). Other studies have shown that some genes seem to confer increased susceptibility to diabetes in Indians (Vimaleswaran et al. 2005). Europeans have some type of protective genes which do not appear to protect Indians (Radha et al. 2006; Radha and Mohan 2007). It is evident that the abdominal or central/regional obesity is closely linked with insulin resistance, enhanced lipolysis and release of free fatty acids which inhibits insulin stimulated peripheral glucose uptake in dose dependent manner while simultaneously inhibiting insulin secretion (Mohan and Rao 2007; Prasad et al. 2010). These features have been referred to as the Asian Indian Phenotype or Paradox (Vimaleswaran et al. 2016; Little 2017). Several studies on neonates have suggested that Indian babies are smaller born but relatively fatter compared to Caucasian babies and are referred to as "the thin fat Indian baby" (Yajnik et al. 2003; Krishnaveni et al. 2005). Neck circumference (NC) is also observed to be associated with the occurrence of MetDs (Hingorjo et al. 2016). Anthropometric measures which have strong association with the occurrence of T2DM can contribute highly in risk detection of T2DM in populations worldwide. Anthropometric measures (e.g., BMI, WHR, WC, NC and CI) can also be used very accurately to control and/or monitor the increasing trend of T2DM/MetDs in population.

Limitation of Anthropometric Measures

Several research studies have reported the associations between anthropometry and MetD, but several questions critical to the use of anthropometry as a direct indicator of MetD or T2DMremain in doubt. It is important to test whether standard metrics of adiposity used in clinical settings (e.g., BMI, WC, WHR and CI) adequately reflect the accurate level of visceral (or subcutaneous) adiposity and the subsequent risks of MetD as well as T2DM. Whether only the high adiposity levels alone explains the cause of MetD or T2DM remains unanswered due to the effect of environmental factors, genetic predisposition to the disease as well as other external factors (viz., socioeconomic, occupation, migration, lifestyle effect, predisposition to other diseases and early life experiences). In this context anthropometry has its limitation because biochemical and genetic methods can give much greater accurate measure of MetD as well as T2DM.

CONCLUSION

The prevalence of T2DM is reaching potentially epidemic proportions in India. The mortality and morbidity associated with T2DM and the potential complications associated with T2DM are enormous, and pose significant burdens of healthcare on both families and society. Therefore, it is very necessary to detect and control the risks of T2DM by using improved intervention techniques and policies. There are evidences from recent studies that strong associations between anthropometric, genetic and biochemical risk for T2DM as a non-communicable disease and MetD are present in populations. Due to the wide population diversity of India based on ethnicity, culture, socioeconomic conditions, resource distribution and nutritional conditions the need for establishing ethnic-specific anthropometric (e.g., BMI, WC and WHR) cut-offs are becoming very much necessary for the proper identification of the relative risks of MetDs and T2DM. Moreover, practical implementations of those cut-off values of anthropometric measures are very necessary. It is possible to minimise the relative risks by only controlling the lifestyles of the individuals and therefore it is very necessary to introduce region/ethnic specific policies to control T2DM and MetDs. Prevention of T2DM and its micro- and macro-vascular complications should be an essential component for future public health strategies for the countries. Collection and reporting of obesity data should be systematically included in all nutrition surveys which are very necessary in prevention of T2DM and MetDs. Extensive studies by researchers are necessary for establishing proper measure for assessing the risk of T2DM in terms of adiposity levels/regional body adiposity as several recent studies have observed significant association between regional adiposity and T2DM and/or MetDs in populations. Moreover, epidemiological and operational information on obesity and T2DM should be integrated into existing international nutrition forums. Proper lifestyle modifications should be induced in populations to minimise the prevalence of T2DM. Also, public/private partnerships are necessary to properly implement the public healthcare policies for controlling the epidemic of T2DM/MetDs. A large proportion of cases of T2DM are preventable therefore initiatives for consumer education to promote a healthy diet could be reinforced by government's involvement towards the problem.

REFERENCES

Ajayi IO, Adebamowo C, Adami HO, Dalal S, Diamond MB, Bajunirwe F, Guwatudde D, Njelekela M, Nankya-Mutyoba J, Chiwanga FS, Volmink J. 2016. Urban–rural and geographic differences in overweight and obesity in four sub-Saharan African adult populations: a multi-country cross-sectional study. *BMC Public Health.* 16:1126.

Akhtar SN, Dhillon P. 2017. Prevalence of diagnosed diabetes and associated risk factors: Evidence from the large-scale surveys in India. *J Soc Health Diabet* 5:28.

Alberti KG, Zimmet P, Shaw J, IDF Epidemiology Task Force Consensus Group. 2005. The metabolic syndrome–a new worldwide definition. *Lancet.* 366:1059-1062.

Alberti KG, Zimmet P, Shaw J. 2007. International Diabetes Federation: a consensus on Type 2 diabetes prevention. *Diabet Med.* 24:451-463.

Ali O. 2013. Genetics of type 2 diabetes. *World J Diabet.* 4:114.

American Diabetes Association. 2005. Expert committee on the diagnosis and classification of diabetes mellitus of the American diabetes association. *Diab Care*. 2005; 28:S4–S36.

Anand SS, Tarnopolsky MA, Rashid S, Schulze KM, Desai D, Mente A, Rao S, Yusuf S, Gerstein HC, Sharma AM. 2011. Adipocyte hypertrophy, fatty liver and metabolic risk factors in South Asians: the Molecular Study of Health and Risk in Ethnic Groups (mol-SHARE). *PloS one*. 6:e22112.

Anoop S, Misra A, Mani K, Pandey RM, Gulati S, Bhatt SP, Mahajan H. 2017. Estimation of liver span using MRI for prediction of type 2 diabetes in non-obese Asian Indians. *J Diabetes Sci Tech.* 11:446-447.

Ashwell M, Gibson S. 2016. Waist-to-height ratio as an indicator of 'early health risk': simpler and more predictive than using a 'matrix' based on BMI and waist circumference. *BMJ Open.* 6:e010159.

Aswathappa J, Garg S, Kutty K, Shankar V. 2013. Neck circumference as an anthropometric measure of obesity in diabetics. *North Am J Med Sci.* 5:.28.

Awasthi A, Rao CR,Hegde DS. 2017. Association between type 2 diabetes mellitus and anthropometric measurements–a case control study in South India. *J Prev Med Hyg.58*:E56.

Banoo H, Nusrat N, Nasir N. 2015. Type 2 Diabetes Mellitus: a review of current trends. *Rama Univ J Med Sci.* 1:50-57.

Barreira TV, Broyles ST, Gupta AK, Katzmarzyk PT. 2014. Relationship of anthropometric indices to abdominal and total body fat in youth: sex and race differences. *Obesity*. 22:1345-1350.

Berghofer A, Pischon T, Reinhold T, Apovian CM, Sharma AM, Willich SN. 2008. Obesity prevalence from a European perspective: a systematic review. *BMC Public Health*. 8:200-10.1186/1471-2458-8-200.

Bhatt SP, Nigam P, Misra A, Guleria R, Luthra K, Jain SK, Pasha MQ. 2012. Association of the Myostatin gene with obesity, abdominal obesity and low lean body mass and in non-diabetic Asian Indians in north India. *PloS one.* 7:e40977.

Bodicoat DH, Gray LJ, Henson J, Webb D, Guru A, Misra A, Gupta R, Vikram N, Sattar N, Davies MJ, Khunti K. 2014. Body mass index and waist circumference cut-points in multi-ethnic populations from the UK and India: the ADDITION-Leicester, Jaipur heart watch and New Delhi cross-sectional studies. *PLoS One*. 9:e90813.

Chandalia M, Lin P, Seenivasan T, Livingston EH, Snell PG, Grundy SM, Abate N. 2007. Insulin resistance and body fat distribution in South Asian men compared to Caucasian men. *PloS one*. 2:e812.

Chatterjee S, Khunti K, Davies MJ. 2017. Type 2 diabetes. *Lancet*. 389:2239-2251.

Cnop M, Welsh N, Jonas JC, Jörns A, Lenzen S, Eizirik DL. 2005. Mechanisms of pancreatic β-cell death in type 1 and type 2 diabetes: many differences, few similarities. *Diabetes*. 54:S97-107.

Deaton C. 2017. Reducing premature mortality from non-communicable diseases. *Nursing Standard*.31:40-43.

Deepa M, Anjana RM, Mohan V. 2017. Role of lifestyle factors in the epidemic of diabetes: lessons learnt from India. *Eur J Clin Nutr*. 71:825.

Després JP. Overweight: The Body Mass Index Category with an Identity Crisis Overweight: The BMI Category With an Identity Crisis. *Annals of Internal Medicine*. 166:671-672.

Deurenberg-Yap M, Chew SK, Deurenberg P. 2002. Elevated body fat percentage and cardiovascular risks at low body mass index levels among Singaporean Chinese, Malays and Indians. *Obes Rev*. 3:209-215.

Dudeja P, Singh G, Gadekar T, Mukherji S. 2017. Performance of Indian Diabetes Risk Score (IDRS) as screening tool for diabetes in an urban slum. *Med J Armed Forces India*. 73:123-128.

Eastwood SV, Tillin T, Wright A, Mayet J, Godsland I, Forouhi NG, Whincup P, Hughes AD, Chaturvedi N. 2014. Thigh fat and muscle each contribute to excess cardio metabolic risk in South Asians, independent of visceral adipose tissue. *Obesity*. 22:2071-2079.

Freedman DS: Obesity - United States, 1988–2008. 2011. *MMWR Surveill Summ*. 60:73-77.

Gamit ST, Gamit AL, Patel TC, Bhatt P, Chaudhari VP. 2017. WHR (waist hip ratio) as risk factor irrespective of body mass index (BMI) among patients of noninsulin dependent diabetes mellitus (NIDDM). *Int J Res Med.* 5:68-72.

Girardi E, Schepisi MS, Goletti D, Bates M, Mwaba P, Yeboah-Manu D, Ntoumi F, Palmieri F, Maeurer M, Zumla A, Ippolito G. The global dynamics of diabetes and tuberculosis: the impact of migration and policy implications. *Int J Infec Diseases.* 56:45-53.

Girdhar S, Sharma S, Chaudhary A, Bansal P, Satija M. 2016. An Epidemiological Study of Overweight and Obesity among Women in an Urban Area of North India. *Ind J Comm Med.* 41:154-157.

Grundy SM, Brewer HB Jr, Cleeman JI, Smith SC Jr, Lenfant C. 2004. Definition of metabolic syndrome: report of the National Heart, Lung, and Blood Institute/American Heart Association conference on scientific issues related to definition. *Circulation.* 109:433-438.

Grundy SM. 2016. Metabolic syndrome update. *Trends Cardiovascular Med.* 26:364-373.

Gulati S, Misra A. 2017. Abdominal obesity and type 2 diabetes in Asian Indians: dietary strategies including edible oils, cooking practices and sugar intake. *Eur J Clin Nutr.* 71:850.

Gupta R, Agrawal A, Misra A, Guptha S, Vikram NK. 2012. Metabolic cardiovascular risk factors worsen continuously across the spectrum of body mass index in Asian Indians. *Indian Heart J.* 64:236-244.

Hardy DS, Stallings DT, Garvin JT, Xu H, Racette SB. 2017. Best anthropometric discriminators of incident type 2 diabetes among white and black adults: A longitudinal ARIC study. *PloS one.* 12:e0168282.

Heindel JJ, Blumberg B, Cave M, Machtinger R, Mantovani A, Mendez MA, Nadal A, Palanza P, Panzica G, Sargis R, Vandenberg LN. 2017. Metabolism disrupting chemicals and metabolic disorders. *Reproductive Toxicol.* 68:3-33.

Horikawa Y, Oda N, Cox NJ, Li X, Orho-Melander M, Hara M, Hinokio Y, Lindner TH, Mashima H, Schwarz PE, del Bosque-Plata L. 2000. Genetic variation in the gene encoding calpain-10 is associated with type 2 diabetes mellitus. *Nature Genetics.* 26:163-175.

Hsu WC, Araneta MR, Kanaya AM, Chiang JL, Fujimoto W. 2015. BMI cut points to identify at-risk Asian Americans for type 2 diabetes screening. *Diabetes Care*. 38:150-158.

Hudda MT, Nightingale CM, Donin AS, Fewtrell MS, Haroun D, Lum S, Williams JE, Owen CG, Rudnicka AR, Wells JC, Cook DG. 2017. Body mass index adjustments to increase the validity of body fatness assessment in UK Black African and South Asian children. *Int J Obesity*. 41:1048.

Hung SP, Chen CY, Guo FR, Chang CI, Jan CF. 2017. Combine body mass index and body fat percentage measures to improve the accuracy of obesity screening in young adults. *Obesity Res Clin Prac*. 11:11-18.

IDF. 2005. *IDF Clinical Guidelines Task Force: Global Guideline for Type 2 Diabetes*. Brussels: International Diabetes Federation.

Jain SC, Gupta RP, Gupta D, Jain MK. 2017. A study on body mass index and its correlation with type 2 *diabetes. Int J ResMed Sci.* 2:1638-1641.

Jayawardana NW, Jayalath WA, Madhujith WM, Ralapanawa U, Jayasekera RS, Alagiyawanna SA, Bandara AM, Kalupahana NS. 2017. Aging and obesity are associated with undiagnosed hypertension in a cohort of males in the Central Province of Sri Lanka: a cross-sectional descriptive study. *BMC Cardiovascular Disorders*. 17:165.

Jayawardana R, Ranasinghe P, Sheriff MH, Matthews DR, Katulanda P. 2013. Waist to height ratio: a better anthropometric marker of diabetes and cardio-metabolic risks in South Asian adults. *Diabetes Res ClinPrac*. 99:292-299.

Joshi SR, Anjana RM, Deepa M, Pradeepa R, Bhansali A, Dhandania VK, Joshi PP, Unnikrishnan R, Nirmal E, Subashini R, Madhu SV. 2014. Prevalence of dyslipidemia in urban and rural India: the ICMR–INDIAB study. *PloS one*. 9:e96808.

Joshi SR, Parikh RM. 2007. India - diabetes capital of the world: now heading towards hypertension. *J Assoc Physicians India*. 55:323–324.

Kautzky-Willer A, Harreiter J, Pacini G. 2016. Sex and gender differences in risk, pathophysiology and complications of type 2 diabetes mellitus. *Endocrine Rev*. 37:278-316.

Khandelwal A, Mathur HN, Jain J, Dixit M, Singhal G, Khandelwal N. 2017. A study of knowledge about the diabetes type I and II, among diabetic patients in Geetanjali medical college and hospital, Udaipur, Rajasthan, India. *Int J Comm Med Pub Health.* 3:1278-1281.

Khanna N, Sharma RS. 2015. Positive correlation of genetic transmittance of type 2 diabetes mellitus with anthropometric indices in adults of Majha region of Punjab, India. *Int J Bioassays.* 4:3926-3930.

Kharroubi AT, Darwish HM. 2015. Diabetes mellitus: The epidemic of the century. *World J Diabetes.* 6:850.

Khullar K, Agarwal A, du Plessis SS. 2014. BMI and Obesity. In Du Plessis SS, Agarwal A, Sabanegh Jr ES, editors. *Male infertility: a complete guide to lifestyle and environmental factors*. Springer New York. 31p-45.

Kruger HS, Schutte AE, Walsh CM, Kruger A, Rennie KL. 2017. Body mass index cut-points to identify cardio metabolic risk in black South Africans. *Eur J Nutr.* 56:193-202.

Kumar A, Goel MK, Jain RB, Khanna P, Chaudhary V. 2013. India towards diabetes control: Key issues. *Australias Med J.* 6:524-531.

Little M. 2017. *Type 2 diabetes and the double burden of malnutrition in rural south India: A mixed-methods examination of a public health crisis* (Doctoral dissertation).

Liu LL, Kahn HS, Pettitt DJ, Fino NF, Morgan T, Maahs DM, Crimmins NA, Lamichhane AP, Liese AD, D'Agostino Jr RB, Bell RA. 2016. Comparing Two Waist-to-Height Ratio Measurements with Cardiometabolic Risk Factors among Youth with Diabetes. *Int J Child Health Nutr.* 5:87.

Mahajan A, Go MJ, Zhang W, Below JE, Gaulton KJ, Ferreira T, Horikoshi M, Johnson AD, Ng MC, Prokopenko I, Saleheen D. 2014. Genome-wide trans-ancestry meta-analysis provides insight into the genetic architecture of type 2 diabetes susceptibility. *Nature Genetics.* 46:234.

Mahalakshmi MM, Bhavadharini B, Kumar M, Anjana RM, Shah SS, Bridgette A, Choudhury M, Henderson M, Desborough L, Viswanathan M, Ranjani H. 2014. Clinical profile, outcomes, and progression to type 2 diabetes among Indian women with gestational diabetes mellitus seen at a diabetes center in south India. *Indian J Endocrinol Metabol.* 18:400.

Mandal A. 2014. Study of prevalence of type 2 diabetes mellitus and hypertension in overweight and obese people. *J Family Med Primary care.* 3:25.

Marcadenti A, Fuchs FD, Moreira LB, Gus M, Fuchs SC. 2017. Adiposity phenotypes are associated with type-2 diabetes: LAP index, body adiposity index, and neck circumference. *Atherosclerosis.* 266:145-150.

Marinou K, Hodson L, Vasan SK, Fielding BA, Banerjee R, Brismar K, Koutsilieris M, Clark A, Neville MJ, Karpe F. 2014. Structural and functional properties of deep abdominal subcutaneous adipose tissue explain its association with insulin resistance and cardiovascular risk in men. *Diabetes care.* 37:821-829.

Marques CL, Beretta MV, Prates RE, Nascimento FV, Nascimento C, de Almeida JC, da Costa Rodrigues T. 2015. Adiponectin levels and waist circumference, waist-hip ratio and conicity index in type 1 diabetes patients. *BMC Diabetol Metabol Syndr.* 7:A86.

Mastorci F, Vassalle C, Chatzianagnostou K, Marabotti C, Siddiqui K, Eba AO, Mhamed SA, Bandopadhyay A, Nazzaro MS, Passera M, Pingitore A. 2017. Undernutrition and overnutrition burden for diseases in developing countries: The role of oxidative stress biomarkers to assess disease risk and interventional strategies. *Antioxidants.* 6:41.

McMurry HS, Shivashankar R, Mendenhall E, Prabhakaran D. 2017. Insights on Overweight and Obesity. *Economic Political Weekly.* 52:85.

Meigs JB, Wilson PW, Fox CS, Vasan RS, Nathan DM, Sullivan LM, D'agostino RB. 2006. Body mass index, metabolic syndrome, and risk of type 2 diabetes or cardiovascular disease. *J Clin Endocrinol Metabol.* 91:2906-2912.

Meshram A, Agrawal U, Dhok A, Adole P, Meshram K, Khare R. 2013. HbA1c, hs-CRP and anthropometric parameters evaluation in the patients of Diabetes Mellitus of Central Rural India. *Int J Med Sci Pub Health*. 2:293-296.

Misra A, Bhardwaj S. 2014. Obesity and the metabolic syndrome in developing countries: focus on South Asians. In *International Nutrition: Achieving Millennium Goals and Beyond.* Karger Publishers.78:133-1440.

Misra A, Ganda OP. 2007. Migration and its impact on adiposity and type 2 diabetes. *Nutr.* 23:696–708.

Misra A, Khurana L. 2011. Obesity-related non-communicable diseases: South Asians vs White Caucasians. *Int J Obes* (Lond). 35:167-1887.

Mohan V, Deepa M. 2007. Measuring Obesity to Assess Cardiovascular Risk -Inch Tape, Weighing Machine, or Both? *JAPI.* 55:617-619.

Mohan V, Sandeep S, Deepa R, Shah B, Varghese C. 2007. Epidemiology of type 2 diabetes: Indian scenario. *Indian J Med Res*. 125:217.

Mohan V, Amutha A, Ranjani H, Unnikrishnan R, Datta M, Anjana RM, Staimez L, Ali MK, Narayan KV. 2013. Associations of β-cell function and insulin resistance with youth-onset type 2 diabetes and prediabetes among Asian Indians. *Diabetes Tech Therap.* 15:315-322.

Mondal N, Sen J. 2014. Role of anthropometry in assessment of excess adiposity and metabolic disorders in Asian Indians. *Public Health in 21st Century: Health consequences of human central obesity*. New York: Nova Biomedical. 71p-83p.

Montesi L, Caletti MT, Marchesini G. 2016. Diabetes in migrants and ethnic minorities in a changing World. *World J Diabetes.* 7:34–44.

Nagar SR, Jain M. 2017. Study to assess predictive value of waist to height ratio and body mass index as a risk factor of hypertension and type 2 diabetes mellitus. *Int J Comm Med Pub Health*. 4:1099-1103.

Nandimath VA, Swamy CS, Nandimath SA, Jatti G, Jadhav S. 2016. Evaluation of certain risk factors of type 2 diabetes mellitus: a case–control study.*Int J Med Sci Pub Health.*5:1334-1339.

NCEP. 2001. Executive Summary of the Third Report of The National Cholesterol Education Program (NCEP) Expert Panel on Detection, Evaluation, and Treatment of High Blood Cholesterol in Adults (Adult Treatment Panel III). *JAMA.* 285:2486–2497.

Nsiah K, Shang VO, Boateng KA, Mensah FO. 2015. Prevalence of metabolic syndrome in type 2 diabetes mellitus patients. *Int J Appl Basic Med Res.* 5:133.

O'Keefe EL, Di Nicolantonio JJ, Patil H, Helzberg JH, Lavie CJ. 2016. Lifestyle choices fuel epidemics of diabetes and cardiovascular disease among Asian Indians. *Prog Cardiovasc Dis* 58:505-513.

Ogden CL, Carroll MD, Kit BK, Flegal KM. 2012. Prevalence of obesity in the United States, 2009–2010. *NCHS Data Brief.* 1-8.

Olokoba AB, Obateru OA, Olokoba LB. 2012. Type 2 diabetes mellitus: a review of current trends. *Oman Med J.* 27:269.

Pandey U, Midha T, Rao YK, Katiyar P, Wal P, Kaur S, Martolia DS. 2017. Anthropometric indicators as predictor of pre-diabetes in Indian adolescents. *Indian Heart J.* 69:474-479.

Papazafiropoulou A, Anagnostopoulou K, Papanas N, Petropoulou K, Melidonis A. 2016. Neck Circumference as a Simple Tool for Assessing Central Obesity in Patients with Type 2 Diabetes Mellitus in Greece-A Descriptive Study.*Rev Diabetic Stud.* 13:215.

Parikh RM, Mohan V. 2012. Changing definitions of metabolic syndrome. *Indian J Endocrinol Metabol.* 16:7.

Perreault L. 2018. Prevention of Type 2 Diabetes. In *Diabetes and Exercise.* Humana Press, Cham. 17p-29p.

Phua KH, Yap MT, Khilji SS, Lee HP. 2017. Development of public health in economic transition: the middle-income countries. Oxford Textbook of Global Public Health. 28:48.

Popkin BM, Adair LS, Ng SW. 2012.Global nutrition transition and the pandemic of obesity in developing countries. *Nutr Rev.* 70:3-21.

Pozza C, Isidori AM. 2018. What's Behind the Obesity Epidemic. In *Imaging in Bariatric Surgery.* Springer, Cham. 1p-8p.

Prasad DS, Kabir Z, Dash AK, Das BC. 2010. Cardiovascular risk factors in developing countries: A review of clinico-epidemiological evidence. *CVD Prev Contr.* 5:115-123.

Pratyush DD, Tiwari S, Singh S, Singh SK. 2012. Waist circumference cut-off and its importance for diagnosis of metabolic syndrome in

Asian Indians: a preliminary study. *Indian J Endocrinol Metabol.* 16:112.

Rabin BA, Boehmer TK, Brownson RC. 2007. Cross-national comparison of environmental and policy correlates of obesity in Europe. *Eur J Pub Health.*17:53-61. 10.1093/eurpub/ckl073.

Radha V, Mohan V. 2007. Genetic predisposition of type 2 diabetes among Asian Indians. *Indian J Med Res.* 125:259-274.

Radha V, Vimaleswaran KS, Babu HN, Abate N, Chandalia M, Satija P, Grundy SM, Ghosh S, Majumder PP, Deepa R, Rao SM. 2006. Role of Genetic Polymorphism Peroxisome Proliferator–Activated Receptor-γ2 Pro12Ala on Ethnic Susceptibility to Diabetes in South-Asian and Caucasian Subjects: Evidence for heterogeneity. *Diabetes Care.* 29:1046-1051.

Raji A, Seely EW, Arky RA, Simonson DC. 2001. Body fat distribution and insulin resistance in healthy Asian Indians and Caucasians. *J Clin Endocrinol Metabol.* 86:5366-5371.

Ramachandran A, Snehalatha C, Kapur A, Vijay V, Mohan V, Das AK, Yajnik CS, Prasanna Kumar KM, Nair JD. 2001. Diabetes Epidemiology Study Group in India (DESI). High prevalence of diabetes and impaired glucose tolerance in India. National Urban Diabetes Survey. *Diabetologia.* 44:1094-1101.

Ramachandran A, Snehalatha C, Ma RC. 2014. Diabetes in South-East Asia: an update. *Diabetes Res Clin Prac.* 103:231-237.

Roriz AK, Passos LC, Oliveira CC, Eickemberg M, Moreira PD, Ramos LB. 2016. Anthropometric clinical indicators in the assessment of visceral obesity: an update. *Nutr Clin Diet Hosp.* 36:168-79.DOI: 10.12873/362carneirororiz.

Ruderman NB, Carling D, Prentki M, Cacicedo JM. 2013. AMPK, insulin resistance, and the metabolic syndrome. *J Clin Investigation.* 123:2764.

Saltiel AR, Olefsky JM. 2017. Inflammatory mechanisms linking obesity and metabolic disease. *J Clin Investigation.* 127:1-4.

Sen J, Mondal N, Dutta S. 2013. Factors affecting overweight and obesity among urban adults: a cross-sectional study. *Epidemiol Biostat Pub Health.* 10:e8741–1-8.

Sengupta A, Angeli F, Syamala TS, Van Schayck CP, Dagnelie P. 2014. State-wise dynamics of the doubleburden of malnutrition among 15-49 year-old women in India: how much does the scenario change considering Asian population-specific BMI cut-off values. *Ecol Food Nutr.* 53:618-638.

Shrestha A. 2015. *Diet, Obesity, and Diabetes in Suburban Nepal-A Community-Based Study* (Doctoral dissertation).

Snehalatha C, Viswanathan V, Ramachandran A. 2003. Cutoff values for normal anthropometric variables in Asian Indian adults. *Diabet Care.* 26:1380-1384.

Soares M, Müller MJ. 2017. *Type 2 diabetes in Asia: where do we go from here?.* 71:801-802.

Staiger H, Machicao F, Fritsche A, Häring HU. 2009. Patho mechanisms of type 2 diabetes genes. *Endocr Rev.* 30:557-585.

Sullivan CA, Kahn SE, Fujimoto WY, Hayashi T, Leonetti DL, Boyko EJ. 2015. Change in intra-abdominal fat predicts the risk of hypertension in Japanese Americans. *Hypertension.* 114. DOI: 10.1161/HYPERTENSIONAHA.114.04990.

Uday S, Gorman S, Feltbower RG, Mathai M. 2017. Ethnic variation in the correlation between waist to height ratio and total daily insulin requirement in children with type 1 diabetes: a cross-sectional study. *Pediatr Diabetes.* 18:128-135.

van Vliet-Ostaptchouk JV, Nuotio ML, Slagter SN, Doiron D, Fischer K, Foco L, Gaye A, Gögele M, Heier M, Hiekkalinna T, Joensuu A. 2014. The prevalence of metabolic syndrome and metabolically healthy obesity in Europe: a collaborative analysis of ten large cohort studies. *BMC Endocrine Disord.* 14:9.

Vazquez G, Duval S, Jacobs DR, Silventoinen K. 2007. Comparison of body mass index, waist circumference, and waist/hip ratio in predicting incident diabetes: a meta-analysis. *Epidemiol Rev.* 29:115-128.

Vimaleswaran KS, Bodhini D, Lakshmipriya N, Ramya K, Anjana RM, Sudha V, Lovegrove JA, Kinra S, Mohan V, Radha V. 2016. Interaction between FTO gene variants and lifestyle factors on metabolic traits in an Asian Indian population. *NutrMetabol.* 13:39.

Vimaleswaran KS, Radha V, Ghosh S, Majumder PP, Deepa R, Babu HN, Rao MR, Mohan V. 2005. Peroxisome proliferator-activated receptor-γ co-activator-1α (PGC-1α) gene polymorphisms and their relationship to Type 2 diabetes in Asian Indians. *Diabetic Med.* 22:1516-1521.

Visscher TL, Kromhout D, Seidell JC. 2002. Long-term and recent time trends in the prevalence of obesity among Dutch men and women. *Int J Obes Relat Metab Disord.* 26:1218-1224.

Wang Y, Rimm EB, Stampfer MJ, Willett WC, Hu FB. 2005. Comparison of abdominal adiposity and overall obesity in predicting risk of type 2 diabetes among men. *Am J Clin Nutr.* 81:555-563.

WHO Expert Consultation. 2004. Appropriate Body Mass Index for Asian populations and its implications for policy and intervention strategies. *Lancet.* 363:157-163.

WHO. 1995. *The use and interpretation of anthropometry.* Geneva CH. WHO 1995, technical report 854.

Wilson PW, D'Agostino RB, Parise H, Sullivan L, Meigs JB. 2005. Metabolic syndrome as a precursor of cardiovascular disease and type 2 diabetes mellitus. *Circulation.* 112:3066-3072.

World Health Organization. 1999. Definition, Diagnosis and Classification of Diabetes Mellitus and its Complications. *Diagnosis and Classification of Diabetes Mellitus.* Provisional Report of a WHO Consultation Geneva.

World Health Organization. 2000. *The Asia Pacific Perspective, Redefining obesity and its treatment.* Geneva: World Health Organization.

Wu TS, Ding LW, Chen HL, Chang YY, Lan YP. 2016. Relationship of neck circumference to metabolic syndrome and central obesity in regional hospital employees. *Diabetes Res Clin Prac.* 120:S72.

Xiao J, Huang JP, Xu GF, Chen DX, Wu GY, Zhang M, Shen Y, Cai H. 2015. Association of alcohol consumption and components of metabolic syndrome among people in rural China. *Nutr Metabol.* 12:5.

Yajnik CS, Fall CH, Coyaji KJ, Hirve SS, Rao S, Barker DJ, Joglekar C, Kellingray S. 2003. Neonatal anthropometry: the thin–fat Indian baby. The Pune maternal nutrition study. *Int J Obes.* 27:173-180.

Yajnik CS. 2004. Early life origins of insulin resistance and type 2 diabetes in India and other Asian countries. *J Nutr.*134: 205-210.

Yang GR, Yuan SY, Fu HJ, Wan G, Zhu LX, Bu XL. 2010. Neck circumference positively related with central obesity, overweight, and metabolic syndrome in Chinese subjects with type 2 diabetes: Beijing community diabetes study 4. *Diabetes Care.* 33:2465-2467.

Yankey BA, Rothenberg R, Strasser S, White KR, Okosun IS. 2017. Relationship between Years of Marijuana Use and the Four Main Diagnostic Criteria for Metabolic Syndrome among United States Adults. *J Addict Res Ther S.* 11:2.Zhao J, Pang ZC, Zhang L, Gao WG, Wang SJ, Ning F, Nan HR, Ren J, Qiao Q. 2011. Prevalence of metabolic syndrome in rural and urban Chinese population in Qingdao. *J Endocrinol Investigation.* 34:444-448.

Zhao W, Rasheed A, Tikkanen E, Lee JJ, Butterworth AS, Howson JM, Assimes TL, Chowdhury R, Orho-Melander M, Damrauer S, Small A. 2017. Identification of new susceptibility loci for type 2 diabetes and shared etiological pathways with coronary heart disease. *Nature Genetics.* 49:1450.

In: Obesity and Syndrome X
Editors: M. Das and K. Bose
ISBN: 978-1-53614-669-1

Chapter 9

C-Reactive Protein and Family History: A Future Threat towards Diabetes and Syndrome X

Riddhi Goswami[1,*], Mithun Das[2] and Indrani Lodh[3]
[1]Department of Biotechnology,
Heritage Institute of Technology, Kolkata, India
[2]Department of Anthropology, Sree Chaitanya College,
Habra, West Bengal, India
[3]Urvaraa IVF Clinic, Kolkata, India

Introduction

Type II Diabetes: A Global Menace

Type II diabetes mellitus is a long term metabolic disorder that consists of an array of dysfunctions characterized by hyperglycemia and resulting from the combination of resistance to insulin action, inadequate insulin

* Corresponding Author Email: rgoswami77@gmail.com.

secretion, and excessive or inappropriate glucagon secretion. Common symptoms include increased thirst, frequent urination, and unexplained weight loss. Symptoms may also include increased hunger, feeling tired, and sores that do not heal (NIDDKD, 2014). Long-term complications from high blood sugar include heart disease, strokes, diabetic retinopathy which can result in blindness, kidney failure, and poor blood flow in the limbs which may lead to amputations (WHO 2011).

Globally, an estimated 422 million adults are living with diabetes mellitus, according to the latest 2016 data from the World Health Organization (WHO 2016). Diabetes prevalence is increasing rapidly; previous 2013 estimates from the International Diabetes Federation put the number at 381 million people having diabetes. The number is projected to almost double by 2030. Type II diabetes makes up about 85-90% of all cases (New York Times 2006). Increases in the overall diabetes prevalence rates largely reflect an increase in risk factors for Type II, notably greater longevity and being overweight or obese (Melmed et al., 2011).

Indian Scenario

Until recently, India had more diabetics than any other country in the world, according to the International Diabetes Foundation, although the country has now been surpassed in the top spot by China, Diabetes currently affects more than 62 million Indians, which is more than 7.1% of the adult population. The average age on onset is 42.5 years. Nearly 1 million Indians die due to diabetes every year (Gale 2010).

According to the Indian Heart Association, India is projected to be home to 109 million individuals with diabetes by 2035 (IHA 2016). A study by the American Diabetes Association reports that India will see the greatest increase in people diagnosed with diabetes by 2030. The high incidence is attributed to a combination of genetic susceptibility plus adoption of a high-calorie, low-activity lifestyle by India's growing middle class (New York Times 2006).

A considerable variability in the incidence and prevalence of Type II diabetes (T2D) coheres with an important contribution of multigenetic predisposition in the development of T2D. Some genes, which probably participate in the pathogenesis of Type II diabetes, also play a role in the regulation of blood pressure, familial hyperlipidemia, familial hypertension and other diseases of the cardiovascular system Demova et al., 2012.

Human C-reactive protein (CRP) is an acute phase reactant involved in chronic and acute inflammation. CRP production is rapidly stimulated in response to infection, tissue injury or inflammation. In a recent study, increased levels of CRP are reported to be associated with metabolic syndrome, obesity, atherosclerosis, unstable angina, insulin resistance and diabetes. Family and twin studies suggest that genetic factors account for 40% of the variance in plasma CRP levels + 1059 G > C (rs1800947) is a single nucleotide polymorphism (SNP) in exon 2 of the *CRP* gene. + 1059 G > C is a silent or synonymous polymorphism at the amino acid level (CTG → CTC, Leu → Leu at codon 184) which has been reported to affect the protein levels of CRP and contribute towards the progression of CAD (coronary artery disease) and T2D Kaur et al., 2013.

METHODS

Study Population

This is a longitudinal follow-up study and present study was being done in continuation with the earlier work. The medical history of the patient's family was recorded. Determination of presence or absence of other risk factors – high cholesterol levels, cigarette smoking, hypertension, and diabetes in first-degree relatives (biological parents, siblings, and offspring) – was recorded. The present study was conducted on 160 healthy (non-diabetic, normotensive) adult Asian Indian women [including 90 with and 70 without family history of diabetes (FHD)] living in and around Kolkata, India. This sample size was sufficient to test all the research hypotheses at the 5% level of significance. During the gestation period they were studied twice, first within 12 weeks and second by 30 weeks. They were then followed up till delivery. During delivery both mothers' venous blood and cord blood were collected to estimate the metabolic variables and genetic polymorphisms of the respective mothers and their new born babies. All the experiments were done according to the "Ethical guidelines for Biomedical Research on Human Participants" published by Indian Council of Medical Research (2006). The Institutional Ethics Committee (IEC) of Heritage Institute of Technology, Kolkata, approved the study. Written consent was obtained from the subjects prior to actual commencement of the study.

Anthropometric Measurements

Demographic profiles including name and age were obtained from participants. Informed consent was obtained from participants prior to the actual commencement of the study. Height was measured to nearest 0.1 cm with a Martin's Anthropometer and weight to the nearest 0.5 kg with a portable weighing machine in light clothing and bare feet.

Blood Pressure Measurements

Left arm systolic (SBP) and diastolic (DBP) blood pressure was taken from each participant with the help of an Omron M1 digital electronic blood pressure/pulse monitor (Omron Corporation, Tokyo, Japan). Two blood pressure measurements were taken and averaged for analysis. A third measurement was taken when the difference between the two measurements was $\geq$ 5 mmHg, and a subsequent mean was calculated. A five minute relaxation period between measurements was maintained for all participants. The working condition of the instrument was checked periodically using a mercury sphygmomanometer and stethoscope (auscultator procedure). Subjects with SBP/DBP values > 130/85 mm Hg were considered as Hypertensive, according to NCEP and ATPIII guidelines, 2005 (NCEP 2005).

Estimation of Metabolic Profiles

A fasting blood sample (7 ml) was collected from each subject for the determination of fasting blood glucose (FBG), Total cholesterol (TC), Triglycerides (TG), and High density lipoproteins (HDL). All subjects maintained an overnight fast of $\geq$12 h prior to blood collection. The plasma was separated within 2 h of blood collection using a microcentrifuge at 1000 rpm for about 20 min at room temperature. Estimation of FBG, TC, TG, CRP and HDL were carried out using a Robonik Biochemistry Analyzer (Robonik India, Mumbai, India). Low-density lipoprotein (LDL) and very low density lipoprotein (VLDL) were then calculated by using the standard formula: $LDL = TC - (HDL + TG/5)$ and $VLDL = TG/5$. All the metabolic profiles were estimated according to NCEP and ATPIII guidelines 2005 (NCEP 2005).

Genotyping of CRP

- The DNA was isolated from whole blood by HiPurA™ Blood Genomic DNA Miniprep Purification Spin Kit. The DNA was amplified by PCR (ABI Biosystems, USA).
- Amplification refractory mutation system-polymerase chain reaction (ARMS-PCR) which is based on allele specific amplification of desired fragment using primers corresponding to the alleles has been used for genotyping of +1059 G > C SNP in the CRP gene.
- The sequences of specific primers used are:
  1. Constant forward:
     5′-CATTTGTACAAGCTGGGAGT-3′,
  2. Allele C-specific reverse:

5′-ATGGTGTTAATCTCATCTGGTGGG-3′,

3. Allele G-specific reverse:
   5′-ATGGTGTTAATCTCATCTGGTGGC-3′.

- The conditions included initial denaturation (95°C for 5 min) following a touchdown PCR with denaturation at 94°C for 45 secs, annealing at 66°C to 62°C with 1°C decrease in temperature for the first 4 cycles followed by 29 cycles at 61°C for 45 secs, extension at 72°C for 45 secs each cycle and final extension at 72°C for 10 min (Cao & Hegele 2000).
- CRP+1059 G > C genotypes were assessed from the presence/ absence of PCR amplicon (237 bp), corresponding to the specific allele (C/G) on 1.5% agarose gel stained with Ethidium bromide.
- The genotyping of CRP genes yielded PCR products of size 744 bp. Digestion of the less common 1059C allele produced two smaller fragments, with sizes of 434 and 310 bp. Digestion of the more common 1059G allele produced three fragments, with sizes of 310, 233, and 201 bp.

Statistical Analyses

Mean and SD for all the metabolic variables, hormones and blood pressure measurements were calculated by conventional statistical methods. Group differences (with and without FHD) for all the variables (18 and 30 months) were tested by One-way ANOVA ($p \pm 0.05$). Differences in CRP values by FHD were estimated by 2X2 Contingency Chi-square analysis ($p \pm 0.05$). Differences in birth outcomes by FHD and CRP values of mothers was estimated by Chi-square analysis ($p \pm 0.05$). All statistical tests weew performed on Statistical Package for Social Sciences (IBM-SPSS version 16) and significance was set at $p < 0.05$ two tailed.

RESULTS

Biochemical Analyses of Metabolic Risk Factors

Statistical Analyses of the comparison of the Group differences (with and without FHD) for all the variables (12 and 30 weeks) were tested by One-way ANOVA ($p = < 0.05$). Table 1 shows the anthropometric measurements and biochemical parameters which were considered during the study.

A comparison of the metabolic variables among the subjects with and without FHD revealed that there were significant differences among them with respect to Waist circumference, Triglycerides, HDL-Cholesterol, VLDL-Cholesterol, Fasting Blood Glucose and Blood pressure, both at the gestational period of 12 weeks and 30 weeks. It indicates that family history plays an influencing metabolic factors and triggering the risk factors early in the gestational phase leading to complications in adult life.

Table 1. Baseline characteristics of the study population by family history (n = 160)

Variables	By 12 Weeks			By 30 Weeks		
	Both/Either*	None**	ANOVA	Both/Either	None	ANOVA
	(n = 90)	(n = 70)	P	(n = 90)	(n = 70)	P
AGE (yrs)	31 (6.3)	27 (3.2)	0.258	32 (6)	30 (6)	0.323
WEIGHT (kg)	68 (13)	63 (8)	0.240	74 (10)	72 (10)	0.061
BMI (kg/m^2)	25.4 (3.8)	27.3 (3.7)	0.415	36.5 (4.1)	32.5 (3.9)	0.416
WC (cm)	91 (13)	79 (9)	<0.001	132 (14)	110 (12)	<0.001
TC (mg/dl)	211 (16)	155 (14)	0.122	217 (21)	210 (20)	0.069
TG (mg/dl)	159 (27)	124 (21)	<0.001	243 (32)	176 (29)	<0.001
HDLc (mg/dl)	54 (9)	44 (10)	<0.001	53 (8)	42 (9)	<0.001
LDLc (mg/dl)	115 (11)	100 (12)	0.001	117 (13)	108 (10)	0.009
VLDLc (mg/dl)	35 (5)	28 (4)	<0.001	55 (10)	34(7)	<0.001
FBG (mg/dl)	117 (10)	98 (12)	<0.001	110 (12)	94 (11)	<0.001
SBP (mmHg)	122 (11)	108 (12)	<0.001	138 (14)	118(16)	<0.001
DBP (mmHg)	83 (10)	77 (9)	<0.001	95 (8)	88 (6)	<0.001

Read as Mean and ± SD within parentheses; *Both/Either - Participants having positive FHD present in both or either parents; **None - No FHD.

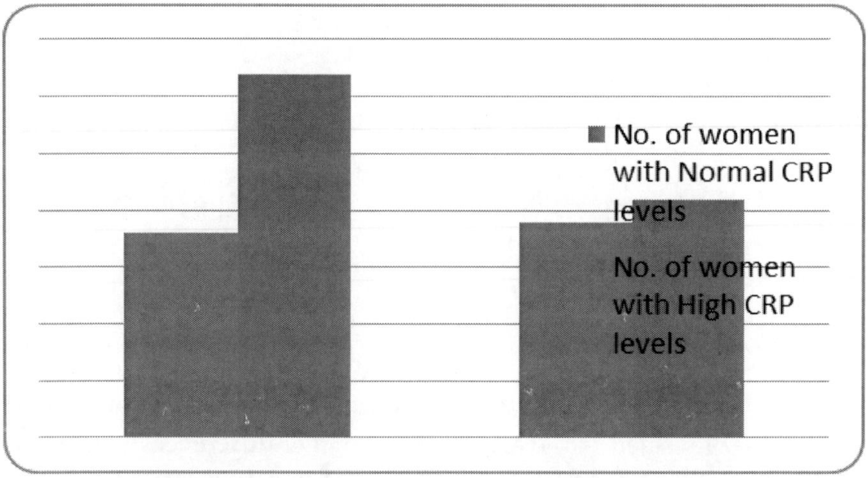

Figure 1. Showing statistically significant difference in C-reactive protein (CRP) levels by FHD ($p = 0.0109$).

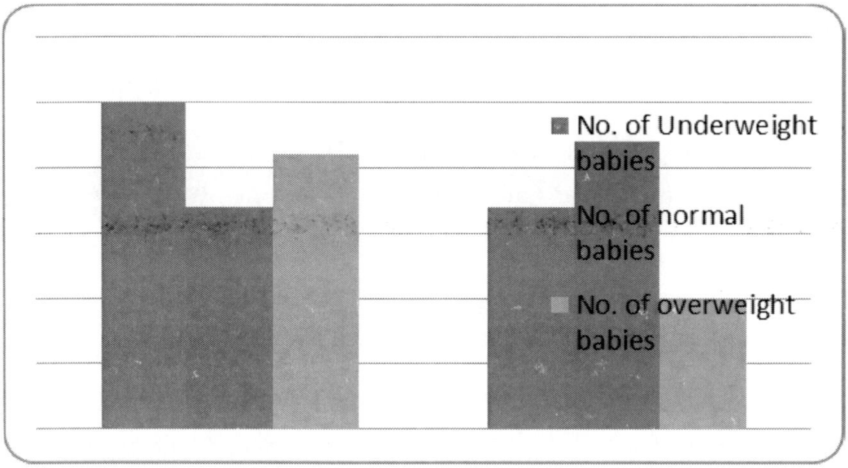

Figure 2. Showing statistically significant differences in birth outcomes (birth weight in kg) by FHD and CRP of the mothers ($p = 0.0252$).

Comparison of subjects in the CRP levels between the same groups also revealed a statistically significant difference in subjects with a positive FHD and high CRP levels in comparison to normal cases (Figure 1 & 2).

Table 2. Differences in C-reactive protein (CRP) of the babies by mothers' CRP and FHD

CRP of the Babies	Mothers with +FHD and high CRP (n = 66)	Mothers with -FHD and normal CRP (n = 45)	ANOVA
Mean	0.45	0.25	P < 0.001
SD	± 0.087	± 0.025	

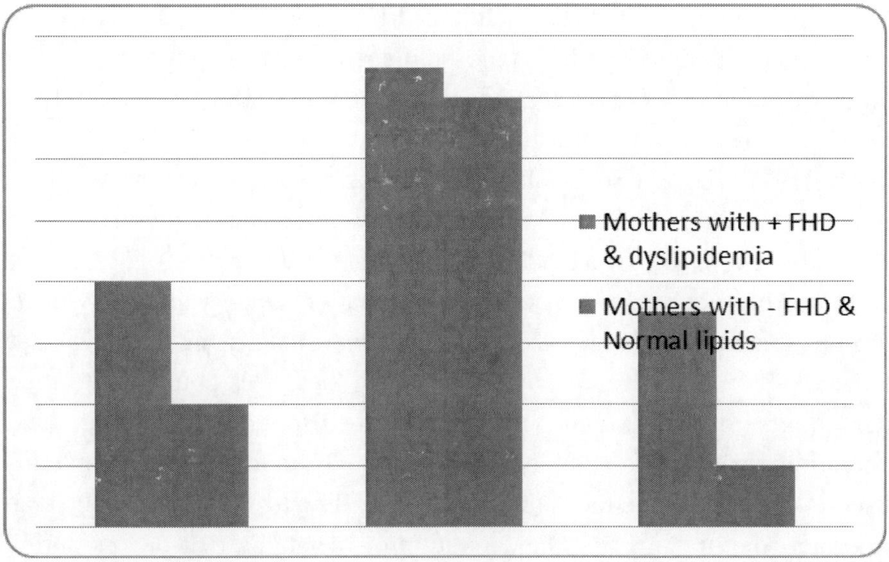

Figure 3. Showing genotyping results of CRP genes of newborn babies, w.r.t their mother's health status.

Comparison of birth outcomes in terms of birth weights was done between subjects with and without a positive family history of T2DM and high CRP levels (Figure 1), which revealed a significant difference between the two groups. This shows that family history and perturbations in the gestational period are reflected in the birth outcomes, affecting the next generation (Table 2). It is evident from the results that there is a significant difference in inflammatory status in those newborns whose mothers have a positive FHD compared to their normal counterparts.

DISCUSSION

The Family History of Diabetes (FHD), evidently, has been found to be most useful for predicting T2DM when the disease is premature, that is, it occurs at younger ages than would be expected. This FHD information in combination with other known risk factors could be used to provide more personalized information about our risk for such diseases. Yang et al., (2010) further suggested that adding FHD could provide significant improvements in detecting undiagnosed diabetes; however, it needs further validation with larger cross-sections of population. In an another study, it was found that not only the adults but even the young population with a positive FHD showed signs of increased risk for these conditions which indicates the importance of family history approach to screening for children at risk of T2DM and CVD (Valdez et al., 2007).

In our present study, we noticed a population trend where individuals with positive family history of diabetes had significantly higher prevalence of metabolic risk factors and its confounding factors as compared to their counterparts during pregnancy, which is also affecting their next generation leading to childhood obesity. Therefore, based on this observation, it can be stated that positive FHD and CRP status plays an important role in triggering the activation of metabolic risk factors during the pregnancy period, and this could be one of the major factors for development of T2DM and metabolic syndrome in the next generations. These findings suggest that family history could be used as a tool for genomic studies among the Asian Indians.

CRP is a potential biomarker for prediction of future risk of cardiovascular disease (CVD) both in diabetic and non-diabetic individuals, because even a small rise in plasma CRP levels leads to cardiovascular events. In the present investigation of the association of CRP+1059 G>C polymorphism with the progression to T2D, we have observed that the frequency of G-allele is high in the Asian Indian population (70%). Similarly high frequency for the G-allele (~90.0%–96.3%) has been reported in studies conducted on other world populations (Pasalic et al., 2009; Tanja et al., 2008).

Heterozygous carriers of C allele (GC) in the present studied population have shown protection towards the disease manifestation. The GC genotype is highest in controls (9.8%) as compared to cases (2.3%–3.4%) suggesting that some kind of selection pressure is operating on the GC genotype. Considering the thrifty genotype hypothesis, the ancestral version of the alleles proves to be deleterious in the present day environment while the rarer alleles which may have protective effects against the disease have evolved lately (Sharma 1998). Fernandez-Real and Ricart have implicated the role of genes encoding for cytokine synthesis as thrifty genes (Fernandez-Real & Ricart, 1999). The hypothesis suggested that higher secretion of cytokines and increased acute phase response were an evolutionary adaptation to phases of acute infections and trauma. In the ancestral period, outbreaks due to infections were higher. Simultaneously due to exposure to famines, metabolic pathways favored insulin resistance to survive in low food situations. It has been proposed that insulin resistance and cytokine responder genotypes were favorable adaptations to low fat, high fiber and high physical activity environment. The genomes of the present day human are still genetically adapted to ancestral conditions which are designed to fight against infection with minimal food intakes and high physical activity. However, environmental transition is more rapid, and evolution being a slow process, our genotypes have not modified according to the present day environments of lower infections, availability of surplus food and low physical activity. In the absence of the favorable conditions and with advancement of age, insulin resistance ensues which further activates inflammatory cascade that eventually results in atherosclerosis. Thus, in the presence of insulin resistance genotypes and western lifestyle, a high cytokine responder genotype would be more prone to develop T2D and atherosclerosis. Although+1059 G > C polymorphism is a silent polymorphism, yet the ancestral allele of the polymorphism (G-allele) has been associated with higher CRP levels in various studies as discussed above. Higher CRP levels are suggestive of inflammatory response which may get accentuated in the background of obesity and insulin resistance condition in T2D. The higher frequency of the G-allele in most of the populations and the protective effect of GC genotype in the present study could be viewed in the background of its role as a thrifty genotype.

CONCLUSION

From our study, we therefore can conclude that the CRP +1059 G > C polymorphism seem to have functional effects on protein production (Eklund et al., 2005). It has also been proposed that silent SNPs can lead to protein product with the same amino acid sequence, but with different structural and functional properties which might play an important role in defining the protein levels (Radha & Mohan 2007). The reason for discrepancies in association studies across populations may be explained by diverse ethnic background of different populations as different ethnic groups have different susceptibility towards the disease (Komar 2007).

Taken together, these observations raise the possibility that these polymorphisms in combination with both family history and environmental factors may account for the phenotype of peripheral insulin resistance and impaired insulin secretion, the two typical features of Type II diabetes.

Also, having observed that family history of diabetes (FHD) is indeed an important and independent risk factor for genomic studies of complex diseases like T2DM, efforts should be made toward translating this knowledge for use in public health programmes designed to detect and prevent diabetes. Once this is achieved, FHD should be incorporated into the screening and prevention programmes for T2DM as rigorously as possible to make these programmes significant and cost-effective.

However, the present study has several limitations. In the limitations of the present study, firstly, the association of polymorphism with the protein levels needs to be established. Secondly further studies relating the protein levels with studied polymorphism and other functionally relevant polymorphisms which may be in LD with the studied SNP are required on larger sample size to validate the findings of the present study with more statistical power.

References

Cao H and Hegele RA. 2000. Human C-reactive protein (CRP) 1059G/C polymorphism. *J Hum Genet*. 45: 100-101.

Demova H, Boleckova J, Rose D, Koeppel H, Prochazka B, Brunerova L, Rychlik I, Marie C. 2012. Gene polymorphisms in patients with Type II diabetes and diabetic nephropathy. *Central European Journal of Biology*. 7(2): 210–218.

Eklund C, Lehtimaki T, Hurme M. Epistatic effect of C-reactive protein (CRP) single nucleotide polymorphism (SNP) + 1059 and interleukin-1B SNP + 3954 on CRP concentration in healthy male blood donors. *Int. J. Immunogenet*. 2005; 32:229–232.

Fernandez-Real J. M., Ricart W. Insulin resistance and inflammation in an evolutionary perspective: the contribution of cytokine genotype/phenotype to thriftiness. *Diabetologia*. 1999; 42:1367–1374.

Gale J. 2010. "India's Diabetes Epidemic Cuts Down Millions Who Escape Poverty". *Bloomberg.com.* November 7, 2010. https://www.bloomberg.com/news/articles/2010-11-07/india-s-deadly-diabetesscourge-cuts-down-millions-rising-tomiddle-class.

IHA, Indian heart Association 2016. *IHA*. http://indianheart association.org/whyindians-why-south-asians/overview/.

Kaur R, Matharoo K, Sharma R, Bhanwer AJS. 2013. C-reactive protein + 1059 G > C polymorphism in Type II diabetes and coronary artery disease patients. *Meta Gene*. 1: 82–92.

Komar AA. Silent SNPs: impact on gene function and phenotype. *Pharmacogenomics*. 2007; 8:1075–1080.

Melmed S, Polonsky KS, Larsen PR, Kronenberg HM. 2011. *Williams textbook of endocrinology* (12th ed.). Philadelphia: Elsevier/Saunders. 1371–1435.

National Cholesterol Education Program (NCEP). 2005. Expert Panel on detection, evaluation, and the treatment of high blood cholesterol in adults (Adult Treatment Program III). *Circulation*. 106: 3134-3421.

New York Times 2006. "Modern Ways Open India's Doors to Diabetes." *New York Times*. Kleinfield, N. R. September 13,

NIDDKD - National Institute of Diabetes and Digestive and Kidney Diseases. "Diagnosis of Diabetes and Prediabetes." *NIDDKD.* June 2014. https://www.niddk.nih.gov/healthinformation/.

Pasalic D, Marinkovic N, Grskovic B, Ferencak G, Bernat R, Stavljenic-Rukavina A. C (2009). Reactive protein gene polymorphisms affect plasma CRP and homocysteine concentrations in subjects with and without angiographically confirmed coronary artery disease. *Mol. Biol. Rep*. 2009; 36:775–780.

Radha V., Mohan V. Genetic predisposition to Type II diabetes among Asian Indians. *Indian J. Med. Res*. 2007; 125: 259–274.

Sharma AM. The thrifty-genotype hypothesis and its implications for the study of complex genetic disorders in man. *J. Mol. Med*. 1998; 76:568–571.

Tanja BG, Winfried M, Wilfried R, Bernhard OB, Michael MH. C-reactive protein genotypes associated with circulating C-reactive protein but not with angiographic coronary artery disease: the LURIC study. *Eur. Heart J*. 2008; 30:170–182.

Valdez R, Greenlund KJ, Khoury MJ, Yoon PW. 2007. Is family history a useful tool for detecting children at risk for diabetes and cardiovascular diseases. A public health perspective? *Pediatrics*; 120 (2):S78–86.

World Health Organization. 2011. "Diabetes Fact sheet." *WHO.* https://web.archive.org/web/20130826174444/http:/www.who.int/mediacentre/factsheets/fs312/en.

World Health Organization. 2016. Global Report on Diabetes. *WHO.* Geneva, Accessed 30 August 2016.

Yang Q, Liu T, Valdez R, Moonesinghe R, Khoury MJ. 2010. Improvements in ability to detect undiagnosed diabetes by using information on family history among adults in the United States. *Am J Epidemiol*; 171:1079–89.

In: Obesity and Syndrome X
Editors: M. Das and K. Bose
ISBN: 978-1-53614-669-1

Chapter 10

SENSITIVITY AND SPECIFICITY OF BODY MASS INDEX TO ASSESS EXCESS ADIPOSITY

Jyoti Ratan Ghosh*
Department of Anthropology, Visva-Bharati,
Santiniketan, West Bengal, India

INTRODUCTION

Since the introduction of the Quetelet index (QI) {body mass index (BMI)} in 1832 (Eknoyan, 2008), it was widely used as a measure of excess adiposity or obesity (Price et al., 2018; Volkovicher et al., 2018). Not only that, BMI was also found to be associated with different metabolic and physiological abnormalities (Ghosh and Bandyopadhyay, 2007; Xu et al., 2008; Kaplan et al., 2014; Leonska-Duniec et al., 2018). However, epidemiological studies in Asian populations, especially in Indians revealed higher prevalence of cardiovascular disease and type 2 diabetes with a lower mean BMI, but interestingly had higher percent body fat (PBF) at a corresponding BMI value than Europeans (Razak et al.,

* Corresponding Author Email: jrghosh@visva-bharati.ac.in.

2007; Xu et al., 2008). Therefore, using a BMI cut-off value based on adult Europeans may not truly identify Asian Indians with excess adiposity, as the relationship between BMI and PBF varied among different ethnic groups (Gurrici et al., 1998; Deurenberg et al., 2000).

As a consequence, in 2000 a WHO expert consultation on the obesity issues in Asia–Pacific region suggested redefining the criteria for obesity, recognizing the necessity for ethnic specific cut-off points. However, they recommended that the conventional (WHO, 1995) BMI cut-off point of $\geq$30 kg/m^2 should be retained as an international classification for obesity. In a publication of this WHO consultation, the proposed BMI cut-off point for overweight was 23–24.9 kg/m^2, and that for obesity was $\geq$25 kg/m^2 (WHO, 2000).

In a succeeding publication in 2004, another WHO consultation resolved that the available data do not necessarily indicate one clear BMI cut-off for all Asian Indians for overweight and obesity. No attempt was made therefore to redefine cutoff points for each population separately (WHO, 2004).

In the present study, an attempted has been made to test the ability of different BMI cut-off points to predict high percent body fat by sensitivity/specificity analysis. This would help to develop population specific BMI cut-off value for identifying individuals with truly excess adiposity. This was more important for Asian populations, because for every level of BMI the predicted fat mass was higher in Asian populations (Dudeja et al., 2001; Deurenberg et al., 2002). Thus, the purpose of this study was to examine the sensitivity and specificity of BMI in adult Asian Indian women to detect excess adiposity.

Materials and Methods

The present community-based cross-sectional study comprised adult Asian Indian women living in and around Kolkata, India. A total of 364 participants aged 18–70 years took part in the study. Pregnant and lactating women, women undergoing hormone therapy as well as under medication or with chronic disease were not included in the study. Prior to participation, individuals were informed by public advertisement and oral communication about the study with the help of the local officials. Individuals who responded to the advertisement were selected randomly. Informed verbal consent was obtained from each participant before commencement of the study. Age was obtained by interview and verified with horoscope or birth certificate whenever possible.

Anthropometric measurements namely height (HT) and weight (WT) were measured using standard procedures (Lohman et al., 1988). HT was measured to the nearest 0.1 cm using moveable anthropometer. WT was measured to the nearest 0.5 kg using weighing machine. BMI (kg/m^2) was derived subsequently. Percent body fat (PBF) was measured using bioelectrical impedance analysis (BIA) (OMRON HBF-302). Several studies have shown a strong correlation between PBF, FM, and FFM as measured by BIA and dual-energy-X-ray-absorptiometry (DEXA) (Goldfield et al., 2006; Boneva-Asiova and Boyanov, 2008). The BIA has also been validated for Asian Indians (Vasudev et al., 2004).

Descriptive statistics for anthropometric variables were computed by mean and standard deviation (SD). Pearson correlation coefficient was used to quantify the relation between BMI and PBF. The receiver operating characteristic (ROC) curve analysis was used to evaluate the ability of BMI for assessing excess adiposity and the accuracy was determined by examining the sensitivity, specificity, positive predictive value (PPV), negative predictive value (NPV), Youden's index and overall misclassification. Excess adiposity was defined as total body fat greater than thirty percent (Hortobagyi et al., 1994; Dudeja et al., 2001). Statistical analyses were performed using the Statistical Package for Social Sciences (SPSS). A p value of <0.05 was considered as significant.

RESULTS

Characteristics of the studied population are shown in Table I. The mean age was 31.88 years (SD 14.26 years), with a range of 18 to 70 years.

The mean BMI and PBF was 23.61 kg/m^2 (SD 4.43) and 28.47 (SD 6.45), respectively. When conventional BMI cut-off value of ≥ 30 kg/m^2 was applied, 30 (8.2%) women were obese or have excess adiposity. However, the result varied considerably when PBF was used as the measurement of excess adiposity. Based on PBF, 132 (36.3%) women had excess adiposity. Result of the Pearson correlation analysis revealed significant positive correlation between BMI and PBF (r = 0.561) and BMI explained 31.4% of variance of PBF ($p < 0.01$). Table II shows the results of the ROC curve analysis for the BMI cut-off values in relation to excess adiposity by PBF. The results revealed that the sensitivity and specificity as well as the PPV and NPV of the conventional BMI cut-off value for excess adiposity were 18.93%, 97.84%, 83.32% and 67.93%, respectively. However, based on the ROC curve (Figure 1) and the trade-offs between improving BMI's sensitivity and specificity, the optimal cut-off value was BMI $\geq$ 23.4 kg/m^2 with a sensitivity and specificity 77.27% and 72.84%, respectively in assessing excess adiposity. With this cut-off value, the sensitivity of BMI in relation to PBF increased but the PPV was low. Moreover, lowering the BMI cut-off value from $\geq$ 30 kg/m^2 to $\geq$ 23.4 kg/m^2 increased Youden's index from 0.17 to 0.50 and decreased overall misclassification 5.22%.

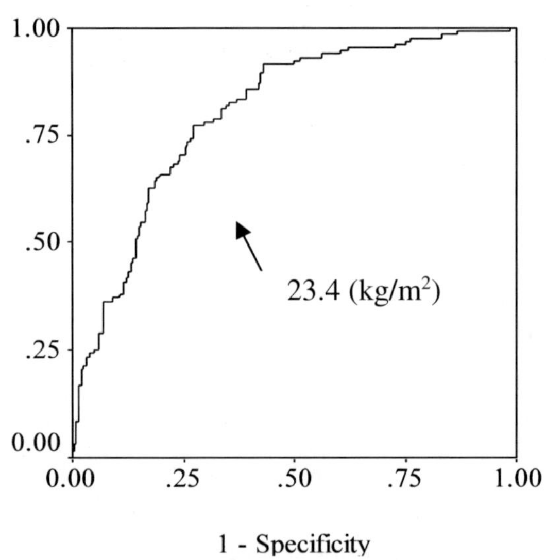

Figure 1. Receiver operating characteristic curve of BMI (kg/m^2) in assessing obesity.

ACKNOWLEDGMENT

ıthor is grateful to all individuals who participated in the study.

REFERENCES

siova, Z. & Boyanov, M. A. (2008). Body composition analysis g-to-leg bioelectrical impedance and dual-energy X-ray tiometry in non-obese and obese individuals. *Diabetes Obes* *10*, 1012-8.

., Ertorer, M. E., Bakiner, O., Tutuncu, N. B. & Demirag, N. G. . The validity of the World Health Organisation's obesity body ndex criteria in a Turkish population: a hospital-based study. *ac J Clin Nutr*, *16*, 443-7.

C. L., Yan, E., Chen, S., Hong, K., Arechiga, A., Kim, W. S., M., Li, Z. & Heber, D. (2013). Body fat and body-mass index a multiethnic sample of college-age men and women. *J Obes*, /10.1155/2013/790654.

au-Roberts, G., Saudny-Unterberger, H., Kuhnlein, G. V. & l, G. M. (2005). Body mass index may overestimate the nce of overweight and obesity among the Inuit. *Int J polar Health*, *64*, 163-9.

, P., Andreoli, A., Borg, P., Kukkonen-Harjula, K., de Lorenzo, htenbelt, W. D. V., Testolin, G., Vigano, R. & Vollaard, N. The validity of predicted body fat percentage from body mass nd from impedance in samples of five European populations. *in Nutr*, *55*, 973-9.

, P., Deurenberg-Yap, M. & Guricci, S. (2002). Asians are t from Caucasians and from each other in their body mass ɔdy fat per cent relationship. *Obes Rev*, *3*, 141-6.

Table I. Characteristics of the study population

Variables	Mean	SD
Age (year)	31.88	14.26
Height (cm)	152.81	6.14
Weight (kg)	55.19	11.13
Percent body fat	28.47	6.45
Body mass index (kg/m^2)	23.61	4.43

SD, standard deviation.

DISCUSSION

The present study examined the sensitivity and specificity of BMI to detect excess adiposity in adult Asian Indian women. In epidemiological studies and in clinical practice BMI was widely used as a proxy measure of excess adiposity. However, the efficiency of BMI is depends on its sensitivity and specificity to detect excess adiposity. This varied with ethnicity, due to the biological variation in body shape and composition. However, the ROC curve analysis in the present study demonstrated low sensitivity (18.93%) and high specificity (97.84%) of the conventional BMI cut-off value to detect excess adiposity. Such a low value of sensitivity and high specificity suggested that this BMI cut-off value failed to detect excess adiposity in ~ 80% of subjects who had truly excess adiposity. In other words, conventional BMI cut-off value was not useful to detect individuals with excess adiposity. A recent study in Saudi adults also revealed low sensitivity and high specificity of BMI in assessing excess adiposity (Habib, 2013). Study in Asian-American women also revealed poor sensitivity of BMI to detect PBF (Carpenter et al., 2013). Dudeja et al. (2001) and Hortobagyi et al. (1994) also observed similar results.

The ROC analysis revealed that the best compromise between sensitivity and specificity for optimal BMI cut-off value to detect excess adiposity was 23.4 kg/m^2, and the corresponding sensitivity and specificity was 77.27% and 72.84%, respectively. However, this cut-off value was lower than the conventional cut-off value to detect excess adiposity and thus, could identify individuals who would otherwise be considered as normal by the conventional cut-off value. In relation to the conventional cut-off value for excess adiposity, a lower BMI cut-off of 23.4 kg/m^2 produced increased sensitivity (18.93% vs. 77.27%) and moderately decreased specificity (97.84% vs. 72.84%). In reality, it was difficult to achieve high sensitivity and specificity simultaneously, thus relative importance of sensitivity vs. specificity was taken into consideration. However, the BMI cut-off value of 23.4 kg/m^2 instead of 30 kg/m^2 increased the likelihood (Youden's index 0.50 vs. 0.17) ~ three times for detecting individuals with excess adiposity, who had truly excess adiposity. Additionally, this lower BMI cut-off value decreased 5.22% overall misclassification. However, it is noteworthy to mention that for women in our sample, the proposed BMI cut-off value (≥25 kg/m^2) of WHO (2000) revealed only 44.7% sensitivity and 83.6% specificity. In a study, Bozkirli et al. (2007) also observed that the conventional BMI cut-off value underestimated the prevalence of excess adiposity in Turkish population. Moreover, several other studies also revealed that lowering the BMI cut-off value improved its ability to assess excess adiposity (Dudeja et al., 2001; Ko et al., 2001; Ghosh and Bandyopadhyay, 2007).

Table II. Sensitivity and specificity of BMI (kg/m^2) as a measure of obesity

Cut-off points	Sensitivity (95%CI)	Specificity (95%CI)	PPV	NPV	Youden's index	Overall misclassification
BMI ≥ 30 kg/m^2	18.93% (14.9-22.9)	97.84% (96.4-99.3)	83.32%	67.93%	0.17	30.78%
BMI ≥ 25 kg/m^2	44.7% (39.6-49.8)	83.6% (79.8-87.4)	60.83%	72.62%	0.28	26.64%
BMI ≥ 23.4 kg/m^2	77.27% (73.8-80.8)	72.84% (68.3-77.4)	61.81%	84.91%	0.50	25.56%

PPP, positive predictive value; NPV, negative predictive value; BMI, body mass index

The cardinal feature of the present study was the predictive values (i.e., PPV and NPV) of BMI in relation to the PBF. As shown by the PPV of the conventional BMI cut-off value, almost 17% of women with high PBF

(PBF >30%) had BMI < 30 kg/m^2. On the oth
that almost one out of three (~32%) women w
high BMI (≥30) kg/m^2. However, the PPV
value in our sample was 61.81%. Indicated
women who had a BMI ≥ 23.4 kg/m^2 did not h
the results indicated that BMI was a relativ
adiposity in the studied population. One p
weaker association between BMI and PBF
Because, BMI as a proxy measure of adipo
variance of PBF. A recent study by Carpent
weak association between BMI and PBF amo

Moreover, the weak association betweer
to the fact that BMI does not measure fat m
measures both fat mass and fat free mass wit
(Garn et al., 1986; Hortobagyi et al., 1994
2005; Rona et al., 2011). Therefore, indivic
have different proportions of fat mass. Furt
that BMI underestimate excess adiposity ar
overestimate excess adiposity among those
length (Garn et al., 1986; Charbonneau-Rob

CONCLUSIC

Therefore, measuring body fat instead
way to categorize individuals with excess
validated measure of body composition,
more accurate measures like DEXA wou
However, this preliminary finding warrant
ethnic groups to understand whether the s
is the amount of excess body fat, rather th
that determines the health risks of obe
Deurenberg et al., 2001).

The a

Boneva-A
by l
absor
Metab
Bozkirli, E
(2007)
mass i
Asia P
Carpenter,
Deng,
among
doi: or
Charbonne
Egelan
prevale
Circum
Deurenberg
A., Lic
(2001).
index a
Eu J Cl
Deurenberg
differen
index/b

Table I. Characteristics of the study population

Variables	Mean	SD
Age (year)	31.88	14.26
Height (cm)	152.81	6.14
Weight (kg)	55.19	11.13
Percent body fat	28.47	6.45
Body mass index (kg/m^2)	23.61	4.43

SD, standard deviation.

DISCUSSION

The present study examined the sensitivity and specificity of BMI to detect excess adiposity in adult Asian Indian women. In epidemiological studies and in clinical practice BMI was widely used as a proxy measure of excess adiposity. However, the efficiency of BMI is depends on its sensitivity and specificity to detect excess adiposity. This varied with ethnicity, due to the biological variation in body shape and composition. However, the ROC curve analysis in the present study demonstrated low sensitivity (18.93%) and high specificity (97.84%) of the conventional BMI cut-off value to detect excess adiposity. Such a low value of sensitivity and high specificity suggested that this BMI cut-off value failed to detect excess adiposity in ~ 80% of subjects who had truly excess adiposity. In other words, conventional BMI cut-off value was not useful to detect individuals with excess adiposity. A recent study in Saudi adults also revealed low sensitivity and high specificity of BMI in assessing excess adiposity (Habib, 2013). Study in Asian-American women also revealed poor sensitivity of BMI to detect PBF (Carpenter et al., 2013). Dudeja et al. (2001) and Hortobagyi et al. (1994) also observed similar results.

The ROC analysis revealed that the best compromise between sensitivity and specificity for optimal BMI cut-off value to detect excess adiposity was 23.4 kg/m^2, and the corresponding sensitivity and specificity was 77.27% and 72.84%, respectively. However, this cut-off value was lower than the conventional cut-off value to detect excess adiposity and thus, could identify individuals who would otherwise be considered as normal by the conventional cut-off value. In relation to the conventional cut-off value for excess adiposity, a lower BMI cut-off of 23.4 kg/m^2 produced increased sensitivity (18.93% vs. 77.27%) and moderately decreased specificity (97.84% vs. 72.84%). In reality, it was difficult to achieve high sensitivity and specificity simultaneously, thus relative importance of sensitivity vs. specificity was taken into consideration. However, the BMI cut-off value of 23.4 kg/m^2 instead of 30 kg/m^2 increased the likelihood (Youden's index 0.50 vs. 0.17) ~ three times for detecting individuals with excess adiposity, who had truly excess adiposity. Additionally, this lower BMI cut-off value decreased 5.22% overall misclassification. However, it is noteworthy to mention that for women in our sample, the proposed BMI cut-off value (≥25 kg/m^2) of WHO (2000) revealed only 44.7% sensitivity and 83.6% specificity. In a study, Bozkirli et al. (2007) also observed that the conventional BMI cut-off value underestimated the prevalence of excess adiposity in Turkish population. Moreover, several other studies also revealed that lowering the BMI cut-off value improved its ability to assess excess adiposity (Dudeja et al., 2001; Ko et al., 2001; Ghosh and Bandyopadhyay, 2007).

Table II. Sensitivity and specificity of BMI (kg/m^2) as a measure of obesity

Cut-off points	Sensitivity (95%CI)	Specificity (95%CI)	PPV	NPV	Youden's index	Overall misclassification
BMI ≥ 30 kg/m^2	18.93% (14.9-22.9)	97.84% (96.4-99.3)	83.32%	67.93%	0.17	30.78%
BMI ≥ 25 kg/m^2	44.7% (39.6-49.8)	83.6% (79.8-87.4)	60.83%	72.62%	0.28	26.64%
BMI ≥ 23.4 kg/m^2	77.27% (73.8-80.8)	72.84% (68.3-77.4)	61.81%	84.91%	0.50	25.56%

PPP, positive predictive value; NPV, negative predictive value; BMI, body mass index

The cardinal feature of the present study was the predictive values (i.e., PPV and NPV) of BMI in relation to the PBF. As shown by the PPV of the conventional BMI cut-off value, almost 17% of women with high PBF

(PBF >30%) had BMI < 30 kg/m^2. On the other hand, high NPV indicates that almost one out of three (~32%) women with normal PBF (<30%) had high BMI (≥30) kg/m^2. However, the PPV of the optimal BMI cut-off value in our sample was 61.81%. Indicated that approximately 38% of women who had a BMI ≥ 23.4 kg/m^2 did not have high PBF (<30%). Thus, the results indicated that BMI was a relatively poor predictor of excess adiposity in the studied population. One possible reason might be the weaker association between BMI and PBF in the studied population. Because, BMI as a proxy measure of adiposity explained only 31.4% of variance of PBF. A recent study by Carpenter et al. (2013) also observed weak association between BMI and PBF among Asian-American women.

Moreover, the weak association between BMI and PBF might be due to the fact that BMI does not measure fat mass or percentage fat only, but measures both fat mass and fat free mass without distinguish between them (Garn et al., 1986; Hortobagyi et al., 1994; Charbonneau-Roberts et al., 2005; Rona et al., 2011). Therefore, individuals with the same BMI may have different proportions of fat mass. Furthermore, it has been observed that BMI underestimate excess adiposity among those with long legs and overestimate excess adiposity among those with short legs relative to torso length (Garn et al., 1986; Charbonneau-Roberts et al., 2005).

CONCLUSION

Therefore, measuring body fat instead of BMI could be an appropriate way to categorize individuals with excess adiposity. Although BIA is a validated measure of body composition, acknowledging that the use of more accurate measures like DEXA would have improved our analysis. However, this preliminary finding warranted further studies in other Asian ethnic groups to understand whether the same relationships exist. Since, it is the amount of excess body fat, rather than the amount of excess weight that determines the health risks of obesity (Deurenberg et al., 1998; Deurenberg et al., 2001).

Acknowledgment

The author is grateful to all individuals who participated in the study.

References

Boneva-Asiova, Z. & Boyanov, M. A. (2008). Body composition analysis by leg-to-leg bioelectrical impedance and dual-energy X-ray absorptiometry in non-obese and obese individuals. *Diabetes Obes Metab*, *10*, 1012-8.

Bozkirli, E., Ertorer, M. E., Bakiner, O., Tutuncu, N. B. & Demirag, N. G. (2007). The validity of the World Health Organisation's obesity body mass index criteria in a Turkish population: a hospital-based study. *Asia Pac J Clin Nutr*, *16*, 443-7.

Carpenter, C. L., Yan, E., Chen, S., Hong, K., Arechiga, A., Kim, W. S., Deng, M., Li, Z. & Heber, D. (2013). Body fat and body-mass index among a multiethnic sample of college-age men and women. *J Obes*, doi: org/10.1155/2013/790654.

Charbonneau-Roberts, G., Saudny-Unterberger, H., Kuhnlein, G. V. & Egeland, G. M. (2005). Body mass index may overestimate the prevalence of overweight and obesity among the Inuit. *Int J Circumpolar Health*, *64*, 163-9.

Deurenberg, P., Andreoli, A., Borg, P., Kukkonen-Harjula, K., de Lorenzo, A., Lichtenbelt, W. D. V., Testolin, G., Vigano, R. & Vollaard, N. (2001). The validity of predicted body fat percentage from body mass index and from impedance in samples of five European populations. *Eu J Clin Nutr*, *55*, 973-9.

Deurenberg, P., Deurenberg-Yap, M. & Guricci, S. (2002). Asians are different from Caucasians and from each other in their body mass index/body fat per cent relationship. *Obes Rev*, *3*, 141-6.

Deurenberg, P., Deurenberg-Yap, M. & Van Staveren, W. A. (1998). Body mass index and percent body fat: a meta-analysis among different ethnic groups. *Int J Obes Relat Metab Disord*, 1998, *22*, 1164-71.

Deurenberg-Yap, M., Schmidt, G., van Staveren, W. A. & Deurenberg, P. (2000). The paradox of low body mass index and high body fat percentage among Chinese, Malays and Indians in Singapore. *Int J Obes Relat Metab Disord*, *24*, 1011-7.

Dudeja, V., Misra, A., Pandey, R. M., Devina, G., Kumar, G. & Vikram, N. K. (2001). BMI dose not accurately predict overweight in Asian Indians in northern India. *Br J Nutr*, *86*, 105-12.

Eknoyan, G. (2008). Adolphe Quetelet (1796–1874)-the average man and indices of obesity. *Nephrol Dial Transplant*, *23*, 47–51.

Garn, S. M., Leonard, W. R. & Hawthorne, V. M. (1986). Three limitations of the body mass index. *Am J Clin Nutr*, *44*, 996-7.

Ghosh, J. R. & Bandyopadhyay, A. R. (2007). Receiver operating characteristic curve analysis of BMI in assessing obesity among adult Bengalee males in India. *Coll Antropol*, *31*, 315-9.

Goldfield, G. S., Cloutier, P., Mallory, R., Prud'homme, D., Parker, T. & Doucet, E. (2006). Validity of foot-to-foot bioelectrical impedance analysis in overweight and obese children and parents. *J Sports Med Phys Fitness*, *46*, 447-53.

Gurrici, S., Hartriyanti, Y., Hautvast, J. G. & Deurenberg, P. (1998). Relationship between body fat and body mass index: differences between Indonesians and Dutch Caucasians. *Eur J Clin Nutr*, 1998, *52*, 779-83.

Habib, S. S. (2013). Body mass index and body fat percentage in assessment of obesity prevalence in Saudi adults. *Biomed Environ Sci*, 2013, *26*, 94-99.

Hortobagyi, T., Israel, R. G. & O'Brien, K. F. (1994). Sensitivity and specificity of the Quetelet index to assess obesity in men and women. *Eur J Clin Nutr*, 1994, *48*, 369-75.

Kaplan, R. C., Aviles-Santa, M. L., Parrinello, C. M., Hanna, D. B., Jung, M., Castañeda, S. F., Hankinson, A. L., Isasi, C. R., Birnbaum-Weitzman, O., Kim, R. S., Daviglus, M. L., Talavera, G. A.,

Schneiderman, N. & Cai, J. (2014). Body mass index, sex, and cardiovascular disease risk factors among hispanic/latino adults: Hispanic community health study/study of latinos. *J Am Heart Assoc*, *3*, doi: 10.1161/JAHA.114.000923.

Ko, G. T., Tang, J., Chan, J. C., Sung, R., Wu, M. M., Wai, H. P. & Chen, R. (2001). Lower BMI cut-off value to define obesity in Hong Kong Chinese: an analysis based on body fat assessment by bioelectrical impedance. *Br J Nutr*, 2001, *85*, 239-42.

Leonska-Duniec, A., Jastrzebski, Z., Jazdzewska, A., Krzysztof, F. & Cieszczyk, P. (2018). Leptin and leptin receptor genes are associated with obesity-related traits changes in response to aerobic training program. *J Strength Cond Res*, 2018, doi: 10.1519/JSC.0000000000002447.

Lohman, T. G., Roche, A. F. & Martorell, R. (1988). *Anthropometric standardization reference manual.* Chicago: Human kinetics Books.

Price, A. J., Crampin, A. C., Amberbir, A., Kayuni-Chihana, N., Musicha, C., Tafatatha, T., Branson, K., Lawlor, D. A., Mwaiyeghele, E., Nkhwazi, L., Smeeth, L., Pearce, N., Munthali, E., Mwagomba, B. M., Mwansambo, C., Glynn, J. R., Jaffar, S. & Nyirenda, M. (2018). Prevalence of obesity, hypertension, and diabetes, and cascade of care in sub-Saharan Africa: a cross-sectional, population-based study in rural and urban Malawi. *Lancet Diabetes Endocrinol*, doi: 10.1016/S2213-8587(17)30432-1.

Razak, F., Anand, S. S., Shannon, H., Vuksan, V., Davis, B., Jacobs, R., Teo, K. K., McQueen, M. & Yusuf, S. (2007). Defining obesity cut points in a multiethnic population. *Circulation.*, *115*, 2111-8.

Rona, R. J., Sundin, J., Wood, P. & Fear, N. T. (2011). Agreement between body mass index, waist circumference and skin-fold thickness in the United Kingdom Army. *Ann Hum Biol.*, *38*, 257-64.

Vasudev, S., Mohan, A., Mohan, D., Farooq, S., Raj, D. & Mohan, V. (2004). Validation of body fat measurement by skinfolds and two bioelectric impedance methods with DEXA-the Chennai Urban Rural Epidemiology Study [CURES-3]. *J Assoc Physicians India.*, *52*, 877-81.

Volkovicher, N., Kurihara, C., Critsinelis, A., Kawabori, M., Sugiura, T., Manon, M., Civitello, A. B. & Morgan, J. A. (2018). Effect of obesity on outcomes in patients undergoing implantation of continuous-flow left ventricular assist devices. *J Artif Organs*, doi: 10.1007/s10047-017-1013-2.

WHO/IASO/IOTF. (2000). The Asia-Pacific perspective: redefining obesity and its treatment. *WHO*. Health Communications Australia: Melbourne.

World Health Organization Expert Consultation. (2004). Appropriate body-mass index for Asian populations and its implications for policy and intervention strategies. *Lancet*, *363*, 157–63.

World Health Organization. (1995). Physical status: the use and interpretation of anthropometry. Report of a WHO Expert Consultation. *WHO Technical Report Series Number*, *854*, Geneva.

Xu, C., Yang, X., Zu, S., Han, S., Zhang, Z. & Zhu, G. (2008). Association between serum lipids, blood pressure, and simple anthropometric measures in an adult Chinese population. *Arch Med Res.*, *39*, 610-17.

PART III: GLOBAL PUBLIC HEALTH ASPECT

In: Obesity and Syndrome X
Editors: M. Das and K. Bose
ISBN: 978-1-53614-669-1

Chapter 11

Framing Obesity and Undernutrition as Problems for Governments

Stanley Ulijaszek*
Institute of Social and Cultural Anthropology,
Oxford University, UK

Introduction

The epidemiologies of obesity and undernutrition are conducted using standardized metrics in very regulated ways. From the 1950s, anthropometric measures have been used overwhelmingly as measures of social welfare in public health, economics and national statistics (Ulijaszek and Komlos 2010). Their predominant use in most recent decades has been as proxies of human nutritional health (both under- and over-nutrition) and well-being (or lack thereof), as well as of physical productivity and health, in relation to measures of economic productivity, morbidity and mortality risk, where non-normative values of body size, usually height and weight, are interpreted as carrying risk. The procedures and protocols involved in

* Corresponding Author Email: stanley.ulijaszek@anthro.ox.ac.uk.

these specific usages have been critiqued in various ways. For example, measurement in public health practice has been criticized as universalizing the human body when relating individuals to norms (Mol 2009) and of health to measurement (Yates-Duerr 2013). Issue has also been taken with the stigma that accompanies the measurement and medicalization of bodies (Rubin and Joseph 2013). Bodies are physical entities with economic, social and medical correlates, and the standardization of bodily measures of obesity and undernutrition have political and economic implications. This paper describes the now-historical process of nutritional assessment in public health anthropometry, and examines how public health reporting of obesity and undernutrition informs the discourse about nutritional health at governmental level. Examples are predominantly taken from India and the United Kingdom (UK).

Nutritional Classification Using Anthropometry

In nutritional epidemiology, anthropometry can be used as a proxy for nutritional status, or as a measure of exposure to nutritional stress. Anthropometry became a proxy for nutritional status with the World Health Organization Technical Report 'Assessment of the Nutritional Status of the Community' (Jelliffe 1966). This became the standard text for relating anthropometry to nutrition and to social welfare in the subsequent two decades. The use of anthropometry in health and nutritional assessment has a formal scientific basis which stems from life insurance estimation of mortality prediction from the early twentieth century. The publication of 'standard height-weight' tables by the life insurance industry began with the *Medico-Actuarial Mortality Investigations of 1912* (Keys et al., 1972). These tables provided 'ideal' weight for ranges of height for use among insured adults in the United States (US) and Canada, according to sex and three categories of body frame. The first version of these standard tables, based on actuarial data relating to blood pressure (as a proxy for chronic disease risk), was brought into general use for assessing ideal body weight in the US in 1942/43 by the Metropolitan Life Insurance

Company (Weigly 1984). Stature and weight continue to be the most widely used measures of nutritional status and disease risk at both extremes of body size. They give the simplest measure of attained frame, or skeletal size, and of soft tissue mass (Ulijaszek 1997).

Obesity came to be measured with the body mass index (BMI), subsequent to its being described as the least-worst anthropometric measure of this phenomenon. The BMI had its origins in the Metropolitan Life Insurance Company tables. While body weight is always related to stature, the relationship is non-linear, and even direct correction for height does not remove this relationality completely. The height dependency of weight and stature-based measures of nutritional status was of concern for early epidemiological investigation of the health impacts of excess body fatness (Boe et al., 1957), because it made nutritional assessment difficult. After examining the height dependency of a number of weight-height indices and ratios, Boe et al., (1957) concluded that weight over height squared (W/H^2) gave the best height independent measure of relative weight. Subsequent studies in British, Cook Islander and US populations confirmed this view (Ulijaszek 2017). In an analysis of the relative height independence of body fat prediction using different weight to height ratios, Keys et al., (1972) found generally much lower correlations of height with W/H^2 than with either weight over height (W/H) or weight over height cubed (W/H^3). These authors concluded that the ratio W/H^2 was clearly better than other measures of relative weight, and declared that this ratio be named the body mass index.

The cut-offs for ideal weight used in the Metropolitan Life Insurance Company tables are similar to those that were subsequently recommended for nutritional assessment using BMI by the Royal College of Physicians (1983) in the UK. The adoption of the closest whole-number BMI equivalent value to the very lowest and very highest boundaries for healthy weight in the Metropolitan Life Insurance Company tables by the Royal College of Physicians (1983) permitted ideal healthy weight to be determined without having to consider or measure frame-size (an undefined construct within these tables), simplifying anthropometric obesity assessment (James 2004). The BMI cut-offs of 18.5, 17.0 and 16.0

kg/m^2 were accepted for the assessment of different grades of adult undernutrition, or chronic energy deficiency, in 1992 (Shetty and James 1994), while BMI cut-offs of 25 and 30 kg/m^2 were accepted for classifying overweight and obesity by the World Health Organization (WHO) in 1997 (World Health Organization 2000). Alongside the acceptance of BMI as the measure of nutritional status of adults came the standardization of risk of mortality (Flegal et al., 2007) and morbidity (Campbell and Ulijaszek 1994; Canoy et al., 2007) at both lower and higher extremes of BMI.

At the upper end of population distribution, BMI shows strong associations with morbidity and mortality from number of chronic diseases and disorders for adults (World Health Organization 2000), and among a limited number of risk markers for chronic disease among adolescents (Bhargava et al., 2004). Figure 1 shows all-cause mortality according to BMI from the largest meta-analysis of BMI against mortality to date, the Prospective Studies Collaboration (2009), which includes nearly a million adults from 57 prospective studies.

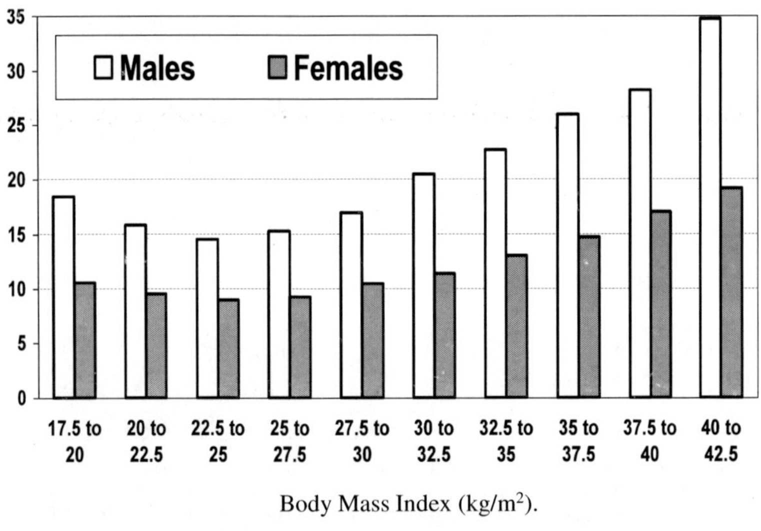

Figure 1. All-cause mortality relative to body mass index, for 894,576 adults in 57 prospective mortality studies in industrialized countries (data from Prospective Studies Collaboration 2009).

Epidemiological studies relating BMI to mortality have methodological biases, however, including reverse causation and confounding by related factors such as smoking (Hu 2008). Epidemiological critiques of BMI include its inconsistent relationship with body fatness (Gallagher et al., 1996; Freedman and Sherry 2009), that it does not distinguish between potentially harmful fat in the liver and viscera (Carroll et al., 2008), and that it does not reflect health risk very well, except at the extremes (Lee et al., 2008).

BMI persists as a standard anthropometric measure of adult obesity, however, for both pragmatic and historical reasons. The BMI has been used for far longer than any other anthropometric measure, and was the first to be appropriated for the assessment of obesity rates in populations, after measures of stature and weight had been formalized for predicting mortality. Furthermore, there is no alternative measure of obesity that is collected nearly as systematically as the BMI. While waist circumference and waist hip ratio show as good, if not better, associations with mortality and morbidity risk (World Health Organization 2011), their possible adoption for international comparison would risk delegitimising programs and policies for obesity control that have used population monitoring of BMI as the measure of success or failure, at a time when adult obesity rates continue to rise (Stevens et al., 2012).

While the BMI has been universally adopted for obesity assessment, it does not have the best fit for all the purposes to which it has been assigned: individual classification; screening and monitoring for medical purposes; population monitoring for public health purposes; and econometric modelling. As the relationships between BMI, fatness and morbidity vary across populations (World Health Organization Expert Consultation 2004), there remain problems of how best to classify obesity using BMI. Relationships with morbidity and mortality vary according to the measure of obesity used, the population under investigation (be it of European, Asian, of African ancestry, whether it is young or old, male or female), and among the various classificatory boundaries that are used in obesity research and practice (World Health Organization 2000). In some Chinese (Li et al., 2002) and Asian (World Health Organization Expert

Consultation 2004) populations, there is increased chronic disease risk at lower levels of BMI than among European populations (Li et al., 2002), and this has prompted recommendations for lower cut-offs for overweight and obesity for people of Asian origin (World Health Organization Expert Consultation 2004). At the other extreme, Pacific Islander populations generally have lower body fatness relative to lean body mass at any level of BMI, prompting the suggestion that higher BMI cut-offs should be used to assess overweight and obesity in these populations (Swinburn et al., 1999).

The BMI is also used to classify childhood obesity. This is more problematic than among adults, because of the variability in the growth rates of children both within- and between-populations which alters the normative range of BMI according to different normative bodily proportions at different ages, making fixed obesity cut-offs inappropriate. Age-specific cut-offs for childhood overweight and obesity that pass through adult classification cut-offs for overweight and obesity have been accepted for international use, however, using normative distributions that vary by age and sex (Cole et al., 2000). Evidence from systematic reviews of adult chronic disease subsequent to childhood obesity shows there to be significantly increased risk of premature mortality with child and adolescent overweight or obesity, as well as significantly increased risk of cardiometabolic morbidity (diabetes, hypertension, ischaemic heart disease, and stroke) in adult life (Reilly and Kelly 2011). Cardiovascular disease risk is, however, dependent on the tracking of BMI from childhood to adulthood, with the risk of raised blood pressure in adult life being highest among those at the lower end of the BMI scale in childhood, but overweight in adulthood (Lloyd et al., 2010).

In the formalization of BMI for international use for the measurement of obesity (World Health Organization 2000), the overarching aim was to provide simplicity for assessment and monitoring of obesity world-wide. Standardized classification of obesity was accepted by the World Health Organization (2000) because it claimed that it allowed meaningful comparisons within and between populations, the identification of individuals and groups at increased risk of morbidity and mortality, the identification of priorities for intervention at individual and community levels, and a firm basis for evaluating interventions.

Reporting Obesity

Both height and BMI are positively associated with socioeconomic status (SES) in India (Som et al., 2014), and a positive secular trend in increased body size has been observed in some populations there (Khanna and Kapoor 2004). There has also been an increase in obesity rates among children and adolescents (Mistry and Puthussery 2015) and among adults in most Indian States (Bharati et al., 2007). While there has been an emergence of the dual burden of undernutrition and obesity across much of India (Bharati et al., 2007) (Table 1), such dual burden does not exist yet among those of low SES, suggesting that transition towards energy-dense, nutrient-poor diets and low physical activity (Popkin 2002) in India is at an early stage (Subramanian et al., 2009).

In the UK, various surveys from the start of the nineteen hundreds onwards show there to have been a secular trend towards increased height and weight until the 1970s (Floud et al., 1990), followed by emergent overweight and obesity among children (Chinn and Rona 2001) and adults (Garrow 1978) especially among those of lower SES (Ulijaszek 2014). In the UK and other high income countries (HICs), rates of childhood overweight and obesity appear to have plateaued (Wabitsch et al., 2014), although this effect has been shown mostly in studies of short duration (Visscher et al., 2015). Where rates of childhood and adolescent obesity have been shown to plateau, socioeconomic inequalities in obesity rates have persisted or increased (Ulijaszek et al., 2016), as in the US (Frederick et al., 2013) and the UK (Stamatakis et al., 2010). Data that is taken to be nationally-representative in England show this effect between 2007 and 2015 (Figure 2) (Public Health England 2016), expressed as percentage differences in obesity rates between the least and most deprived Local Authority Districts.

Table 1. Percent obesity, overweight and undernutrition, India, adult women (data from Bharati et al., 2007)

State	Obesity (BMI>30)	Overweight (BMI 25-30)	Undernourished (BMI<18.5)	Combined burden
Punjab	9.0	21.1	16.4	46.5
New Delhi	8.9	24.1	12.2	45.2
Goa	4.4	16.7	26.8	47.9
Gujarat	4.3	11.3	36.3	51.9
Maharashtra	4.1	12.6	33.2	49.9
Kerala	3.8	17.0	18.0	38.8
Haryana	3.7	12.3	25.6	41.6
Himachal Pradesh	3.3	13.2	26.5	43.0
Jammu	3.3	11.7	24.7	36.4
Tamil Nadu	3.1	13.4	26.1	42.6
Karnataka	2.8	10.3	38.2	51.3
All India	**2.6**	**9.4**	**31.2**	**43.2**
Sikkim	2.3	12.1	10.9	25.3
West Bengal	2.3	10.3	37.9	50.5
Andhra Pradesh	2.2	9.9	36.5	48.6
Tripura	1.8	6.5	34.5	42.8
Uttar Pradesh	1.5	5.8	34.7	42.0
Rajasthan	1.4	5.0	35.2	41.6

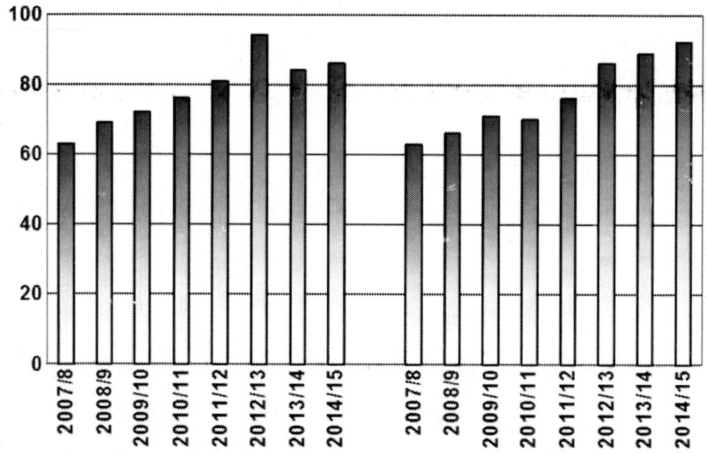

Figure 2. Percentage difference in obesity rates between the least (1st decile) and most (10th decile) deprived Index of Multiple Deprivation Local Authority Districts based on school postcode, England, between 2007/8 and 2013/14, children aged between four and five years, and between ten and eleven years (data from Public Health England 2016).

Anthropometry as Evidence in Policy Making

The most basic form of evidence for policy on nutritional status is nationally-representative data across administrative units and across time. The use of the concept of human capital, which includes adult height, educational achievement, income and birth weight, expresses the economic logics that underpin the intervention, that good nutrition is a prerequisite for economic development (Bryce et al., 2008). Nutrition came to the policy forefront in India in the 1990s, with the National Nutrition Policy (1993) and the 1995 National Plan of Action on Nutrition (Mohmand 2012). With respect to undernutrition in India, two data sources for nationally-assessed nutritional status for policy purposes have predominated. The first of these, the National Family Health Survey (NFHS) is collected periodically by the International Institute for Population Sciences, and is a large-scale, household level sample survey conducted across India that provides information on the main outcome indicators of malnutrition - underweight, stunting and wasting, along with a host of other health indicators. This survey has been repeated periodically, with NFHS-1 having been conducted in 1992-93, NFHS-2 in 1998-99 and NFHS-3 in 2005-06. The second of these, the Integrated Child Development Services (ICDS) scheme of the Ministry of Women and Child Development carries out regular monitoring of the weight of children under the age of 6 years, among its many functions. Anthropometric nutritional assessment has been used in both NFHS and ICDS surveys to identify the regions of India with highest burdens of undernutrition. Obesity has never been measured or reported systematically using the NFHS or ICDS surveys. However, at the national level, obesity policy in India is observed in the reporting of data to the WHO and some compliance to WHO obesity policy (World Health Organization 2000; 2016).

As with measures of anthropometric undernutrition, the measurement of obesity rates and its reporting provides evidence for the existence of population obesity and its changing patterns across time, and for identifying possible governmental interventions against it. Speaking to the importance of data collection for childhood obesity policy, Nathan et al., (2005) assert that policy can be made in the absence of strong research evidence, but where powerful and competing groups contest possible policy options, the evidence required needs to be substantial. Nationally-representative data on obesity rates are often illustrated using obesity prevalence maps, where obesity rates are shown according to administrative units within-nation. Figure 3 shows such a map for England, according to Local Authority. Such maps have been used to illustrate inequalities in rates of obesity according to social class, gender, ethnicity and geography across the country and within cities. By combining categories, such mapping has also been used to demonstrate regional differences due to variations in proportions of the population of low SES across the country and according to levels of deprivation (Moon et al., 2007).

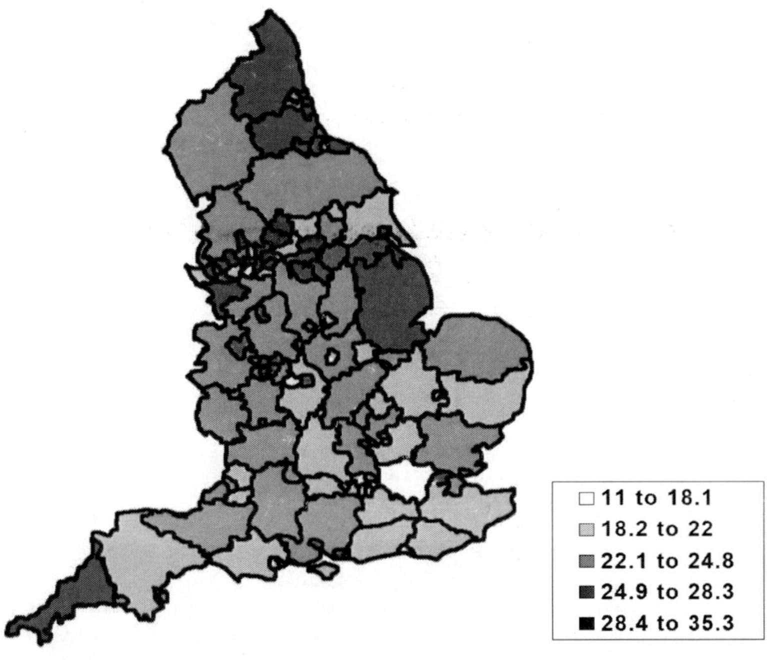

Figure 3. Obesity rates in adults, England 2012.

Epidemiological data collection and reporting, and the use of obesity epidemiology in econometric modelling of the impacts of obesity, are usually starting points for state-led obesity interventions (Malik et al., 2013). The spur to policy action by most nation-states is overwhelmingly economic (Ulijaszek 2017). The most persuasive political arguments usually involve framing obesity as a significant burden to the economy and health service, usually through costs to employers, its medical management, and of the chronic diseases associated with it (Wang et al., 2011). In the UK, obesity has also been compellingly depicted as a drag on the economy, both in terms of lost productivity and in terms of costs to state-provided health care provision (House of Commons Health Committee 2004). Obesity assessment from annual data collection of adult heights and weights by Health Survey for England (HSE) was initiated in 1993, while the National Child Measurement Programme (NCMP) was set up to monitor childhood obesity in 2007 by the National Obesity Observatory (NOO). The NCMP continues as an annual programme of measurement of heights and weights of the vast majority of children in the first and final years of State-funded primary schools in England. Both HSE and NCMP obesity monitoring hold UK National Statistics status in the same way that the reporting of births, deaths and marriages does.

The categorization of obesity as a disease in the US and by the WHO has aimed to raise the profile of obesity for medical intervention, but this categorization continues to be contested (Rich et al., 2011). Obesity as risk factor also has a place in the framing of health policy, because it sits among other risk categories such as smoking, unhealthy diet, and physical inactivity for chronic disease onset and progression (Erlichman et al., 2002). Categories of risk have ambivalent status in policy-making, however. For example, smoking damages health and human productivity, but its taxation gives a steady stream of reliable income to governments (Chaloupka and Warner 2000). Similarly, unhealthy diet is damaging, but the food industry, which supplies uncontaminated and affordable food to large populations, primarily seeks to continue its operations without undue regulation (Ulijaszek and McLennan 2016).

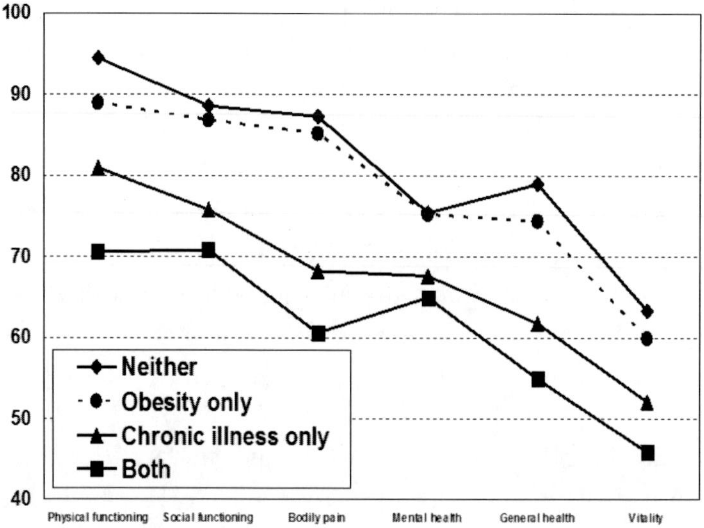

Figure 4. Distribution of self-reported health scores (the higher the healthier) according to obesity (according to body mass index) and chronic illness, after adjusting for age, gender, and frequency of health service utilization, United Kingdom (data from Doll et al., 2000).

Discussion

Undernutrition reduces work capacity and productivity among adults, reducing earning capacity and aggravating poverty, as well as enhancing mortality and morbidity among children (Anish et al., 2013). Furthermore, poverty in childhood increases risk of non-communicable diseases in adult life (Conroy et al., 2010). While nutrition policy in India remains focused on undernutrition, the collection of nationally-representative data on anthropometric nutritional status has highlighted the decline in nutritional stunting, if not of wasting (Mohmand 2012), and the rise in obesity in more recent years (Bharati et al., 2007). The emergence of the dual burden of both undernutrition and obesity across the nation, even if not yet located among those of low SES (Subramanian et al., 2009), has led to calls for national nutrition policy that can address this new problem (Mohmand 2012). The economic costs of obesity to India include those of lost productivity, but increasingly the costs of treating the rapidly rising rates of type two diabetes (Mohan et al., 2007).

While BMI cut-offs for obesity classification are viewed as being meaningful according to epidemiological analyses (World Health Organization Expert Consultation 2004), they can differ from individual health perceptions of health and well-being. For example, self-reported health status of adults in the UK among obese people who have not experienced chronic disease is similar to that of people categorized as being of normal weight (Figure 4), with respect to physical function, bodily pain, general health and vitality, social functioning and mental health (Doll et al., 2000).

Obesity may not be perceived as a problem among those carrying excess body fatness prior to experiencing any of the chronic diseases associated with it. Anthropometric measurement of obesity has been critiqued by social scientists for its medical distancing of the individual experience of living with a fat body (Yates-Doerr 2013), whether or not such experience has been linked to chronic disease experience. It has also been viewed by social scientists as a way of universalizing the human body by governmental institutions through epidemiological reporting, by relating individuals to norms and health to measurement (McCullough and Hardin 2013). Brewis et al., (2011) note the stigma that accompanies the measurement and medicalization of fat bodies, while Puhl and Brownell (2001) have reported the widespread stigma attached to obesity. The stigma attached to undernutrition has also been reported to be a barrier to the uptake of medical treatment and nutritional rehabilitation by mothers and young children in Pakistan (Mull 1991), Tanzania (Howard and Millard 1997) and Kenya (Bliss et al., 2016).

The policy uses of anthropometric nutritional status combine it with other nationally-oriented data such as birth, death, disease and economics. The reported numbers and their use in policy are a long way from the individuals that data collection is designed to serve. Undernutrition in India persists, and is framed as an object for policy intervention, as good nutrition is seen as a prerequisite of economic development in low income countries. In HICs, obese people are shamed and obesity is viewed as a drag on the economy. Through reporting nutritional status, ideal citizen-bodies are constructed through growth and body size references, not in relation to individual well-bring, but in relation to the best economic functioning of the State. Neoliberal politics forces ideal body citizenship on the individual, however, despite individuals and populations being urged, in the case of India, to develop (Berg 1973), and in the case of the UK, to consume (Ulijaszek and McLennan 2016). Thus measuring and reporting nutritional status and obesity raises questions about differing forms of biological citizenship.

REFERENCES

Analysing Nutrition Governance: *India Country Report.* Institute of Development Studies. http://www.ids.ac.uk/idsproject/analysing-nutrition-governance.

Anish TSN, Sreelakshmi PRN, Soumya G. et al., 2013. Recommendations for a new nutrition policy for India. *Acad Med J India* 1: 9-16.

Bharati S, Pal M, Bhattacharaya BN, Bharati P. 2007. Prevalence and causes of chronic energy deficiency and obesity in Indian women. *Hum Biol* 79:395-412.

Bhargava SK, Sachdev HS, Fall CHD et al., 2004. Relation of serial changes in childhood body-mass index to impaired glucose tolerance in young adulthood. *N Engl J Med* 350:865-875.

Berg A, 1973. *The Nutrition Factor; its Role in National Development.* Washington, The Brookings Institution.

Bliss JR, Njenga M, Stoltzfus RJ, Pelletier DL. 2016. Stigma as a barrier to treatment for child acute malnutrition in Marsabit County, Kenya. *Maternal Child Health* 12: 125-138.

Boe J, Humerfelt S, Wedervang F. 1957. The blood pressure in a population: blood pressure readings and height and weight determinations in the adult population of the city of Bergen. *Acta Med Scandinavica* 321: 1-336.

Brewis AA, Wutich A, Falletta-Cowden A, Rodriguez-Soto I. 2011. Body norms and fat stigma in global perspective. *Curr Anthropol* 52: 269-276.

Bryce J, Coitinho D, Darnton-Hill I, Pelletier D, Pinstrup-Andersen P. 2008. Maternal and child undernutrition: effective action at national level. *Lancet* 371: 510-526.

Campbell P, Ulijaszek SJ. 1994. Relationships between anthropometry and retrospective morbidity in poor men in Calcutta, India. *Eur J Clin Nutr* 48: 507-512.

Canoy D, Boekholdt SM, Wareham N. et al., 2007. Body fat distribution and risk of coronary heart disease in men and women in the European prospective investigation into cancer and nutrition in Norfolk cohort: a population-based prospective study. *Circulation* 116: 2933-2943.

Carroll JF, Chiapa AL, Rodriquez M. et al., 2008. Visceral fat, waist circumference, and BMI: impact of race/ethnicity. *Obesity* 16: 600-607.

Chaloupka FJ, Warner KE. 2000. The economics of smoking. In: *Handbook of Health Economics Volume 1, Part B*, ed. A.J. Culyer & J. P. Newhouse. Amsterdam: Elsevier Science, pp. 1539-1627.

Chinn S, Rona RJ. 2001. Prevalence and trends in overweight and obesity in three cross sectional studies of British children, 1974-94. *BMJ* 322 doi: https://doi.org/10.1136/bmj.322.7277.24

Cole TJ, Bellizzi MC, Flegal KM, Dietz WH. 2000. Establishing a standard definition for child overweight and obesity worldwide: international survey. *Br Med J* 320: 1240-1245.

Conroy K, Sandel M, Zuckerman B. (2010). Poverty grown up: how childhood socioeconomic status impacts adult health. *J Dev Beh Pediatr* 31:154-160.

Doll HA, Peterson SEK, Stewart-Brown SL. 2000. Obesity and physical and emotional well-being: associations between body mass index, chronic illness, and the physical and mental components of the SF-36 questionnaire. *Obes Res* 8: 160-170.

Erlichman J, Kerbey AL, James WPT. 2002. Physical activity and its impact on health outcomes. Paper 2: Prevention of unhealthy weight gain and obesity by physical activity: an analysis of the evidence. *Obes Rev* 3: 273-287.

Flegal KM, Graubard BI, Williamson DF, Gail MH. 2007. Cause-specific excess deaths associated with underweight, overweight, and obesity. *J Am Med Assoc* 298: 2028-2037.

Floud R, Wachter K, Gregory A. 1990. *Height, Health and History.* Cambridge, Cambridge University Press.

Freedman DS, Sherry B. 2009. The validity of BMI as an indicator of body fatness and risk among children. *Pediatr* 124 Suppl 1: 1338-1342.

Frederick CB, Snellman K, Putnam RD. 2013. Increasing socioeconomic disparities in adolescent obesity. *Proc Nat Acad Sci* 111: 1338-1342.

Gallagher D, Visser M, Sepulveda D. et al., 1996. How useful Is body mass index for comparison of body fatness across age, sex, and ethnic groups? *Am J Epidemiol* 143: 228-239.

Garrow JS. 1978. *Energy Balance and Obesity in Man*, 2nd edition. Amsterdam: Elsevier.

González D, Nazmi A, Victora CG. 2009. Childhood poverty and abdominal obesity in adulthood: a systematic review. *Cadernos de Saude Publica*. 25 Suppl 3: S427-440.

House of Commons Health Committee, 2004. Obesity. *Third Report of Session 2003-04. Volume I.* Report, together with formal minutes. London: The Stationery Office Limited.

Howard M, Millard A. 1997. *Hunger and Shame: Child Malnutrition and Poverty on Mount Kilimanjaro. Routledge:* London.

Hu FB. 2008. Obesity and mortality. In: *Obesity Epidemiology*, ed. F. Hu, pp. 216-233. Oxford: Oxford University Press.

James WPT. 2004. Obesity: The worldwide epidemic. *Clin Dermatol* 22: 276-280.

Jelliffe DB. 1966. Assessment of Nutritional Status of the Community. *Monograph Series Number 53.* Geneva: World Health Organization.

Keys A, Fidanza F, Karvonen MJ, Kimura N, Taylor HL. 1972. Indices of relative weight and obesity. *J Chron Dis* 25: 329-243.

Khanna G, Kapoor S. 2004. Secular trend in stature and age at menarche among Punjabi Aroras residing in New Delhi, India. *Colleg Antropologicum* 28: 571-575.

Lee CMY, Huxley RR, Wildman RP, Woodward M. 2008. Indices of abdominal obesity are better discriminators of cardiovascular risk factors than BMI: a meta-analysis. *J Clin Epidemiol* 61: 646-653.

Li G, Chen X, Jang Y. et al., 2002. Obesity, coronary heart disease risk factors and diabetes in Chinese: an approach to the criteria of obesity in the Chinese population. *Obes Rev* 3: 167-172.

Lloyd LJ, Langley-Evans SC, McMullen S. 2010. Childhood obesity and adult cardiovascular disease risk: a systematic review. *Int J Obes* 34: 18-28.

Malik VS, Willett WC, Hu FB. 2013. Global obesity: trends, risk factors and policy implications. *Nature Rev Endocrinol* 9: 13-27.

McCullough MB, Hardin JA. 2013. *Reconstructing Obesity. The Meaning of Measures and the Measure of Meanings.* Oxford: Berghahn Books.

Mistry SK, Puthussery S. 2015. Risk factors of overweight and obesity in childhood and adolescence in South Asian countries: a systematic review of the evidence. *Publ Health* 129: 200-209.

Mohan V, Sandeep S, Deepa R, Shah B, Varghese C. 2007. Epidemiology of type 2 diabetes: Indian scenario. *Indian J Med Res* 125: 217-230.

Mohmand SK. 2012. *Policies Without Politics: Analysing Nutrition Governance in India.*

Mol A. 2009. Good taste: the embodied normativity of the consumer-citizen. *J Cult Econ* 2: 269-283.

Moon G, Quarendon G, Barnard S, Twigg L, Blyth B. 2007. Fat nation: deciphering geographies of obesity in England. *Soc Sci Med* 65: 20-31.

Mull D. (1991) Traditional perceptions of marasmus in Pakistan. *Soc Sci Med* 32: 175-191.

Nathan SA, Develin E, Grove N, Zwi AB. 2005. An Australian childhood obesity summit: the role of data and evidence in 'public' policy making. *Australia and New Zealand Health Pol* 2:17. Doi: 10.1186/1743-8462-2-17.

National Nutrition Policy, 1993. Department of women and child development; *Ministry of human resource development.* Government of India 1993. http://wcd.nic.in/nnp.pdf. Accessed 25th January 2018.

Popkin BM. 2002. Part II. What is unique about the experience in lower- and middleincome less-industrialised countries compared with the very-high income industrialised countries? The shift in stages of the nutrition transition in the developing world differs from past experiences! *Publ Health Nutr* 5: 205-214.

Prospective Studies Collaboration, 2009. Body mass index and cause-specific mortality in 900 000 adults: collaborative analyses of 57 prospective studies. *Lancet* 373: 1083-1096.

Public Health England, 2016. *PHE Obesity.* http://www.noo.org.uk/ accessed December 20th 2017.

Puhl R, Brownell KD. 2001. Bias, discrimination, and obesity. *Obes R*es 9: 788-805.

Reilly JJ, Kelly J. 2011. Long-term impact of overweight and obesity in childhood and adolescence on morbidity and premature mortality in adulthood: systematic review. *Int J Obes* 35: 891-898.

Rich E, Monaghan L, Aphramor L. (eds), 2011. *Debating Obesity: Critical Perspectives.* Basingstoke, Hampshire: Palgrave Macmillan.

Royal College of Physicians, 1983. Obesity: Report of the Royal College of Physicians. *Journal Royal College of Physicians* 17: 1-58.

Rubin L, Joseph JA. 2013. An ounce of prevention, a ton of controversy. Exploring tensions in the fields of obesity and eating disorder prevention. In: *Reconstructing Obesity. The Meaning of Measures and the Measure of Meanings*, ed. M. B. McCullough & J. A. Hardin. Oxford: Berghahn Books, pp. 199-214.

Shetty PS, James WPT. 1994. Body Mass Index. A Measure of Chronic Energy Deficiency in Adults. *FAO Food and Nutrition Paper 56.* Rome: Food and Agriculture Organization.

Sinalko AR, Steinberger J, Moran A. et al., 2005. Relation of body mass index and insulin resistance to cardiovascular risk factors, inflammatory factors, and oxidative stress during adolescence. *Circulation* 111:1985-91.

Stamatakis E, Wardle J, Cole T. 2010. Childhood obesity and overweight prevalence trends in England: evidence for growing socioeconomic disparities. *Int J Obes* 34: 41-47.

Som S, Ulijaszek SJ, Pal M, Bharati S, Bharati P. 2014. Variation in height and weight of adult Indians, *J Biosoc Sci* 46: 47-65,

Stevens GA, Singh GM, Lu Y. et al., 2012. National, regional, and global trends in adult overweight and obesity prevalences. *Population Health Metrics* 10: 22. Doi: 10.1186/1478-7954-10-22.

Subramanian SV, Perkins JM, Khan KT. 2009. Do burdens of underweight and overweight coexist among lower socioeconomic groups in India? *Am J Clin Nutr* 90: 369-376.

Swinburn BA, Ley SJ, Carmichael MHE, Plank LD. 1999. Body size and composition of Polynesians. *Int J Obes* 23: 1178-1183.

Ulijaszek SJ. 1997. *Anthropometric measures. In Design Concepts in Nutritional Epidemiology*, ed. B. M. Margetts and M. Nelson, pp. 289-311. Oxford: Oxford University Press.

Ulijaszek SJ 2017. *Models of Obesity. From ecology to complexity in science and policy.* Cambridge: Cambridge University Press.

Ulijaszek SJ. 2014. Do adult obesity rates in England vary by insecurity as well as by inequality? An ecological cross-sectional study. *BMJ Open* 4:e004430. doi:10.1136/bmjopen-2013-004430.

Ulijaszek SJ, Komlos J. 2010. From a history of anthropometry to anthropometric history. In *Human Variation, from Laboratory to the Field* (ed. C. G. N. Mascie-Taylor, A Yasukouchi and S. J. Ulijaszek, pp. 183-97). Boca Raton: CRC Press.

Ulijaszek SJ,McLennan AK. 2016. Framing obesity in UK policy from the Blair years, 1997-2015: persistent individualistic approaches despite overwhelming evidence of societal and economic factors, and the need for collective responsibility. *Obes Rev* 17: 397-411.

Visscher TLS, Seidell JC. 2001. The public health impact of obesity. *Annu Rev Public Health* 22: 355-375.

Wabitsch M, Moss A, Kromeyer-Hauschild K. 2014. Unexpected plateauing of childhood obesity rates in developed countries. *BMC Med* 12:17.

Wang YC, McPherson K, Marsh T, Gortmaker SL, Brown M. 2011. Health and economic burden of the projected obesity trends in the USA and the UK. *Lancet*, 378: 815-25.

Weigly ES. 1984. Average? Ideal? Desirable? A brief overview of weight tables in the United States. *J Am Dietet Assoc* 84: 417-423.

World Health Organization, 2000. Obesity: Preventing and Managing the Global Epidemic. Report of a WHO Consultation. Geneva: World Health Organization.

World Health Organization, 2011. Waist circumference and Waist–Hip Ratio: Report of a WHO Expert Consultation. Geneva: World Health Organization.

World Health Organization, 2016. Consideration of the evidence on childhood obesity for the Commission on Ending Childhood Obesity. *Report of the Ad hoc Working Group on Science and Evidence for Ending Childhood Obesity*. Geneva: World Health Organization.

World Health Organization Expert Consultation, 2004. Appropriate body-mass index for Asian populations and its implications for policy and intervention strategies. *Lancet* 363: 157-63.

Yates Doerr E. 2013. The mismeasure of obesity. In: Reconstructing Obesity. *The Meaning of Measures and the Measure of Meanings*, ed. M. B. McCullough & J. A. Hardin. Oxford: Berghahn Books, pp. 49-70.

In: Obesity and Syndrome X
Editors: M. Das and K. Bose
ISBN: 978-1-53614-669-1

Chapter 12

MODERNIZATION AND OBESITY: A PANDEMIC ISSUE

***Soibam Jibonkumar Singh*[1,*]**
***and Thoudam Bedita Devi*[2,†]**
[1]Department of Anthropology, Manipur University, Manipur, India
[2]Department of Anatomy,
Sikkim Manipal Institute of Medical Sciences, Sikkim, India

OBESITY: CONCEPT AND EPIDEMIOLOGY

Overweight and obesity are defined as abnormal or excessive fat accumulation that may impair health. Body Mass Index (BMI) is a simple index of weight-for-height that is commonly used to classify overweight and obesity in adults. It is defined as a person's weight in kilograms divided by the square of his height in meters (kg/m2) i.e., BMI = Wt in Kg/Ht in m^2. The WHO defines overweight as BMI greater than or equal to 25kg/m2 but less than 29.9kg/m2; and obesity as BMI greater than or equal

*Corresponding Author Email: drjibonkumar@yahoo.com.
†Corresponding Author Email: thnoubi@gmail.com.

to 30 kg/m2(WHO, 2017a).Though for the Asian population a BMI of 27kg/m2 is equivalent to a value of 30 kg/m2 in other groups (WHO, 1998). Overweight means excess in body weight and may be the resultant of higher lean body mass(muscle, bone, or body water content) but not only because of the weight of the total body fat. Obesity, on the other hand, denotes the presence of excess body fat. All obese persons are overweight, but all overweight persons are not necessarily obese as the excess body weight may arise from the lean body mass as well (Mandal, 2010). The adverse health outcomes associated with overweight and obesity range from an increase risk of mortality to a non-fatal debilitating disease (WHO, 1998). Obesity therefore is a medical condition of excess of body weight due to the accumulation of fat leading to an adverse effect on health, reduced life expectancy and/or increased health problems.

Genetics, environmental, metabolic, behavioral, and socio-cultural factors play major roles in pre disposing a person to obesity. Genetics plays an important role in shaping the BMI status of an individual. How much variation in weight gain among individuals can be accounted for by genetic factors? Obesity frequently begins in childhood and generally the obese parents may likely have overweight children. Familial association is not a proof of genetic inheritance for families having shared eating and exercise habits. However, familial association cannot be considered as a proof of genetic inheritance-as families share common lifestyle pattern such as dietary pattern and exercise habit. It is claimed that about 200 different genes or loci have been linked with controlling obesity in humans (Lau, 1999). However, the pattern of inheritance of obesity suggests that the effect is polygenic, with each variant of many different genes making a small difference in effect (Sorensen and Soren, 2001). Apart from this, both age and sex have role to play in causing obesity. Many studies have shown that excessive weight gain leading to overweight and obese condition usually develops slowly through adulthood and most weight gain occurs between the age of 25 to 44 years. Again females are more prone to obesity as compared to males because of their anatomical structure and physiological features such as not losing the weight they have gained during pregnancy and gaining body weight by about 12-15 pounds with the attainment of menopause.

When we talk of the environmental factors, it encompasses the totality of the surrounding in which we find ourselves. Gaining excessive body weight leading to overweight and obese condition is a long term process brought about by a number of socio-cultural practices and habits. The way of eating during childhood can affect the way one eats as adults. The way of eating over many years becomes a habit. What we eat, when we eat, and how much we eat is certainly a determinant of weight gain and obesity. Certain habits such as eating more food than our body can use, drinking too much alcohol, not getting enough exercise, quit smoking, stress, anxiety, feeling sad, or not sleeping well are said to be important contributory factors for gaining excessive weight and obesity. At the same time certain medical problems or treatments cause weight gain including underactive thyroid gland (hypothyroidism), medicines such as birth control pills, antidepressants, and antipsychotics.

On the whole, the potential contributory factors culminating to global increase in overweight and obesity in the past three decades are changing lifestyle patterns such as increase in calorie intake, changes in the composition of diet, decreasing levels of physical activity, and changes in the gut microbiome as well (Bleichet al., 2008, Astrup and Brand-Miller J, 2012, Drewnowski and Popkin, 1997, Popkin, 2001, Blair, 2013). Though there are multiple causal factors associated with the rise in obesity in developing countries, the two most important factors are urbanization and globalization (Benjamin Caballero, 2007, Nanan, 2002). In short, urbanization and globalization have resulted in modernization which is the key causal factor for overweight and obesity. The urban lifestyle as compared to the rural setting has difference in energy balance as a result of difference in energy intake and energy expenditure. The energy consuming manual labor, long walks to work places for earning their livelihood and also procuring their subsistence typical of rural areas are replaced by sedentary lifestyle characterized by mechanized system of transportation, machineries and desk or sidewalk job. In short the urban lifestyle demands much lower energy expenditure as compared to the rural way of living in rural settings. On the other hand, the urban dwellers consume more energy dense food readily available in the urban market in contrast with low energy expenditure thus culminating to gradual weight gain. Whereas the reverse is the condition of the rural dwellers as they expend more energy and consume low nutrient and less energy content food conditioned by low economy on one hand, and unavailability of energy dense food on the other. As such the children in rural areas cannot achieve normal growth thus resulting into underweight adults. As economic development bring some characteristics of urban lifestyle to rural communities, these populations also begin to show increasing rates of obesity, particularly among women these days (Mendez, 2005). Unhealthy deitary habits and less physical activity are likely to endure thereby increasing the risk among today's youth for obesity and chronic diseases in future unless the public health initiatives are designed to be multilevel and take into consideration the multiple correlations that influence behaviour surrounding dietary intake and physical activity (Sandra et al., 2012).

Obesity is a major risk factor for cardiovascular disease (CVD) and Type 2 diabetes mellitus (DM) and in the presence of other risk factors for non-communicable diseases (NCDs) such as smoking, hypertension, elevated blood cholesterol and it has a multiplicative effect (Thorkhildet al., 2000, Blackburn and Luepker, 1986). A number of literatures reveals that the consequences of obesity include various diseases and morbid conditions which increase the chances of mortality such as Diabetes, Coronary Heart Disease, Peripheral Artery Disease, Stroke, Hypertension, Hyperlipidemia, Arthritis, Obstructive sleep apnea, Pulmonary disease, PCOS/infertility, Dysmenorrhea, Pregnancy complications, Gallbladder disease, Skin infections, Urinary incontinence, Depression, Eating disorders, social stigma, Cancers: breast, endometrial, colon, prostate, gallbladder, kidney, esophagus, etc.

OBESITY: GLOBAL SCENARIO

The worldwide prevalence obesity has nearly tripled since 1975. In 2016, more than 1.9 billion adults, 18 years and older, were overweight. Of these over 650 million were obese. As many as 39% of adults aged 18 years and above were overweight in 2016, and 13% were obese. Most of the world's population live in countries where overweight and obesity kill more people than underweight. As many as 41 million children under the age of 5 were overweight or obese in 2016. Over 340 million children and adolescents aged 5-19 were overweight or obese in 2016 (WHO, 2017a). Obesity has reached pandemic proportions globally with at least 2.8 million people dying each year as a result of being overweight or obese. Once associated with high-income countries, obesity is now also prevalent in low- and middle-income countries (WHO, 2017b). It has been reported that number of overweight and obese individuals increased from 857 million in 1980, to 2.1 billion in 2013. The worldwide prevalence of overweight and obesity combined rose by 27.5% for adults and 47.1% for children between 1980 and 2013 (Emmanuelaet al., 2014).

It is a well-established and known fact that the prevalence of overweight and obesity is overwhelmingly increasing globally during the last few decades. Several studies have revealed that it has become a global pandemic issue (Roth et al., 2004, Swinburnet al., 2011, Popkin and Adair, 2012). In 2010, a worldwide estimate reveals that overweight and obesity resulted in 3.4 million deaths, 4% of years of life lost, and 4% of disability-adjusted life-years (Lim SS, 2010), thus resulting in future fall of life expectancy.

Getting little bit acquaintance with the numerical figure, the total population of the world is 7,505,257,673 while 774,000,000 of them are obese thus constituting almost 10.5%. New research suggests that, there are about 775 million obese people in the world including adults, children, and adolescents. Our research suggests that, there are nearly 650 million obese adults on the planet, as defined as a body mass index (BMI) over 30.

There are also about 125 million obese children and adolescents in the entire world according to a BMI over 30 kg/m^2. The majority of the obesity on the planet resides in a few countries. The following data will reveal top ranking status in relation to obesity parameter.

Top 10 Countries with most obese population size in order of ranking as of July 1st, 2017

1.	US	–	109,342,839
2.	China	–	97,256,700
3.	India	–	65,619,826
4.	Brazil	–	41,857,656
5.	Mexico	–	36,294,881
6.	Russia	–	34,701,531
7.	Egypt	–	28,192,861
8.	Turkey	–	23,819,781
9.	Iran	–	21,183,488
10.	Nigeria	–	20,997,494

Source of Data; Renew Bariatrics, 2017.

Top 10 Countries with most obese population percentage in order of ranking as of July 1st, 2017

1	Cook Islands	–	50.80%
2	Palau	–	47.60%
3	Nauru	–	45.60%
4	Samoa	–	43.40%
5	Tonga	–	43.30%
6	Niue	–	43.20%
7	Marshal Islands	–	42.80%
8	Qatar	–	42.30%
9	Kiribati	–	40.60%
10	Tuvalu	–	40.30%

Source of Data; Renew Bariatrics, 2017.

Top 10 Countries with least obese population percentage in order of ranking as of July 1st, 2017

1.	Central African Repoublic	–	5.10%
2.	India	–	4.90%
3.	Uganda	–	4.90%
4.	Somalia	–	4.60%
5.	Democratic Republic of the Congo	–	4.40%
6.	Niger	–	4.30%
7.	Eritrea	–	4.10%
8.	Rwanda	–	4.00%
9.	Bangladesh	–	4.00%
10.		–	3.60%

Source of Data; Renew Bariatrics, 2017.

The health risks associated with rising obesity being well aware universally; member states of WHO have introduced a voluntary target to stop the rise in obesity by 2025, (WHO 66.10, 2013) and also to address the issue by regular monitoring and assessing the trend in the prevalence of overweight and obesity in all populations (Swinburn BA, 2008, Cole TJ et al., 2000, Gortmaker SL et al., 2011).

Substantial rise in the prevalence of overweight and obesity with marked variations and distinct regional patterns across countries has been observed in the past three decades. Though the trend of increasing overweight and obesity is expected to continue in developing countries, as suggested by the fact that two in three of the world's obese people live in such countries, it has started gradually attenuating in the past 8 years in developed countries where increase in obesity that began in the 1980s (Emmanuela et al., 2014).

Excess adiposity/body weight is now widely recognized as one of today's leading health threats in most countries around the world and as a major risk factor for type 2 diabetes, cardiovascular disease, and hypertension (Fogel, 1986). Until the last decades of the 19th century, developed countries were still struggling with poverty, malnutrition, and communicable diseases. These health problems were considered a major cause of low industrial productivity (Fogel, 1997).

Until relatively recently, obesity was considered a condition associated with high socio-economic status. Indeed, early in the 20th century, most populations in which obesity became a public health problem were in the developed world primarily the United States and Europe. In more recent decades, available data shows that the most dramatic increases in obesity are in developing countries such as Mexico, China, and Thailand (Popkin and Gordon, 2004). The global nature of the obesity epidemic was formally recognized by a World Health Organization consultation in 1997 (WHO, 2004).

OBESITY: INDIAN SCENARIO

According to a study published in the noted journal *Lancet*, India is just behind the US and China in this global hazard list of top 10 countries with highest number of obese people (Emmanuela, 2014, Sharma, 2014)). Report of the first phase of the National Family Health Survey (NFHS-4) 2015-16 shows that among the males the highest obesity is observed in the population of Andaman and Nicober Union territory, followed by Goa, Andhra Pradesh, Sikkim, Punjab, Dadra & Nagar Haveli, Daman and Diu, Puducherry, Mizoram and Telangana in order of ranking. As for female population is concerned, the top 10 ranking States and Union territories are Chandigarh, Lakshadweep, Andhra Pradesh, Puducherry, Delhi, Goa, Punjab, Telangana, Tamil Nadu and Daman and Diu. The report also clearly reveals that in all the states and Union Territories, the number of obese women almost doubled that of males. On comparing the report of NHFS 4 with that of NFHS 3 and NFHS 2, the percentage of overweight and obese population has risen substantially in India during the last one and a half decade among the female population. The overweight and obese population increased by almost 60% and 80% respectively among the females during the said period. As for male population is concerned, a marked increase of almost 90% for overweight population and 400% for obese population is seen during the last decade.

Top 10 States/Union Territory of India with most obese population Percent in order of ranking, 2015-2016

Ranking	Most obese male population		Most obese female population	
	State/ Union Territory	Percentage	State/ Union Territory	Percentage
1	Andaman & Nicobar	8.1	Chandigarh	14.9
2	Goa	7.7	Lakshadweep	14.6
3	Andhra Pradesh	7.7	Andhra Pradesh	10.3
4	Sikkim	5.9	Puducherry	10.2
5	Punjab	5.1	Delhi	10.1
6	Dadra & Nagar Haveli	4.8	Goa	9.9
7	Daman & Diu	4.8	Punjab	9.2
8	Puducherry	4.8	Telangana	8.6
9	Mizoram	4.8	Tamil Nadu	8.3
10	Telangana	4.8	Daman & Diu	8.1

Source: NFHS data.

Top 10 States/Union Territory of India with least obese population Percent in order of ranking, 2015-2016

Ranking	Least obese male population		Least obese female population	
	State/ Union Territory	Percentage	State/ Union Territory	Percentage
1	Jharkhand	1.2	Meghalaya	1.7
2	Nagaland	1.3	Jharkhand	2.1
3	Bihar	1.3	Assam	2.1
4	Meghalaya	1.4	Bihar	2.2
5	Chhattisgarh	1.4	Tripura	2.4
6	Uttar Pradesh	1.6	Chhattisgarh	2.4
7	Madhya Pradesh	1.6	Nagaland	2.7
8	Tripura	1.7	Arunachal Pradesh	2.9
9	Assam	1.7	Madhya Pradesh	3.1
10	West Bengal	1.8	Rajasthan	3.3

Source: NFHS data.

Top 10 States/Union Territory of India with Normal BMI population Percent in order of ranking, 2015-2016

Ranking	Normal BMI male population		Normal BMI female population	
	State/ Union Territory	Percentage	State/ Union Territory	Percentage
1	Meghalaya	78.4	Meghalaya	75.7
2	Nagaland	74.7	Arunachal Pradesh	72.7
3	Mizoram	71.9	Nagaland	71.6
4	Arunachal Pradesh	71.1	Mizoram	70.6
5	Manipur	69.1	Sikkim	66.9
6	Haryana	68.7	Manipur	65.2
7	Tripura	68.4	Tripura	65.0
8	Jammu and Kashmir	68.0	Haryana	63.2
9	Lakshadweep	67.7	Chhattisgarh	61.4
10	Assam	66.4	Uttarakhand	61.1

Source: NFHS data.

While considering the Union territory and State-wise distribution of least obese population among the males, it is observed that Jharkhand has the least obese population followed by Nagaland, Bihar and Meghalaya. As for female population, the least is observed in Meghalaya followed by Jharkhand, Assam and Bihar. Interestingly almost all the States of North East India has a very high percentage of normal BMI ranging from 66.4% to 78.4% among the males and 65% to 75.8% among the females.

According to World Health Organization (WHO), many low-and middle-income countries are now facing a double burden of disease which means that while they continue to struggle with infectious disease and under-nutrition, they are also experiencing a sharp rise in non-communicable disease risk factors such as obesity and overweight. Several research findings reveals that obesity is rising during the last few decades and NFHS, 1998-199, 2005-2006 and 2015-2016 data confirms the trend. This could be a result of lifestyles changing over the years and is a confounder of a large number of non-communicable diseases," said Sutapa Agrawal, an epidemiologist with Public Health Foundation of India, a public-private initiative involving Indian and international academics, and state and central governments (Live Mint, 2016).

Obesity: Strategy for Management and Prevention

It is globally known fact that, excessive weight gain carries significant high mortality health risks diseases - cancers, diabetes, heart diseases and strokes. And it is not a time to keep watching the menace, allowing ourselves to be controlled by a "pandemic" but to address it through timely intervention. Swinging back the pendulum for achieving a healthier bodyweight and desirable BMI level is the need of the hour so as to prevent from undesirable morbid condition. For the last few decades, numerous scientists and organizations around the world have worked tirelessly to address the issue of obesity though with only modest success. Continuous efforts are needed for improving and standardizing strategic planning for fighting this pandemic issue.

One of the most effective steps is changing the "obesogenic" environment toward reducing obesity. Reducing the excess caloric intake and equalizing it with energy expenditure by way of increasing physical activities is one of the best ways to fight obesity. There is no single or simple solution to the obesity epidemic. So this complex problem can be addressed by a multifaceted approach. Policy makers, state and local organizations, business and community leaders, civil society organizations, educational institutions, childcare and healthcare professionals, and individuals must put their heads together and work together to create an environment that supports a healthy lifestyle. To reverse the obesity epidemic, community efforts should focus on supporting healthy eating and active living in a variety of settings. Learn about different efforts that can be used in early childhood care, hospitals, schools, and food service venues (CDC, 2015). There are several ways by which state and local organizations and NGOs and Government allied system can create a supportive environment and awareness to the general public to promote healthy living behaviours that prevent obesity. The etiology of obesity is multifaceted; there are factors from multiple contexts, and interactions between factors that led to obesity are not yet well understood (Jhanet al.,

2010). Indeed, a comprehensive approach is needed to potentially reverse the global pandemic of obesity (Jhanet al., 2010, Reed, 2011). Globally, there is also solid consensus on the steps taken up to stop the obesity epidemic which were outlined in the Food and Agriculture Organization/World Health Organization global strategy for the prevention of diet-related chronic diseases (WHO, 2003). Researchers and medical scientists can also play major roles by researching the epidemiology and etiology of obesity in order to fight this pandemic issue.

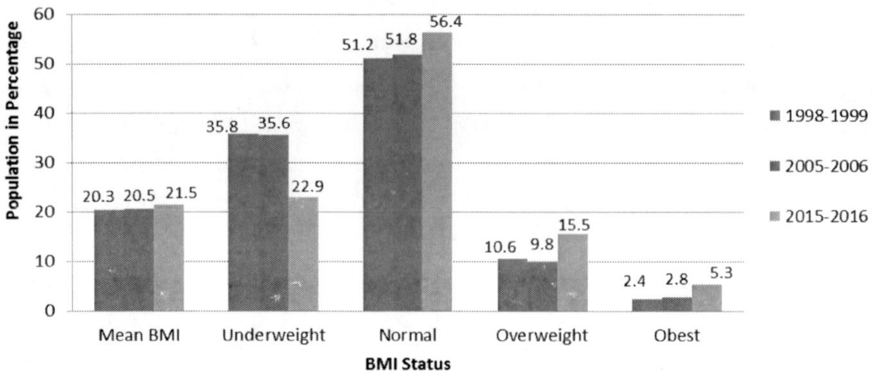

Source of Data: NFHS.

Figure 1. BMI Trend of Indian Women Population Observed from 1998 to 2016.

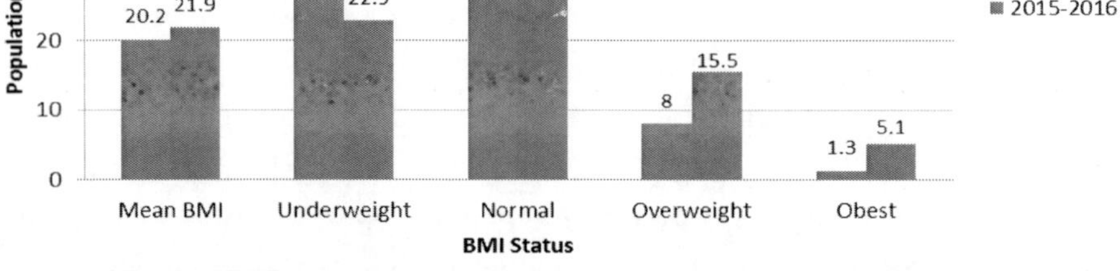

Source of Data: NFHS.

Figure 2. BMI Trend of Indian Male Population Observed from 2005 to 2016.

REFERENCES

Astrup A, Brand-Miller J. Diet composition and obesity. *Lancet* 2012; 379: 1100–01.

Benjamin Caballero. *The Global Epidemic of Obesity*: An Overview *Epidemiologic Reviews*, 2007, 29(1) 1–5.

Blackburn H, Luepker R. Heart disease. In: Last, SM (ed). *Maxcy-Rosenau Public Health and Preventive Medicine. 12th ed.* Norwalk, Conn. Appleton Century-Crofts, 1986, 1159-93.

Blair SN, Archer E, Hand GA. Commentary: Luke and Cooper are wrong: physical activity has a crucial role in weight management and determinants of obesity. *Int J Epidemiol*2013; 42: 1836–38.

Bleich S, Cutler D, Murray C, Adams A. Why is the developed world obese? *Annu Rev Public Health* 2008; 29: 273–95.

CDC, Overweight and Obesity: Strategies to Prevent Obesity, Centre for Disease Control and Prevention, 2015. https://www.cdc.gov/obesity/strategies/index.html?s_cid=tw_ob063 (Retrieved on 2/7/18, 11.30 pm).

Cole TJ, Bellizzi MC, Flegal KM, Dietz WH. Establishing a standard definition for child overweight and obesity worldwide: international survey. *BMJ* 2000; 320: 1240–43.

Drewnowski A, Popkin BM. The nutrition transition: new trends in the global diet. *Nutr Rev* 1997; 55: 31–43.

Emmanuela Gakidout, Murray J L, Lopez A Det. al; Global, regional, and national prevalence of overweight and obesity in children and adults during 1980–2013: a systematic analysis for the Global Burden of Disease Study 2013, *The Lancet*, 2014, 384(766-781).

Fogel RW, Engerman SL, Gallman RE; Nutrition and the decline in mortality since 1700: somepreliminary findings *Long-term Factors in American Economic Growth* 1986 Chicago, IL University of Chicago Press (439-555).

Fogel RW. The global struggle to escape from chronic malnutrition since 1700, Rome, Italy, *Proceedings of the World Food Programme/United Nations University Seminar. 1997.*

Gortmaker SL, Swinburn BA, Levy D, et al., Changing the future of obesity: science, policy, and action. *Lancet* 2011; 378: 838–47.

Haslam D (March 2007). "Obesity: a medical history." *Obes Rev* 8 Suppl 1: 31–6 https://www.livemint.com/Politics (retrieved on 4/7/18. 4.30 pm).

Jhan, J C, Lawlor, D A and Kimm, S Y. "Childhood obesity," *The Lancet*, 2010, 375(9727), 1737–1748.

Lau DCW. Call for action: preventing and managing the expansive and expensive obesity epidemic. *Can. Med. Assoc. J.*, 1999; 160:503-5.

Lim SS, Vos T, Flaxman AD, et al., A comparative risk assessment of burden of disease and injury attributable to 67 risk factors and risk factor clusters in 21 regions, 1990–2010: a systematic analysis for the Global Burden of Disease Study 2010. *Lancet* 2012; 380: 2224–60.

Live Mint. Obesity rising in most states covered by *National Family Health Survey*, 2016.

Mandal, S K. Obesity: An invited disease, *Everyman's Science*, 2010, XLV(3) 161-165.

Mendez MA, Monteiro CA, Popkin BM. Overweight exceeds underweight among women in most developing countries, *Am J ClinNutr*, 2005, vol. 81 (pg. 714-21).

Nanan D J. The Obesity Pandemic - Implications for Pakistan, *Journal of Pakistan Medical Association*, 2002, http://www.jpma.org.pk/full_article_text.php?article_id=2356 (retrieved on 5/7/2018, 3.35 pm).

NFHS-2 (1998-1999); *National Family Health Survey – 2*, International Institute for Population Sciences, Mumbai.

NFHS-3 (2005-2006); *National Family Health Survey –3*, International Institute for Population Sciences, Mumbai.

NFHS-4 (2015-2016); *National Family Health Survey – 4*, International Institute for Population Sciences, Mumbai.

Olshansky SJ, Passaro DJ, Hershow RC, et al., A potential decline in life expectancy in the United States in the 21st century. *N Engl J Med* 2005; 352: 1138–45.

Popkin BM, Gordon-Larsen P. The nutrition transition: worldwide obesity dynamics and their determinants, *Int J Obes Relat Metab Disord*, 2004, 28 supp l (S2-9).

Popkin BM, Adair LS, Ng SW. Global nutrition transition and the pandemic of obesity in developing countries. *Nutr Rev,* 2012; 70: 3–21.

Popkin BM. The nutrition transition and obesity in the developing world. *J Nutr* 2001; 131: 871S–73S.

Reed, D B, Patterson, P J and Wasserman, N. "Obesity in rural youth: looking beyond nutrition and physical activity," *Journal of Nutrition Education and Behavior*, 2011, 439(50), 401–408.

Renew Bariatrics. *Report: Obesity Rates by Country*, 2017, https://renewbariatrics.com/obesity-rank-by-countries/ (retrieved on 4/7/18 10 am).

Roth J, Qiang X, Marban SL, Redelt H, Lowell BC. The obesity pandemic: where have we been and where are we going? *Obes Res* 2004; 12 (suppl 2): 88S–101S.

Sandra G. Affenito, Debra L. Franko, Ruth H. Striegel-Moore, Douglas Thompson, Behavioral Determinants of Obesity: Research Findings and Policy Implications. *Journal of Obesity,* 2012, (1-4).

Sharma Neetu Chandra https. I*ndia the third most obese country in the world, 2014* www.indiatoday.in/mail-today/story/obesity-india-weighs-third-on-obesity-scale-196126-2014-06-08 (Retrieved on 2/7/18, 11.50 pm).

Sorensen TIA, Soren ME. Obesity genes: identifying single genes involved in polygenic inheritance is not easy. *Br. Med. J.,* 2001; 322: 630-3 1.

Swinburn BA, Sacks G, Hall KD, et al., The global obesity pandemic: shaped by global drivers and local environments. *Lancet* 2011; 378: 804–14.

Swinburn BA. Obesity prevention: the role of policies, laws and regulations. *Aust N Z Health Policy* 2008; 5: 12.

Thorkhild I A, Sorinsen, DERMEDSCI. Changing lifestyle in the world, *Diabetes Care* 2000. 23(2) B1-B4.

WHO 66.10. *Follow-up to the Political Declaration of the High-level Meeting of the General Assembly on the Prevention and Control of Non-Communicable Diseases. Geneva, Switzerland, World Health Assembly, 2013*, http://http://apps.who.int/gb/ebwha/pdf_files/WHA66/A66_R10-en.pdf (retrieved on July 4, 2018, 10.30 pm).

WHO. *Consultation on Obesity*. Geneva, WHO, 1998.

WHO. *10 Facts on Obesity. World Health Organization* 2017b, http://www.who.int/features/factfiles/obesity/en/ (retrieved on2/7/18,11pm).

WHO. *Obesity and Overweight: World Health Organization* 2017a, http://www.who.int/news-room/fact-sheets/detail/obesity-and-overweight, (retrieved on 2/7/18, 11 pm).

WHO. Obesity: preventing and managing the global epidemic. Report of a WHO consultation. *World Health Organ Tech Rep Ser* 2000; 894: i–xii, 1–253. www. who.int /nutrition /publications /obesity /WHO_TRS_894/en /(retrieved on July 4, 2018, 9.30 pm).

World Health Organization. *Obesity: Preventing and managing the global epidemic*. Report of a World Health Organization. *Obesity: preventing and managing the global epidemic, Report of a WHO Consultation*, 2000 Geneva, Switzerland World Health Organization (WHO technical report series 894).

World Health Organization/Food and Agriculture Organization of the United Nations. *Diet, nutrition and the prevention of chronic diseases, Report of a Joint WHO/FAO Consultation*, 2003 Geneva, Switzerland World Health Organization (WHO technical report series 916).

In: Obesity and Syndrome X
Editors: M. Das and K. Bose
ISBN: 978-1-53614-669-1

Chapter 13

OBESITY AND SYNDROME X

Anup Adhikari*
Anthropometrica, Toronto, Canada

Metabolic Syndrome is a group of health conditions like obesity, high blood pressure, high blood sugar, high serum triglycerides and low high density lipoprotein (HDL) level. This combination is also known as Syndrome X. Hence, metabolic syndrome is a group of risk factors but not a disease. The main sign of metabolic syndrome is obesity. Obesity goes together with unhealthy level of cholesterol, high blood pressure and excess blood sugar (Ganong 2008).

Obesity turned into epidemic and became a public health challenge throughout the world. In past few years, the prevalence of obesity has been increased significantly across the world no matter whether it is a developed or developing or underdeveloped country. According to World health Organization, more than 1.9 billion adults aged 18 or older were reported overweight. Of these, over 650 million were obese. 39% of adults aged 18 year and over were overweight and 13% were obese in 2016 according to WHO report. 41 million children under the age of 5 were overweight or

* Corresponding Author Email: dranupadhikari@yahoo.com.

obese, whereas 340 million children and adolescent aged 5-19 were overweight or obese in 2016. Once considered to be a high-income country problem, overweight and obesity are now on the rise in low, and middle income countries also, particularly in urban settings (WHO 2012; Adhikari 2014; WHO 2018).

Obesity is a health problem associated with accelerated atherosclerosis and increased incidence of gall bladder and other diseases like type two diabetes. Not only that, recent studies reported death from many kinds of cancer in obese people. The causes for obesity in general population are due to multiple reasons. The primary cause of obesity is excess intake of energy over energy expenditure. The other causes are genetic and decrease sensitivity to leptin. Genetic factors are also responsible for obesity in some cases and causes excessive accumulation of body fat.Though, genetic tendency does not necessarily cause obesity, but it helps to accumulate more fat in right environment for the genetically susceptible individuals. A faulty gene or obese gene inside the fat cell produce Leptin, which after entering into blood, stimulates the hypothalamic area which controls the appetite and metabolism, causing fat accumulation. But genetic factors are not the reason for worldwide obesity epidemic. Instead, misbalance between energy intake and energy expenditure is the main reason for obesity (Frisch et al. 1987; Frisch et al. 1989; Bouchard et al. 1990; Stager & Halter 1995; Bouchard 1997; Fogelholm et al. 1998; Elchebly 1999).

While expressing body composition and related health risks of excessive body fat, three terms are used -over weight, overfat and obese. There is a confusion over the meaning of precise terms for overweight, overfat, and obese. Each term has a different meaning when using in different circumstances. Still there is a need to make a distinction between overweight, overfat and obese during interpretation. In most cases the term overweight is meant for an overfat condition even in the absence of accompanying body fat. Within this context, obesity then refers at the extreme of overweight continuum. This is precisely the frame of reference which is used to define the body fat range by means of BMI. Thus, weight -for-height at a given age has provided the most suitable index to express body fat and accompanying health risks. However, the overweight refers to a body weight greater than the average for stature. Overweight is not always due to presence of fat, it may be due to presence of muscle mass. For example, man with more muscle mass will be overweight (male power athletes). The overweight condition may or may not go with glucose intolerance, insulin resistance, dyslipidemia, and hypertension (e.g., physically fit overfat men and women). But obesity or overfat condition will go with one or all of the following components of the syndrome X like insulin resistance, glucose intolerance, dyslipidemia, type 2 diabetes, hypertension, high serum triglycerides, elevated plasma leptin concentrations, increased visceral adipose tissue, and increased risk of coronary heart disease and cancer etc. Syndrome X is related with excess body fat not with excess body weight which is due to more muscle mass or having more mesomorphic component which was revealed by different studies. Person may be overweight or overfat but does not have the syndrome X sign and symptoms. Men above 20% and women above 30% may be considered as overfat but it may vary population to population.

There are two types of regional fat distribution. When fat deposits more in abdominal area causing obesity, is called Android type obesity. This is particularly internal visceral deposition which is due to catecholamine secretion resulting lively lipolysis of tissues. The other type of deposition where fat deposit more in gluteal and femoral region, is called as Gynoid type obesity. The Android type obesity which causes deposition of more fat in central region causes heart disease. For men, percentage of visceral fat increases gradually with age, whereas in women, it starts at the onset of menopause. In Android-type obesity where fat deposits centrally, results risk of hyperinsulinemia, glucose intolerance, type 2 diabetics, hypertriglyceridemia, endometrial cancer, hypercholesterolemia and negative altered lipoprotein profile, hypertension, and atherosclerosis. The waist to hip ratio can be considered as an indicator of health risk when the ratio exceeds 0.80 for women and 0.95 for men. Excess fat distribution in abdomen area also increases the risk for colorectal cancer. Thus Android -type obesity has a greater risk than gynoid-type obesity where fat deposit at thighs and buttocks instead of central region of the body.

Less energy expenditure than energy intake causes fat accumulation which results body weight gain. Similarly when energy expenditure is more than energy intake causes weight loss. Thus three ways can reduce body weight. If calorie intake goes down below the daily energy requirement by dieting, it causes weight loss. Similarly, when energy expenditure exceed than normal calorie intake by means of physical activities causes weight loss. One more method, when reducing the daily calorie intake by dieting but increasing the daily energy expenditure by means of physical activities, causes weight loss.

Weight loss through dietary restriction for short period results more water and carbohydrate loss per unit weight loss than the loss of fat. But dieting by low carbohydrate for long period may have some adverse effects which are dehydration, frequent urination, muscle cramp, constipation, irregular menstruation etc. Studies reveal that long term maintenance of weight loss through dietary restriction could be followed by return of lost weight within few years once restriction is stopped. Though careful dieting results weight loss but it may cause loss of Fat Free Mass (FFM), lethargy, possible malnutrition, and depressed resting metabolism (Miller 1999; Jeffrey et al. 2000; National Task Force 2000).

The best way to reduce body weight or excess body fat is regular physical exercise. Increased physical activity with dietary restriction causes weight loss more effectively than long term caloric restriction alone. Aerobic exercise and resistance training are more effective for weight loss for obese population. Aerobic exercise reduces the amount of fat and resistance training increase muscle strength and muscle mass which ultimately increase Fat Free Mass (FFM). Studies revealed that 40 -50 min aerobic exercise comprises of running and jogging for five days a week for 3-4 months significantly reduces excess body fat for obese population (vanEtten et al. 1994; Kraemer et al. 1995; Owens et al. 1999). Active children gain more Fat Free Mass (FFM) and loss total fat compare to their inactive children. Similarly, adolescent males who do regular aerobic exercise, reduce total body fat significantly faster than their sedentary counterparts.

Aerobic exercise or endurance run very effective for the obese population to reduce excess body weight by burning excess body fat. Endurance run or aerobic exercises increase the aerobic metabolism where energy releases from the breakdown of carbohydrate and fat in the presence of oxygen.. Walking, jogging, running, biking, aerobic dances are the best examples of aerobic exercises which help the obese people to reduce fat as well improve cardiovascular fitness, reduce syndrome X risk factors. While walking, it is recommended for more than one hours walking with fast pace for 3-4 days in a week. If someone wants jogging, it is recommended to walk first, then after few weeks start jogging and then running gradually. Biking is also very good aerobic exercise. Obese people also can join with aerobic dance program in a gymnasium which is also an effective aerobic exercise for reducing excess body fat. Dancing is also an effective aerobic exercise. But before starting any exercise program, one must see the family physician if they already have syndrome X rich factors and should take the physicians advice before any aerobic exercise program.

To fight against the obesity epidemic, promotion of aerobic exercise is needed which will increase the total energy expenditure significantly and regularly rather than increase exercise intensity.An obese person can expend more calories if he or she starts with slow walking or jogging with simply extending for long duration as duration of exercise significantly affects fat loss. It is important to note that recommended aerobic exercise should be minimum 3 days in week to have a good impact on fat loss. Regular aerobic exercise delay lean tissue loss, while resistance training increases Fat Free Mass. To combat against obesity and syndrome X, aerobic exercise should be popularized more and more across the world.

References

Adhikari A. 2014. Prevalence of obesity among immigrants living in Canada. *American Journal of Sports Science and Medicine.* 2; 35-39.

Bouchard C. et al. 1990. The response to long term feeding in identical twins. *N Engl J Med.* 322; 1447.

Bouchard C. 1997. Human variation in body mass: evidence for a role of the genes. *Nutr Rev*. 55:S21.

Elchebly M.et al. 1999. Increased insulin sensitivity and obesity resistance in mice lacking the tryosine phosphate-1B gene. *Science*. 283; 1544.

Fogelholm M. et al. 1998. Addictive effects of mutations in the beta-adrenergic receptor and uncoupling protein-1 genes on weight loss and weight maintenance of Finish women. *J.Clin Endocrinol Metabol*. 8:42.

Frisch, RE. et al. 1987. Lower life time occurrence or breast cancer and cancer of the reproductive system among former college athletes. *American Journal of Clinical Nutrition*. 45:328.

Frisch RE, et al. 1989. Lower prevalence of non-reproductive cancer among female former college athletes. *Med Sci Sports Exerc*. 21:250.

Jeffrey RW, et al. 2000. Long-term maintenance of weight loss: current status. *Health Psychol* 19(1 suppl):5.

Kraemer WJ, et al. 1995. Compatibility of high intensity strength and endurance training on hormonal and skeletal muscle adaptations. *J. Appl Physiol*, 78:976.

Miller WC. 1999. How effective are traditional dietary and exercise interventions for weight loss? *Med Sci Sports Exerc*. 31:1129.

National task force on the prevention and treatment of Obesity. 2000. *Obesity, Overweight and Health Risk*. aRCHiNTERM mED,160:898.

Owens S. et al. 1999. Effect of Physical training on total and visceral fat in obese children. *Med Sci Sports Exerc*. 31:143.

Stager JM, Halter LK. 1995. Menarche in athletes: the influence of genetics and prepubertal training. *Med Sci Sports Exerc*. 27:1450.

vanEtten LMLA et al. Effect of body build on weight training induced adaptation in body composition and muscle strength. *Med Sci Sports Exerc*, 26:515, 1994.

William F.Ganong, *Review of Medical Physiology,* Tata McGraw-Hill Publishing Company Limited, New Delhi, 2008.

World Health Organization (WHO), *Global Database on Body Mass Index*. Available from http://www.who.int/mediacentre/factsheets/fs311/en/2018.

World Health Organization (WHO), *Obesity and overweight, Fact sheet No 311,* May 2012. www.who.int/mediacentre/factsheets/fs311/en/index.html, 2012.

In: Obesity and Syndrome X
Editors: M. Das and K. Bose
ISBN: 978-1-53614-669-1

Chapter 14

SYNDROME X: SOME COMMON DETERMINANTS WORLDWIDE

***Mithun Das*[1,*] *and Kaushik Bose*[2]**
[1]Department of Anthropology,
Sree Chaitanya College, Habra, West Bengal, India
[2]Department of Anthropology,
Vidyasagar University, Midnapore, West Bengal, India

Syndrome X or Metabolic Syndrome (MetS) is defined as a constellation of several cardiovascular disease (CVD) risk factors including genetic and environmental factors that is responsible for ultimate predisposition of the disease (Grundy 2005). The constellation of centrally distributed obesity; decreased high density lipoprotein cholesterol (HDLc); elevated triglycerides; elevated blood pressure and hyperglycemia is known as the MetS. Persons with MetS are at twice the risk for CVD compared with those without the syndrome. It further raises the risk for type 2 diabetes mellitus (T2DM) by about five-fold (Zimmet et al., 2005; Grundy et al., 2008). This chapter will highlight the common

* Corresponding Author Email: mithundas01@yahoo.com.

determinants/factors associated with Syndrome X worldwide, which include: Family history of chronic diseases, Physical Inactivity, Dietary Intake of Fatty Acids, and Epigenetic Modifications.

Family History of Chronic Diseases

Most of the common chronic diseases are the result of interactions between multiple genetic variants and environmental vis-à-vis lifestyle factors. Although there have been significant advances in the last decade in the understanding of our genome, there are certain limitations in epidemiological and analytic approaches to studying the effects of chronic diseases. Family history has been shown to be a risk factor for a majority of chronic diseases of public health significance, including Syndrome X, CVD, diabetes etc. Family history of specific diseases reflects the consequences of genetic susceptibility, shared environment and common behaviors (Yoon et al., 2002). Family history has been recognized in clinical medicine as an important, yet non-modifiable, disease risk factor that when present could influence the probability of a suspected diagnosis. However, collection and interpretation of family history has rarely been applied in the practice of preventive medicine to assess disease risk and influence early detection and prevention strategies (Scheuner et al., 1997; Williams et al., 2001). The advantages of family history over other genomic tools include a lower cost, greater acceptability, and a reflection of shared genetic and environmental factors. However, the utility of family history in public health has been poorly explored (Valdez et al., 2010). Professional guidelines usually include family history to assess health risk, initiate interventions, and motivate behavioral changes.

Family history of diabetes is not only a risk factor for the disease but is also positively associated with risk awareness and risk- reducing behaviors. It may provide a useful screening tool for detection and prevention of diabetes (Hariri et al., 2006). In a study among the adult Chinese, it was found that sufficient physical activity and negative family history of diabetes might jointly reduce the risk of developing hyperglycemia and

T2DM (Xu et al., 2011). In the US population, family history of diabetes showed significant, independent, and graded association with the prevalence of diabetes. This association not only highlights the importance of shared genes and environment in diabetes but also opens the possibility of formally adding family history to public health strategies aimed at detecting and preventing the disease (Valdez et al., 2007). In another study on a nationally representative sample of US adults without diabetes, family history of diabetes showed a significant, independent association with syndrome X and its traits. This association supports the idea that shared genes and environment contribute to the expression of complex traits such as diabetes and syndrome X (Ghosh et al., 2010). Evidence suggests that family history by itself is most useful for predicting disease when there are multiple family members affected, the relationship among relatives is close, and disease is premature, that is, it occurs at younger ages than would be expected. It has been mentioned that family history information in combination with other known risk factors could be used to provide more personalized information about our risk for common diseases (Yoon et al., 2002). Moreover, it has been suggested that adding family history of diabetes could provide significant improvements in detecting undiagnosed diabetes (Yang et al., 2010). In an another study, it was found that not only the adults, even the youths with a positive family history showed signs of increased risk for these conditions which indicates the importance of family history approach to screening for children at risk of diabetes and CVD (Valdez et al., 2007). In a study from India, it was found that individuals with positive family history of diabetes had significantly higher prevalence of syndrome X and its confounding factors as compared to their counterparts (Das et al., 2012).

It suggests that family history could be used as a tool for genomic studies among the Asian Indians as well as in other world populations. It is however reasonable to argue that in developing countries including India, a large section of the community remains undiagnosed and therefore accuracy of self-reported family history could be challenging. In addition to risk assessment, family history information can be used to personalize health messages, which are potentially more effective in promoting healthy lifestyles than standardized health messages (Janssens et al., 2012). Having a family history of a disease increases its salience and does not change one's perceived ability to prevent the disease (Acheson et al., 2010). To establish family history as a public health tool, it needs to be evaluated within the ACCE (analytical validity; clinical validity; clinical utility; and ethical, legal, and social issues) framework. These advances will help realize the potential of family history as a public health tool (Valdez et al., 2010). It seems that population screening would be of substantial importance for further research as family history of chronic diseases plays a vital role in better understanding of the etiological factors related to such complex traits, and hence could be used as a tool for preventive strategies.

Physical Inactivity

The identification and modification of the root cause, overweight/obesity, physical inactivity, and the closely associated condition - syndrome X, needs to be one of the initial strategies that are addressed by the clinician (Borgman et al., 2006). Each component of syndrome X predisposes people to atherosclerosis, and when clustered together, these components promote atherosclerosis even more prominently. It has been found that lifestyle modification, such as physical activity level (PAL) and dietary habits reduces the risk of syndrome X (Yao et al., 2003; Katzmarzyk et al., Panagiotakos et al., 2004).

Studies have shown that sedentary lifestyle could predict the development of syndrome X. Both vigorous and moderate leisure-time activities were found to be beneficial to the metabolic syndrome cluster of cardiovascular risk factors among the adult men and women of U.K It was suggested that even modest increases in physical activity was worthwhile in public health targets (Rennie et al., 2003). In a study from India, it was found that individuals with low physical activity level (PAL) had much higher prevalence of MetS than individuals with moderate PAL. The lowest prevalence was observed among the individuals with high PAL (Das et al., 2012). It has been evidenced that Asian Indians who are physically active have a favorable metabolic profile which highlights the need to encourage physical activity in Asian Indian immigrants, particularly women, to reduce prevalence of MetS (Misra et al., 2005). Physical inactivity has also been found to be associated with the components of MetS and coronary artery disease (CAD) among the urban south Indian population. Lifestyle changes focusing on increasing physical activity supposed to prevent the exploding epidemic of MetS and CAD in India (Mohan et al., 2005).

The China National Nutrition and Health Survey (2002) reported that individuals who were active or very active were 40% less likely to have MetS compared with those who were leading sedentary life (Ma et al., 2008). Among the middle-aged and old Chinese adults, physically active individuals were found to have been associated with a better profile of inflammatory factors and adipocytokines and a reduced risk of having MetS (Zhijie et al., 2009). In a Finnish cohort study, baseline total leisure-time physical activity was found to be inversely associated with the risk of developing MetS during a 4-year follow-up (Laaksonen et al., 2002). In an another study among the adult men and women of Chinese Taipei, it was also found high amount of physical activity was inversely correlated with the left ventricular hypertrophy (LVH) and prevalence of MetS (Dao et al., 2009). Moderate and vigorous physical leisure-time activities were each associated with reduced risk of being classified with MetS independently of age, smoking, and high alcohol intake both among the U.S. men and women (Rennie et al., 2003). Total physical activity (measured as habitual energy expenditure) and fitness (measured as maximal oxygen consumption per kilogram) shown to have independent effects on the components of MetS (Wareham et al., 1998). It has been found that insulin action could be modulated by body weight and physical fitness which is a core feature of MetS (Reaven 2001). It therefore seems that modulation of MetS is a plausible biological pathway through which physical inactivity may affect cardiovascular health.

To prevent increasing morbidity and mortality due to obesity-related diabetes and CVD in developing countries, there seems to be an urgent need to initiate large-scale community intervention programs focusing on increased physical activity and healthier food options (Misra & Khurana 2008). In the World Health Survey (2002– 2003), data of 212,021 adults from 51 countries, most of which were from developing countries showed that about 15% of men and 20% of women were at risk for chronic diseases due to physical inactivity (Guthold et al., 2008). Among the Asian Indian immigrants living in U.S (Misra et al., 2005) as well as those living in Indian (Mohan et al., 2005) it was found that physical inactivity was highly associated with MetS phenotypes. Although at what intensity activity may be of benefit in reducing the risk of MetS is not yet clearly understood, but one thing is clear that active lifestyle could curb this epidemic of obesity related metabolic disorders.

DIETARY INTAKE OF FATTY ACIDS

Lack of habitual physical activity and certain dietary patterns, including high saturated fatty acids (SFA) and low vegetable intakes, contribute to weight gain and increase the risk of metabolic disturbances (Feskens et al., 1995). Saturated fat intake is associated with increased risk of coronary heart disease (CHD); the greatest risk reduction is associated with poly unsaturated fatty acids (PUFA) followed by mono unsaturated fatty acids (MUFA) (Kris-Etherton et al., 2001). In Asian Indians, there existed significant inverse association between central obesity measures and intake of unsaturated fatty acids due to recent shift in dietary habits causing an increase in the prevalence of obesity and dyslipidemia in this region. It was that intake of saturated fat may be a major risk factor for the onset of MetS in adult Asian Indians. Moreover, it appears that it is not the total fat but the amount of saturated fat consumed in association with TFA:SFA, SFA:MUFA, and SFA:PUFA was adversely affecting the adiposity level, lipids, blood pressures, and blood glucose levels in this population and in turn cumulatively enhancing the possibility to predispose to MetS phenotypes ((Ghosh 2006; Ghosh 2007; Das et al., 2010). The findings of an adverse impact of TFA:SFA intake and inverse relation of adiposity with PUFA, i.e., protection of polyunsaturated fat concerning the association with MetS is in accordance with the finding of several other investigations (Das et al., 2010).

Certain dietary patterns, including high SFA and low vegetable intake, contribute to weight gain and increase the risk of metabolic disturbances, whereas such potentially modifiable lifestyle factors may reduce cardiovascular risk (Feskens et al., 1995; van Dam et al., 2002). In a study from India revealed that increased dietary ω-6 PUFA and saturated fat intake are significantly associated with fasting hyperinsulinemia and subclinical inflammation, respectively, and found to be responsible for the increasing prevalence of insulin resistance, the MetS and diabetes (Feskens et al., 1995; Misra & Misra 2003; Misra & Khurana 2009; Ghosh 2009). In another study, it was found that the dietary total fat may increase whereas linoleic acid intake may reduce the risk of MetS in Japanese descendants living in Brazil (Cardoso et al., 2005). Study from the United Arab Emirates (UAE) pointed out that poor dietary habits including consumption of high-energy foodstuffs, diets high in total carbohydrates, fat, and simple sugars were associated with MetS (Al-Sarraj et al., 2010). In a multiethnic study (comprising of African-Americans, Whites and Hispanics) on healthy children aged 7–12 years revealed that diet composition was more closely related to the components of the MetS than was physical activity, with carbohydrate intake being adversely related to WC, TG levels, and glucose levels. Moreover, relationships among diet and MetS outcomes were stronger among African-American children (Casazza et al., 2009) reflecting ethnic variation. It seems that while dealing with MetS in Asian Indians, or any world populations, researchers and clinicians should consider obesity measures, metabolic profiles and dietary fatty acids simultaneously. Since it is not the amount of calorie intake but the amount of fatty acids which seems to be associated with obesity related metabolic disorders.

Epigenetic Modifications

The term epigenetics itself describes the concept as 'epi' means above and it was Conrad Waddington who, in 1940, provided the first broad and operational definition of epigenetics as "the causal interactions between genes and their products, which bring the phenotype into being" (Waddington 1940). Epigenetics has been defined as the study of heritable changes in gene expression that occur in the absence of a change in the DNA sequence itself. In mammals, these changes are mediated through DNA methylation, covalent histone modifications, microRNA, and polycomb group complex recruitment (Dolinoy 2008; Schwartz & Pirrotta., 2008). The epigenetic marks either alone or in combination alter the chromatin structure and function, and thereby promote or inhibit gene transcription. Therefore, chromatin is the ideal substrate for nutrient-sensitive transcriptional instructions, existing in multiple permutations leading to multiple phenotypes. In addition, the epigenetic state of chromatin can undergo transgenerational epigenetic inheritance, a process facilitated by the incomplete erasure of epigenetic modifications during gametogenesis and embryogenesis, resulting in a maintained epigenetic state in future generations (Bruce & Hanson 2010).

Susceptibility to Syndrome X has an inherited or familial component. Although some fixed genomic variations have been associated with high risk but such single nucleotide polymorphisms attribute very little to the overall risk in the population (Gluckman et al., 2007). Whereas, subtle alterations in gene expression are responsible for an increased risk of disease outcome in many members of the population to a variable extent, rather than genomic alterations, such as those involved in placental nutrient transport. In recent years, epigenetic regulation leading to such subtle modulations in gene expression (without a change in DNA sequence) of key metabolic genes has emerged as a contributing factor to increased susceptibility to Syndrome X (Bruce & Hanson 2010).

Positive natural selection describes the increase in the prevalence of beneficial traits in a population, and is one of the factors driving evolution. A trait under positive selection must be beneficial, thus increasing survival and reproduction, and the trait must also be heritable. This positive selection has been attributed to particular DNA variants that become more common since of the beneficial effects on those who carry them (Kelley & Swanson 2008). However, a trait that may be advantageous at one point in human history may be detrimental under different environmental conditions. Here comes the classic example of *'thrifty genotype*,' a concept coined by the geneticist James Neel to explain the prevalence of obesity and diabetes (Neel 1962). Neel hypothesized that people with diabetes often have allelic variations in certain genes that enable them to efficiently collect and utilize food. The human variations which were favorable in populations facing challenges of episodic undernutrition might be disadvantageous when food supplies became abundant. It provides a possible explanation for why the propensity to diabetes varies greatly among populations. Carriers of these variations are, therefore, at a high risk of developing obesity and diabetes when exposed to abundant and cheap supply of energy, and a dramatic reduction in energy expenditure. This thrifty genotype would have been beneficial during periods of history characterized by food instability (Stoger 2008). In contrast to the long-term nature of the selective forces that are hypothesized to have positively selected the thrifty genotype, epigenetic changes occur rapidly to alter metabolism. There are ways in which epigenetic changes increase disease risk, perhaps in combination with evolutionarily mediated phenotypes.

Throughout history, humans have had to cope with adverse environmental changes such as periods of plague or famine. Famines provide an ideal setting to examine the biological adaptation and long-term consequences of unfavorable conditions, especially during human development. One of the most well documented events is the Dutch Hunger during the winter of 1944–1945. It was suggested that epigenetic mechanisms underlie the increased incidence of Syndrome X in adults prenatally exposed to the Dutch famine and the transgenerational effects of prenatal exposure to the Dutch famine in the grandchildren of women exposed (Painter et al., 2008). A sex-specific increased risk of obesity, dyslipidemia, and cerebrocardiovascular-related deaths has been observed six decades later among those whose mothers were exposed to famine early in gestation (Kyle & Pichard 2006). The outcomes of these studies strongly support that *in utero* exposure to famine may result in adverse metabolic phenotypes, which depend on the sex of the exposed individual, and the timing of exposure during gestation as the embryo is more vulnerable around the time of conception. Similar observations inspired the Barker's hypothesis almost three decades ago, also known as the '*thrifty phenotype*' that malnutrition acts not as a selection acting over many generations to alter the genetic make-up of the population, rather the early environmental (including prenatal environment) influence acting in an individual to increase the susceptibility of the disease (Hales & Barker 2003).

In Neel's hypothesis, entire populations have an increased predisposition to diabetes due to genetic selection. They are better adapted to different nutritional circumstances than those they experience today. In Baker's hypothesis, maladaptive responses occur as a result of environmentally induced alteration of physiology in the early life of the individual. Both hypotheses offer explanations of why the frequency of diabetes and obesity differ in different populations. People in the Indian subcontinent, for example, have faced undernutrition for many generations, and Indian babies (new born) are among the smallest in the world (Yajnik 2003). However, diabetes epidemic is of recent origin, and it is more common among urban than rural Indians despite the higher birth weight of urban babies. The two explanations (hypotheses) are therefore not necessarily exclusive and may complement each other. Then there is a third hypothesis called the '*common soil*' hypothesis as proposed by Lebovitz (2006) that diabetes and CVD might share underlying cause(s) – hence termed common soil. It was mentioned that insulin resistance is central to the progression from normal glucose tolerance to diabetes and to a constellation of CVD risk factors known as Syndrome X. Changes in adipose tissue and metabolism (perhaps mediated through epigenetic changes) might link insulin resistance and visceral obesity – a condition that is common in diabetes.

Epigenetics may provide a mechanism by which developmental plasticity mediates developmental priming. Therefore, epigenetics may be the interface between nutritional stimuli during development and resulting phenotype, thus being central to the developmental origins of the Syndrome X (Bruce & Hanson 2010). The genomic information is the same in all our cells and during our entire lifespan, whereas, the epigenomic information varies from cell to cell and during the lifetime of the individual. An increased understanding of epigenetic mechanisms may lead to the development of novel and targeted therapies that will act not only at the risk-factor level, but also directly on the vascular system (Ordovas & Smith 2010). This makes epigenomic information more important for pharmacological interventions. In a recent epigenome wide association study (EWAS) it was found that methylation in *CPT1A* was significantly associated with syndrome X and it's confounding factors in both European and African ancestry participants. It indicated a promising epigenetic marker for metabolic disorder which could become useful for treatment target (Das et al., 2016).

Several compounds have been identified that are able to regulate DNA methyl transferase or histone deacetylase activity. DNA methylation is not just the driving force behind the developmental priming of disease but also a channel that transfers information of the transcriptional patterns required in a particular environment. Epigenetic modifications facilitate a transcriptional state, which may be inherited and may impart an increased risk of Syndrome X development in the context of unfavourable environmental conditions. Therefore, it is not the epigenetic landscape that is ultimately causal to the phenotype but the stimulus that it receives at the cellular level. This in part explains tissue-specific epigenetic modulations, because each particular tissue will receive specific stimuli and resides within a unique milieu (Bruce & Hanson 2010). Epigenetic control of key genes is central to the developmental priming of the metabolic syndrome (Syndrome X) phenotype, and provides a likely target for pharmacological therapies in near future.

REFERENCES

Acheson LS, Wang C, Zyzanski SJ, Lynn A, Ruffin MT 4th, Gramling R, et al., 2010. Family history and perceptions about risk and prevention for chronic diseases in primary care: A report from the family healthcare impact trial. *Genet Med.* 12:212-218.

Al-Sarraj T, Saadi H, Volek JS, Fernandez ML. 2010. Metabolic syndrome prevalence, dietary prevalence, dietary intake, and cardiovascular risk profile among overweight and obese adults 18-50 years old from the United Arab Emirates. *Metab Syndr Relat Disord*. 8:39-46.

Borgman M, McErlean E. 2006. What is the metabolic syndrome? Prediabetes and cardiovascular risk. *J Cardiovasc Nurs*. 21: 285-290.

Bruce KD, Hanson MA. 2010. The Developmental Origins, Mechanisms, and Implications of Metabolic Syndrome. *The Journal of Nutrition*. doi:10.3945/jn.109.111179: 648-652.

Cardoso RF, Gimeno SG, Ferreira SR. 2005. Dietary fat is associated with metabolic syndrome in Japanese Brazilians. *Diabetes Care*. 28: 1779-1785.

Casazza K, Dulin-Keita A, Gower BA, Fernandez JR. 2009. Differential influence of diet and physical activity on components of metabolic syndrome in a multiethnic sample of children. *J Am Diet Assoc*. 109: 236-244.

Dao-Fu Dai, Juey-Jen Hwang, Chi-Ling Chen et al., 2010. Effect of Physical Activity on the Prevalence of Metabolic Syndrome and Left Ventricular Hypertrophy in Apparently Healthy Adults. *J Formos Med Assoc*. 109: 716-724.

Das M, Pal S, Ghosh A. 2010. Association of metabolic syndrome with obesity measures, metabolic profiles, and intake of dietary fatty acids in people of Asian Indian origin. *J Cardiovasc Dis Res.* 1:130-135.

Das M, Pal S, Ghosh A. 2012. Interaction of Physical Activity level and Metabolic Syndrome among the adult Asian Indians living in Calcutta, India. *J Nutr Health Ageing*. 15: 539-543.

Das M, Pal S, Ghosh A. 2012. Family history of type 2 diabetes and prevalence of metabolic syndrome in adult Asian Indians. *J Cardiovasc Dis Res*. 3: 104-108.

Das M, Sha J, Hidalgo B et al., 2016. Association of DNA methylation at CPT1A locus with Metabolic Syndrome in the Genetics of Lipid Lowering Drugs and Diet Network (GOLDN) study. *PLoS One*. 11(1): e0145789.

Dolinoy DC. 2008. The agouti mouse model: an epigenetic biosensor for nutritional and environmental alterations on the fetal epigenome. *Nutr Rev*. 66 Suppl 1:S7–S11.

Feskens EJ, Virtanen SM, Räsänen L, Tuomilehto J, Stengård J, Pekkanen J, et al., 1995. Dietary factors determining diabetes and impaired glucose tolerance: A 20-year follow-up of the Finnish and Dutch cohorts of the Seven Countries Study. *Diabetes Care*. 18:1104-1112.

Ghosh A. 2006. Anthropometric, metabolic and dietary fatty acids profiles in lean and obese diabetic Asian Indian subjects. *Asia Pac J Clin Nutr*. 15:189-195.

Ghosh A. 2007. Comparison of anthropometric, metabolic and dietary fatty acids in lean and obese dyslipidemic Asian Indian male subjects. *Eur J Clin Nutr* 2007;61: 412-419.

Ghosh A. 2009. Obesity measures, metabolic syndrome and dietary fatty acids in lean and obese post-menopausal diabetes Asian Indian women. *Anthropol Anz*. 67: 83-93.

Ghosh A, Liu T, Khoury MJ, Valdez R. 2010. Family history of diabetes and prevalence of the metabolic syndrome in U. S. adults without diabetes: 6-year results from the National Health and Nutrition Examination Survey (1999-2004). *Public Health Genomics*. 13:353-259.

Gluckman PD, Hanson MA, Beedle AS. 2007. Non-genomic transgenerational inheritance of disease risk. *Bioessays*. 29: 145–154.

Grundy SM. 2005. A constellation of complications: the metabolic syndrome. *Clin Cornerstone*. 7: 36-45.

Grundy SM, Adams-Huet B, Vega GL. 2008. Variable contributions of fat content and distribution to metabolic syndrome risk factors. *Metab Syndr Relat Disord*. 6: 281-288.

Guthold R, Ono T, Strong KL, Chatterji S, Morabia A. 2008. Worldwide variability in physical inactivity a 51-country survey. *Am J Prev Med* 34: 486-494.

Hales CN, Barker DJP. 1992. Type 2 (non-insulin-dependent) diabetes mellitus: the thrifty phenotype hypothesis. *Diabetologia*. 35: 595-601.

Hariri S, Yoon PW, Qureshi N, Valdez R, Scheuner MT, Khoury MJ. 2006. Family history of type 2 diabetes: A population-based screening tool for prevention? *Genet Med*. 8:102-108.

Janssens AC, Henneman L, Detmar SB, Khoury MJ, Steyerberg EW, Eijkemans MJ, et al., 2012. Accuracy of self-reported family history is strongly influenced by the accuracy of self-reported personal health status of relatives. *J Clin Epidemiol*. 65: 82-89.

Katzmarzyk PT, Leon AS, Wilmore JH, et al., 2003. Targeting the metabolic syndrome with exercise: evidence from the HERITAGE Family Study. *Med Sci Sports Exerc*. 35: 1703–1709.

Kelley JL, Swanson WJ. 2008. Positive selection in the human genome: from genome scans to biological significance. *Annu Rev Genomics Hum Genet*. 9:143–160.

Kris-Etherton P, Daniels SR, Eckel RH, Engler M, Howard BV, Krauss RM, et al., 2001. Summary of the scientific conference on dietary fatty acids and cardiovascular health: Conference summary from the nutrition committee of the American heart association. *Circulation*. 103:1034-1039.

Kyle UG, Pichard C. 2006. The Dutch Famine of 1944–1945: a pathophysiological model of long-term consequences of wasting disease. *Curr Opin Clin Nutr Metab Care*. 9: 388–394.

Laaksonen DE, Lakka HM, Salonen JT et al., 2002. Low levels of leisure-time physical activity and cardiorespiratory fitness predict development of the metabolic syndrome. *Diabetes Care*. 25: 1612–1618.

Lebovitz HE. 2006. Insulin resistance – a common link between type 2 diabetes and cardiovascular disease. *Diabetes Obes Metab*. 8: 237-249.

Ma G, Luan D, Li Y et al., 2008. Physical activity level and its association with metabolic syndrome among an employed population in China. *Obes Rev*. 9(suppl):113–118.

Misra KB, Endemann SW, Ayer M. 2005. Leisure time physical activity and metabolic syndrome in Asian Indian immigrants residing in northern California. *Ethn Dis*.15:627-634.

Misra A, Khurana L. 2008. Obesity and the Metabolic Syndrome in Developing Countries. *J Clin Endocrinol Metab*. 93: s9-s30.

Misra A, Khurana L. 2009. The metabolic syndrome in South Asians: Epidemiology, determinants, and prevention. *Metab Syndr Relat Disord*. 7:497-514.

Misra A, Misra R. 2003. Asian Indians and insulin resistance syndrome: Global perspective. *Metab Syndr Relat Disord*.1:277-285.

Mohan V, Gokulakrishnan K, Deepa R et al., 2005. Association of physical inactivity with components of metabolic syndrome and coronary artery disease--the Chennai Urban Population Study (CUPS no. 15). *Diabet Med*. 22: 1206-1211.

Neel JV. 1962. Diabetes mellitus: a "thrifty" genotype rendered detrimental by "progress"? *Am J Hum Genet*. 14:353–362.

Ordovas JM, Smith CE. 2010. Epigenetics and cardiovascular disease. *Nat Rev Cardiol*. 7: 510-519.

Painter RC, Osmond C, Gluckman P, Hanson M, Phillips DI, Roseboom TJ. 2008. Transgenerational effects of prenatal exposure to the Dutch famine on neonatal adiposity and health in later life. *BJOG*. 115:1243–1249.

Panagiotakos DB, Pitsavos C, Chrysohoou C et al., 2004. Impact of lifestyle habits on the prevalence of the metabolic syndrome among Greek adults from the ATTICA study. *Am Heart J*. 147: 106–112.

Reaven G. 2001. Syndrome X. Current treatment. *Options in Cardiovascular Medicine* 2001; 3: 323–332.

Rennie KL, McCarthy N, Yazdgerdi S et al., 2003. Association of the metabolic syndrome with both vigorous and moderate physical activity. *Int J Epidemiol*. 32: 600-606.

Scheuner MT, Wang SJ, Raffel LJ, Larabell SK, Rotter JI. 1997. Family history: A comprehensive genetic risk assessment method for the chronic conditions of adulthood. *Am J Med Genet*. 71:315-324.

Schwartz YB, Pirrotta V. 2008. Polycomb complexes and epigenetic states. *Curr Opin Cell Biol*. 20:266–273.

Stöger R. 2008. The thrifty epigenotype: an acquired and heritable predisposition for obesity and diabetes? *Bioessays*. 30:156–166.

Valdez R, Yoon PW, Qureshi N, Green RF, Khoury MJ. 2010. Family history in public health practice: A genomic tool for disease prevention and health promotion. *Ann Rev Public Health*. 31:69-87.

Valdez R, Yoon PW, Liu T, Khoury MJ. 2007. Family history and prevalence of diabetes in the U. S. population: The 6-year results from the National Health and Nutrition Examination Survey (1999-2004). *Diabetes Care*. 30:2517-2522.

Valdez R, Greenlund KJ, Khoury MJ, Yoon PW. 2007. Is family history a useful tool for detecting children at risk for diabetes and cardiovascular diseases? A public health perspective. *Pediatrics*. 120 Suppl 2:S78-S86.

van Dam RM, Willett WC, Rimm EB, Stampfer MJ, Hu FB. 2002. Dietary fat and meat intake in relation to risk of type 2 diabetes in men. *Diabetes Care*. 25:417-424.

Waddington, CH. 1940. *Organisers and Genes*. Cambridge University Press; Cambridge.

Wareham NJ, Hennings SJ, Byrne CD et al., 1998. A quantitative analysis of the relationship between habitual energy expenditure, fitness and the metabolic cardiovascular syndrome. *Br J Nutr*. 80: 235–241.

Williams RR, Hunt SX, Heiss G, Province MA, Bensen JT, Higgins M, *e*t al., 2001. Usefulness of cardiovascular family history data for population-based preventive medicine and medical research (the Health Family Tree Study and the NHLBI Family Health Study). *Am J Cardiol*. 87:129-135.

Xu F, Wang Y, Ware RS, Tse LA, Dunstan DW, Liang Y, et al., 2011. Physical activity, family history of diabetes and risk of developing hyperglycaemia and diabetes among adults in mainland China. *Diabet Med*. 29: 593-599.

Yajnik CS. 2003. Early life origins of insulin resistance and type 2 diabetes in India and other Asian countries. *Diabetologia*. 46: 303-304.

Yao M, Lichtenstein AH, Roberts SB, et al., 2003. Relative influence of diet and physical activity on cardiovascular risk factors in urban Chinese adults. *Int J Obes Relat Metab Disord*. 27: 920–932.

Yang Q, Liu T, Valdez R, Moonesinghe R, Khoury MJ. 2010. Improvements in ability to detect undiagnosed diabetes by using information on family history among adults in the United States. *Am J Epidemiol*. 171:1079-1089.

Yoon PW, Scheuner MT, Peterson-Oehlke KL, Gwinn M, Faucett A, Khoury MJ. 2002. Can family history be used as a tool for public health and preventive medicine. *Genet Med*. 4:304-310.

Zhijie Yu, Xingwang Ye, Jing Wang et al., 2009. Associations of Physical Activity with Inflammatory Factors, Adipocytokines, and Metabolic Syndrome in Middle-Aged and Older Chinese People. *Circulation*. 119; 2969-2977.

Zimmet PZ, Alberti KG, Shaw JE. 2005. Mainstreaming the metabolic syndrome: a definitive definition. *Med J Aust*. 183: 175-176.

About the Editors

Mithun Das, PhD

Assistant Professor,
Department of Anthropology,
Sree Chaitanya College, Habra,
West Bengal, India
Email: mithundas01@yahoo.com

Dr. Mithun Das is an Assistant Professor at the Department of Anthropology, Sree Chaitanya College, Habra, West Bengal, India. He obtained his Bachelor of Science in Anthropology in 1998 and Master of Science in Anthropology in 2000 from the University of Calcutta. He obtained in PhD in Anthropology from Visva Bharati University, Santiniketan in 2011.

He was awarded the Raman Post-Doctoral Fellowship (2014-15) to study in the USA from the University Grants Commission, New Delhi, India. He worked as a Visiting Scientist at the Department of Epidemiology, School of Public Health, University of Alabama at Birmingham, AL, USA, under the mentorship of Prof. Donna K. Arnett on epigenetics of metabolic syndrome and related phenotypes.

His current interests include genetic, epigenetic and lifestyle factors related to ethnic variations in susceptibility to complex diseases like cardiovascular diseases, hypertension, diabetes and metabolic syndrome. To date he has over 20 publications in several peer reviewed journals (which include *PLoS One, Frontiers in Genetics, Journal of Nutrition Health and Ageing, Diabetes Research & Clinical Practice, American Journal of Human Biology, Human Biology, Journal of Cardiovascular Disease Research*, etc.*)* and one edited book.

Kaushik Bose, PhD, DSc

Professor,
Department of Anthropology, Vidyasagar University,
Midnapore, West Bengal, India
Email: kaushikbose@cantab.net

Dr. Kaushik Bose is a Professor at the Department of Anthropology, Vidyasagar University, India. He has been the recipient of several scholarships, fellowships and medals. He is a Member/Fellow of several professional bodies including Unit for the Biocultural Variation and Obesity, Oxford University. He was the recipient of a Commonwealth Scholarship and obtained his Ph.D. from Cambridge University in 1996. He was at Queens' College, Cambridge. Earlier he had obtained his PhD degree from Panjab University, India. He also worked as a Post-Doctoral Fellow at the Department of Nutrition and Dietetics, King's College London. He was awarded a DSc degree by Vidyasagar University in 2016.

He has published more than 260 research papers besides editing seven books. He is the editor of the *Journal of Life Sciences*. His research interests are anthropometry and body composition; particularly ethnic variation in health and disease.

He has undertaken collaborative research with several institutes including USAID, Tufts University, FHI360 (Washington, D.C.) and Polish Academy of Sciences, Wroclaw.

List of Contributors

Anup Adhikari, PhD
Exercise Physiologist, Personal Training Specialist and Nutrition & Wellness Specialist, Anthropometrica, Toronto, Canada

Saw Aik, MMed, FRCS
Professor, National Orthopaedic Centre of Excellence for Research and Learning, Department of Orthopaedic Surgery, Faculty of Medicine University of Malaya, Malayasia

Premananda Bharati, PhD
Professor (Retd.)
Biological Anthropology Unit, Indian Statistical Institute, Kolkata, India

Sampriti Debnath, MSc
Research Scholar, Department of Anthropology, University of North Bengal, Darjeeling, West Bengal, India

Thodam Bedita Devi, MSc
Medical Anatomy
Tutor, PhD Research Scholar, Department of Anatomy,
Sikkim Manipal Institute of Medical Sciences
Gangtok, India

Rodolfo F. Florentino, MD
Chairman-President, Nutrition Foundation of the Philippines,
Director, Food and Nutrition Research Institute,
Department of Science and Technology, Manila, Philippines

Jyoti Ratan Ghosh, PhD
Assistant Professor, Department of Anthropology, Visva-Bharati,
Santiniketan, West Bengal, India

Riddhi Goswami, PhD
Assistant Professor,
Department of Biotechnology, Heritage Institute of Technology, Kolkata,
India

Md. Golam Hossain, PhD
Professor, Health Research Group, Department of Statistics,
University of Rajshahi, Rajshahi, Bangladesh

Gabriel V. Jasul (Jr.), MD
Clinical Associate Professor, University of the Philippines College of
Medicine,
Head, Diabetes, Thyroid and Endocrine Center, St. Luke's Medical Center,
Quezon City, Philippines

Sylvia Kirchengast, PhD
Professor, Department of Anthropology, University of Vienna,
Vienna, Austria

Gautam K. Kshatriya, PhD
Professor,
Department of Anthropology,
University of Delhi,
Delhi, India

Rashidul Alam Mahumud, MPH
Senior Research Officer,
Health Economics and Financing Research Group,
Centre for Equity and Health System, International Centre for Diarrhoeal Disease Research, Bangladesh, Dhaka, Bangladesh

Suhaili Mohd., **MD**
National Orthopaedic Centre of Excellence for Research and Learning (NOCERAL)
Department of Orthopaedic Surgery, Faculty of Medicine University of Malaya, Kuala Lumpur, Malayasia

Nitish Mondal, PhD
Assistant Professor, Department of Anthropology, Assam University, Diphu Campus, Karbi-Anglong, Assam, India

Barun Mukhopadhyay, PhD
Professor, Biological Anthropology Unit, Indian Statistical Institute, Kolkata, India

Md. Sadekur Rahman, PhD
Professor, Health Research Group, Department of Statistics, University of Rajshahi, Rajshahi, Bangladesh

Ramanpreet Randhawa, MSc
Research Scholar, Department of Human Genetics, Guru Nanak Dev University, Amritsar, Punjab, India

Yacoob K. Seedat, MD
Emeritus Professor of Medicine, Department of Internal Medicine, University of KwaZulu-Natal,
Durban, South Africa

Jaydip Sen, PhD
Professor,
Department of Anthropology, University of North Bengal, Darjeeling, West Bengal, India

Sharda Sidhu, PhD
Professor (Retd.),
Department of Human Genetics, Guru Nanak Dev University, Amritsar, Punjab, India

Soibam Jibonkumar Singh, PhD
Professor,
Department of Anthropology, Manipur University, Manipur, India

Rosa Allyn G. Sy, MD
Director,
Research Development Innovation Division, Ospital ng Makati, Metro Manila, Head, Endocrinology, Diabetes, Metabolism and Nutrition Specialty Center, Cardinal Santos Medical Center, San Juan, Metro Manila, Philippines

Stanley Ulijaszek, PhD
Professor,
Institute of Social and Cultural Anthropology, Oxford University, UK

INDEX

A

activity level, 78, 81, 276, 286
Adhikari, vii, 265, 266, 269, 293
adipocyte, 181
adiponectin, 107, 185
adipose tissue, 6, 108, 112, 117, 174, 180, 189, 193, 267, 282
adiposity, vi, 14, 26, 28, 30, 31, 42, 49, 61, 66, 68, 71, 73, 75, 76, 82, 84, 89, 91, 92, 97, 99, 101, 103, 104, 106, 107, 112, 114, 115, 116, 117, 144, 169, 171, 172, 174, 175, 176, 177, 180, 184, 186, 187, 193, 194, 198, 215, 216, 217, 218, 219, 221, 255, 278, 287
adolescents, 23, 108, 109, 115, 116, 117, 144, 162, 179, 195, 232, 235, 253
adult obesity, 17, 160, 233, 247
adulthood, 234, 242, 244, 246, 250, 287
adults, 12, 16, 17, 18, 19, 20, 21, 23, 24, 25, 27, 33, 35, 36, 40, 56, 58, 64, 69, 70, 71, 85, 87, 91, 107, 108, 110, 114, 115, 116, 137, 143, 144, 159, 163, 164, 171, 172, 173, 174, 178, 179, 190, 191, 192, 197, 202, 210, 213, 214, 219, 223, 224, 230, 232, 234, 235, 238, 240, 241, 246, 249, 251, 252, 253, 261, 265, 275, 277, 278, 281, 284, 285, 287, 288, 289
Africa, v, 3, 7, 8, 10, 141, 166, 295
African Americans, 108, 279
alcohol consumption, 76, 82, 93, 105, 134, 199
Algeria, 147
angiotensin converting enzyme, 6
Angola, 141
anthropometry, 49, 67, 68, 165, 172, 177, 178, 180, 185, 194, 198, 199, 225, 230, 237, 243, 247, 292
Asia, v, 13, 16, 24, 26, 29, 34, 35, 36, 37, 116, 141, 159, 166, 197, 198, 216, 222, 225, 285
Asian Americans, 30, 31, 32, 34, 35, 191
Asian countries, 199, 288
atherosclerosis, 4, 20, 36, 113, 203, 211, 266, 267, 276
athletes, 267, 270
Australasia, 28
Austria, 143, 148, 149, 156, 165, 294

B

Bangladesh, vi, 117, 121, 123, 124, 128, 132, 134, 135, 136, 137, 141, 147, 165,
Bhutias, v, 73, 75, 76, 83, 84, 86
biological citizenship, 242
birth weight/birthweight, 145, 146, 147, 148, 149, 152, 153, 154, 155, 156, 157, 158, 161, 164, 165, 208, 209, 237, 282
Blacks, 7, 8, 10, 12
blood glucose, 21, 25, 76, 77, 169, 205, 207, 278
blood pressure, 11, 12, 14, 15, 19, 26, 74, 76, 86, 90, 91, 96, 97, 101, 102, 103, 104, 105, 107, 108, 109, 110, 115, 117, 118, 122, 123, 124, 128, 129, 132, 133, 134, 139, 140, 141, 170, 203, 204, 206, 225, 230, 234, 242, 265, 273, 278
body composition, 40, 42, 44, 45, 58, 60, 62, 63, 65, 70, 97, 98, 99, 100, 110, 111, 115, 172, 221, 266, 270
body fat, v, 24, 28, 31, 32, 39, 41, 42, 45, 46, 47, 48, 58, 59, 60, 61, 62, 63, 64, 66, 67, 68, 69, 70, 71, 72, 74, 76, 82, 83, 90, 94, 97, 98, 99, 100, 105, 107, 111, 115, 133, 135, 162, 188, 189, 191, 215, 216, 217, 219, 221, 222, 223, 224, 231, 233, 234, 241, 243, 244, 250, 266, 268, 269
body fatness, 24, 58, 162, 191, 231, 233, 234, 241, 244
body mass index (BMI), v, vi, 8, 18, 21, 22, 24, 26, 27, 28, 29, 30, 31, 32, 33, 34, 35, 39, 41, 42, 44, 45, 46, 48, 49, 51, 52, 53, 54, 56, 61, 62, 64, 65, 66, 67, 68, 69, 71, 72, 82, 83, 90, 92, 95, 97, 98, 99, 100, 101, 102, 104, 109, 110, 111, 112, 113, 114, 116, 117, 122, 123, 124, 128, 131, 133, 134, 141, 144, 151, 152, 154, 155, 157, 168, 169, 170, 171, 172, 173, 174, 175, 177, 178, 179, 180, 189, 190, 191, 192, 194, 197, 198, 207, 215, 216, 217, 218, 219, 220, 221, 222, 223, 224, 231, 232, 233, 234, 235, 240, 241, 243, 244, 249, 250, 253, 254, 258, 259, 260, 266, 270
body size, 62, 173, 229, 231, 235, 242
body weight, 3, 4, 41, 42, 46, 49, 58, 62, 115, 124, 144, 151, 230, 231, 250, 251, 255, 267, 268, 277
Brazil, 147, 254, 279

C

Cambodia, 70
Cancun, 147
carbohydrate, 5, 7, 159, 168, 268, 269, 279
cardiovascular disease, xi, 6, 9, 14, 28, 34, 40, 61, 64, 65, 74, 89, 112, 118, 122, 144, 193, 195, 198, 210, 214, 215, 224, 245, 252, 255, 273, 286, 287, 288
cardiovascular risk, 11, 46, 65, 72, 110, 111, 113, 139, 140, 141, 189, 190, 193, 245, 246, 276, 279, 284, 288
Caucasians, 26, 28, 30, 61, 64, 69, 116, 175, 181, 182, 184, 194, 196, 222, 223
central adiposity, v, 30, 71, 73, 75, 84, 91, 104
Central Europe, 213
children, 23, 65, 67, 91, 109, 114, 117, 144, 161, 162, 166, 191, 197, 210, 214, 223, 234, 235, 236, 237, 239, 240, 241, 243, 244, 250, 252, 253, 261, 265, 268, 270, 275, 279, 284, 288
Chile, 123, 140
China, 17, 28, 29, 74, 87, 118, 147, 163, 166, 171, 180, 199, 202, 254, 256, 277, 286, 288
cholesterol, 9, 15, 18, 19, 22, 110, 144, 169, 170, 180, 185, 203, 205, 252, 265, 273
chronic diseases, 144, 232, 239, 241, 252, 260, 264, 274, 276, 278, 283
chronic illness, 30, 84, 240, 243

cigarette smoking, 63, 125, 128, 133, 134, 203
conicity index, 76, 91, 175, 193
consumption, 82, 83, 85, 154, 155, 157, 279
Cook Islands, 57, 254
coronary artery disease, 203, 213, 214, 277, 287
coronary heart disease, 6, 11, 12, 65, 67, 71, 90, 116, 138, 169, 199, 243, 245, 267, 278
cramp, 268
Croatia, 161

D

Department of Health and Human Services (DHS), 56, 64
Department of Internal Medicine, 3, 295
developed countries, 75, 147, 160, 171, 247, 255
developing countries, 16, 28, 34, 65, 73, 74, 75, 86, 110, 132, 146, 159, 163, 164, 170, 184, 193, 194, 195, 251, 255, 256, 262, 263, 275, 277
developing nations, 75, 83
diabetes, 3, 4, 5, 6, 8, 9, 10, 11, 16, 17, 19, 20, 21, 22, 23, 30, 31, 33, 34, 36, 63, 67, 68, 71, 84, 85, 87, 89, 107, 110, 113, 117, 134, 144, 148, 149, 150, 158, 159, 160, 163, 164, 168, 169, 170, 171, 172, 178, 179, 181, 182, 185, 187, 188, 189, 190, 191, 192, 193, 195, 196, 197, 198, 199, 201, 202, 203, 210, 212, 213, 214, 224, 234, 241, 245, 252, 259, 266, 274, 277, 279, 281, 282, 285, 287, 288, 289
diabetic nephropathy, 4, 213
diabetic patients, 4, 172, 192
diabetic retinopathy, 202
diagnostic criteria, 14, 29
diastolic blood pressure (DBP), 22, 77, 95, 96, 97, 98, 99, 100, 103, 104, 105, 122, 124, 204, 207
diet, 6, 7, 57, 159, 172, 187, 239, 251, 260, 261, 279, 284, 288
dietary fat, 279, 284, 285, 286
dietary habits, 60, 75, 83, 276, 278, 279
dietary intake, 69, 252, 274, 278, 284
Durban, 3, 7, 9, 10, 12, 295
dyslipidemia, 30, 64, 113, 144, 167, 180, 191, 267, 278, 281

E

East Asia, 28, 196
economic productivity, 28, 229
Egypt, 57, 254
energy expenditure, 83, 251, 259, 266, 268, 277, 281, 288
England, 235, 236, 238, 239, 245, 246, 247
environmental conditions, 182, 183, 281, 283
environmental factors, 27, 134, 181, 186, 192, 212, 251, 273, 274
environmental stress, 145
epidemiology, xii, 14, 16, 32, 35, 65, 70, 83, 109, 110, 117, 162, 187, 194, 196, 224, 230, 239, 244, 245, 247, 249, 260, 287, 291
epigenetic modifications, 274, 279, 280
Eritrea, 255
ethnic background, 112, 212
ethnic groups, 28, 31, 32, 36, 64, 105, 182, 183, 212, 216, 221, 223, 244
ethnic Indians, 8
ethnicity, 15, 61, 62, 146, 186, 219, 238, 243
Europe, 56, 144, 150, 196, 197, 256
excess body weight, 250, 267, 269
exercise, 7, 87, 135, 250, 251, 268, 269, 270, 286

F

family history, vi, 178, 201, 203, 207, 209, 210, 212, 214, 274, 275, 286, 288, 289
fast food, 83, 183
fasting, 6, 15, 18, 19, 21, 22, 23, 25, 26, 74, 76, 77, 168, 169, 178, 205, 279
fasting glucose, 15, 21, 23, 74
fat, 5, 6, 7, 29, 30, 31, 32, 40, 42, 45, 46, 47, 49, 58, 59, 60, 61, 62, 67, 69, 70, 71, 76, 83, 90, 91, 92, 94, 96, 97, 98, 99, 100, 104, 105, 107, 109, 116, 146, 158, 168, 173, 174, 176, 181, 185, 189, 196, 197, 199, 211, 216, 221, 222, 231, 233, 241, 242,243, 249, 266, 267, 268, 269, 270, 278, 279, 284, 285, 288
fat free mass, 58, 61, 62, 71, 221, 268, 269
fat intake, 7, 278
fatty acids, 185, 278, 279
Fiji, 8
Filipino, 16, 18, 19, 20, 21, 23, 27, 29, 30, 31, 33, 34, 36, 37
food, 18, 50, 83, 90, 105, 132, 158, 162, 211, 239, 251, 252, 259, 278, 281
food habits, 50, 105, 132
food industry, 239
food intake, 18, 211
France, 148, 158, 165
free, 3, 5, 6, 42, 45, 58, 61, 185, 268

G

genes, 182, 185, 197, 203, 206, 209, 211, 224, 250, 263, 270, 275, 280, 281, 283
genetics, 5, 26, 74, 148, 169, 182, 270
genotype, 211, 213, 214, 281, 287
genotyping, 205, 206, 209
Germany, 57
gestational age, 145, 146, 149, 156, 157, 159, 161, 165
gestational diabetes, 148, 159, 160, 162, 193
glucose, 4, 5, 6, 9, 11, 21, 23, 25, 31, 36, 40, 67, 72, 74, 76, 77, 109, 146, 150, 167, 168, 169, 177, 181, 183, 185, 196, 205, 242, 267, 278, 279, 282, 285
glucose regulation, 169
glucose tolerance, 4, 6, 9, 21, 67, 72, 168, 169, 177, 196, 242, 282, 285

H

health problems, 18, 89, 168, 250, 255
health risks, 58, 107, 118, 158, 173, 174, 175, 221, 255, 259, 266
heart disease, ix, 12, 40, 144, 158, 202, 259, 267
height, 33, 41, 42, 43, 44, 45, 47, 49, 64, 71, 90, 94, 95, 96, 97, 98, 99, 100, 103, 107, 110, 112, 115, 116, 117, 124, 144, 150, 152, 154, 155, 158, 164, 166, 169, 172, 175, 178, 188, 191, 192, 194, 197, 204, 217, 219, 229, 230, 231, 235, 237, 242, 244, 247, 249, 266
high blood pressure, 26, 90, 105, 108, 110, 123, 132, 134, 137, 139, 265
high density lipoprotein, 144, 265, 273
Hispanics, 279
Hong Kong, 17, 224
human body, 66, 133, 230, 241
Hungary, 133
hypercholesterolemia, 267
hyperglycaemia, 9, 74, 168, 288
hyperglycemia, 167, 170, 201, 273, 274
hyperinsulinemia, 167, 267, 279
hyperinsulinism, 4
hyperlipidemia, 180, 203
hypertension, 3, 4, 6, 7, 9, 10, 11, 19, 21, 25, 26, 29, 30, 31, 33, 34, 39, 64, 68, 69, 74, 75, 86, 89, 90, 91, 94, 95, 101, 103, 105, 106, 107, 109, 110, 111, 113, 114, 115, 116, 117, 118, 122, 123, 124, 125, 126, 127, 128, 129, 130, 131, 132, 133,

134, 135, 137, 138, 139, 140, 141, 144, 150, 158, 168, 169, 170, 178, 180, 191, 193, 194, 197, 203, 224, 234, 252, 255, 267
hypertriglyceridemia, 178, 267

I

India, v, vi, x, 17, 39, 40, 49, 51, 52, 63, 64, 66, 67, 68, 69, 70, 71, 73, 74, 75, 83, 85, 86, 89, 90, 91, 103, 104, 105, 106, 107, 108, 109, 110, 111, 112, 113, 114, 115, 116, 117, 122, 123, 147, 162, 167, 171, 172, 177, 178, 179, 183, 186, 187, 188, 189, 190, 191, 192, 193, 194, 196, 197, 199, 201, 202, 203, 205, 213, 215, 216, 223, 224, 230, 235, 236, 237, 240, 241, 242, 243, 244, 245, 246, 247, 249, 254, 255, 256, 257, 258, 263, 273, 275, 276, 279, 284, 288, 291, 292, 293, 294, 295, 296
Indians, vi, 8, 9, 12, 30, 40, 61, 68, 69, 86, 91, 116, 167, 177, 180, 181, 182, 183, 184, 188, 189, 190, 194, 195, 196, 198, 202, 210, 214, 215, 216, 217, 223, 247, 275, 276, 278, 279, 282, 284, 287
Indonesia, 75, 86
industrialized countries, 162, 232
infants, 26, 146, 147, 149, 156, 158, 161, 162, 164, 165
informed consent, 41, 77, 204
insulin, 4, 5, 6, 9, 10, 11, 26, 63, 66, 69, 86, 87, 91, 105, 108, 115, 116, 144, 145, 146, 164, 167, 168, 170, 171, 172, 175, 178, 180, 182, 184, 193, 194, 196, 197, 199, 201, 203, 211, 212, 246, 267, 270, 277, 279, 282, 285, 287, 288
insulin resistance, 9, 11, 63, 66, 69, 86, 87, 91, 105, 108, 116, 144, 145, 164, 167, 168, 170, 171, 172, 175, 180, 185, 193, 194, 196, 199, 203, 211, 212, 246, 267, 279, 282, 287, 288
insulin sensitivity, 6, 270
intervention strategies, 72, 106, 198, 225, 248
Iran, 254
Ireland, 57
Islam, 89, 107, 141, 142
Israel, 223
Italy, 31, 147, 261

J

Japan, 75, 85, 94, 204

K

Kenya, 241, 242
kidney, 90, 122, 202, 252
kidney failure, 90, 202
Korea, 17, 64
Kuwait, 123, 132, 137

L

later life, 145, 146, 148, 149, 157, 160, 161, 184, 287
Latin America, 146, 166
Latvia, 57
lean body mass, 184, 188, 234, 250
lipid profiles, 76
lipids, 108, 225, 278
lipolysis, 6, 185, 267
lipoproteins, 205
logistic regression, 77

M

macrosomia, 146, 147, 148, 149, 152, 153, 154, 155, 156, 157, 158, 159, 160, 161, 162, 163, 164, 165, 166
Malaysia, 123, 139
malnutrition, 103, 105, 143, 145, 192, 197, 237, 242, 255, 261, 268, 282
Mauritius, 8, 114
medicalization, 230, 241
mellitus, 9, 10, 12, 14, 19, 20, 23, 28, 30, 33, 34, 67, 72, 84, 91, 134, 148, 150, 161, 163, 168, 170, 171, 178, 188, 190, 191, 192, 193, 194, 195, 198, 201, 202, 252, 273, 285, 287
menopause, 251, 267
metabolic disorder, 61, 68, 156, 167, 178, 190, 194, 201, 278, 279, 283
metabolic syndrome, v, xi, 13, 14, 15, 16, 17, 18, 19, 20, 21, 24, 27, 28, 29, 30, 32, 33, 34, 35, 36, 40, 63, 64, 65, 66, 67, 68, 69, 73, 74, 78, 84, 85, 86, 87, 91, 96, 109, 116, 117, 122, 138, 144, 162, 164, 187, 190, 193, 194, 195, 196, 197, 198, 199, 203, 210, 265, 273, 276, 283, 284, 285, 286, 287, 289, 291, 292
Mexico, 147, 254, 256
Middle East, 28
Mongoloid, 76
Myanmar, 57, 66

N

National Health and Nutrition Examination Survey (NHANES), 56, 63
Nauru, 57, 254
Nepal, 197
New Zealand, 70, 163, 245
Nigeria, 132, 138, 254
Niue, 254
norms, 230, 241, 242
North Africa, 137
North America, 108
Norway, 57
nutrition, xi, 16, 18, 28, 33, 34, 36, 40, 72, 86, 115, 116, 162, 163, 164, 183, 187, 195, 199, 229, 230, 237, 240, 241, 242, 243, 245, 246, 258, 261, 263, 264, 286
nutritional assessment, 42, 230, 231, 237
nutritional deficiencies, 146
nutritional status, 58, 71, 114, 163, 172, 230, 231, 232, 237, 240, 241, 244

O

overweight, 3, 16, 17, 22, 23, 24, 26, 27, 30, 34, 35, 40, 45, 46, 47, 48, 53, 63, 64, 69, 70, 74, 92, 95, 103, 107, 114, 118, 124, 125, 133, 135, 143, 151, 152, 153, 157, 165, 172, 173, 175, 187, 193, 197, 199, 202, 216, 222, 223, 232, 234, 235, 236, 243, 244, 245,246, 247, 249, 250, 251, 253, 255, 256, 258, 261, 264, 265, 266, 271, 276, 284

P

Pacific Islanders, 160, 165
Pakistan, 29, 75, 85, 241, 245, 262
period, xi, 41, 53, 54, 56, 147, 161, 204, 207, 209, 210, 211, 256, 268
Philippines, v, 13, 14, 17, 18, 23, 24, 25, 28, 29, 33, 34, 36, 294, 296
phosphate, 270
physical activity, 6, 22, 29, 32, 41, 75, 76, 83, 87, 90, 126, 128, 132, 133, 135, 158, 162, 172, 181, 211, 235, 243, 251, 261, 263, 268, 274, 276, 277, 278, 279, 284, 286, 287, 288
physical inactivity, 5, 9, 28, 69, 75, 145, 183, 239, 274, 276, 277, 278, 285, 287

polymorphisms, 182, 198, 203, 204, 211, 212, 213, 214, 280
Portugal, 123, 133
pregnancy, 5, 148, 149, 150, 152, 153, 154, 155, 157, 161, 162, 164, 210, 251
prevention, 32, 42, 65, 108, 133, 138, 139, 145, 172, 187, 212, 246, 260, 263, 264, 270, 274, 283, 286, 287, 288
wareness, 35
public health, vi, ix, xi, xii, 12, 15, 28, 29, 30, 31, 33, 35, 39, 63, 66, 67, 68, 70, 73, 87, 107, 108, 109, 111, 112, 118, 135, 137, 138, 141, 144, 157, 176, 187, 188, 192, 194, 195, 212, 214, 227, 229, 233, 235, 236, 246, 247, 252, 256, 258, 261, 265, 274, 275, 276, 285, 288, 289, 291

Q

questionnaires, 74, 76
Quetelet index, 215, 223

R

regression analysis, 77, 82, 83, 97, 98, 99, 100, 104, 126
Republic of the Congo, 255
revenue block, 76
risk factors, ix, xi, 9, 10, 11, 14, 20, 22, 23, 24, 26, 27, 30, 33, 36, 37, 64, 65, 66, 67, 70, 71, 74, 83, 84, 86, 91, 107, 111, 112, 116, 122, 123, 125, 133, 137, 140, 141, 145, 146, 148, 159, 162, 163, 169, 175, 176, 177, 187, 188, 194, 195, 202, 203, 207, 210, 224, 245, 252, 258, 262, 265, 269, 273, 275, 282, 285
Russia, 147, 158, 165, 254
Rwanda, 255

S

Samoa, 165, 254
Saudi Arabia, 123, 132, 138
sedentary lifestyle, xi, 14, 60, 74, 75, 89, 105, 134, 171, 183, 184, 251, 276
sensitivity, vi, 6, 215, 216, 217, 218, 219, 220, 223, 266, 270
skinfold, 76, 82, 94, 98, 99, 100, 116
Slovakia, 138
smoking, 5, 7, 10, 63, 105, 123, 125, 131, 157, 233, 239, 243, 251, 252, 277
socioeconomic status, 28, 41, 50, 76, 84, 87, 116, 235, 243
Somalia, 255
South Africa, 3, 7, 8, 9, 10, 12, 192, 295
South Asia, 9, 11, 29, 33, 61, 68, 69, 113, 117, 177, 180, 184, 188, 189, 191, 194, 245, 287
South Asian Association for Regional Cooperation, 68
South Korea, 29, 75, 86
Southeast Asia, 16, 28, 35
specificity, vi, 215, 216, 217, 218, 219, 220, 223
sphygmomanometer, 86, 95, 204
Sri Lanka, 75, 85, 191
stature, 114, 150, 152, 154, 155, 159, 165, 231, 233, 244, 267
sub-Saharan Africa, 7, 133, 187, 224
Sweden, 11, 57, 110, 147
Switzerland, 118, 264
Syndrome X, vi, vii, ix, xi, 74, 87, 201, 265, 267, 269, 273, 274, 275, 276, 280, 281, 282, 283, 287
systolic blood pressure, 91, 98, 99, 100, 142

T

Taiwan, 17, 29, 113
Tanzania, 241

Thailand, 17, 63, 256
tobacco, 63, 81, 82
Tonga, 254
triglycerides, 15, 19, 20, 22, 26, 169, 170, 265, 267, 273
t-tests, 77
Turkey, 254
Tuvalu, 254
type 1 diabetes, 193, 197
type 2 diabetes, ix, xi, 8, 14, 16, 28, 30, 31, 33, 34, 36, 67, 72, 91, 114, 161, 163, 164, 187, 188, 189, 190, 191, 192, 193, 194, 195, 196, 197, 198, 199, 215, 245, 255, 267, 273, 284, 286, 288

U

undernutrition, vi, 39, 105, 112, 145, 161, 193, 229, 232, 235, 236, 237, 240, 241, 243, 281, 282
United Kingdom, 8, 224, 230, 240
United Nations, 162, 261, 264
United States (USA), 32, 36, 43, 63, 65, 70, 97, 133, 147, 156, 162, 164, 171, 189, 195, 199, 205, 214, 230, 248, 256, 262, 289
urban areas, 7, 22, 40, 91, 105, 160, 172
urban population, 57, 65, 69, 75, 85, 91, 104, 105, 112

V

visceral adiposity, 31, 180, 185

W

weight, vi, 3, 4, 6, 27, 36, 41, 42, 44, 45, 46, 49, 58, 62, 67, 70, 95, 97, 98, 103, 115, 124, 128, 129, 133, 143, 144, 145, 146, 147, 148, 149, 150, 151, 152, 153, 154, 155, 156, 157, 158, 159, 160, 161, 163, 164, 165, 166, 169, 172, 175, 176, 178, 179, 202, 204, 208, 217, 219, 221, 229, 230, 231, 233, 235, 237, 241, 242, 243, 244, 247, 248, 249, 250, 251, 252, 255, 259, 261, 266, 268, 269, 270, 277, 278, 279, 282
weight gain, 149, 150, 152, 153, 154, 155, 156, 157, 160, 173, 176, 243, 250, 251, 252, 259, 278, 279
weight loss, 202, 268, 270
weight management, 27, 70, 261
weight reduction, 6
weight status, 149, 151, 152, 153, 154, 155, 157, 164
weight-height indices, 231
West Africa, 7, 8, 10
West Bank, 123, 141
Western countries, 123, 147

Y

young adults, 37, 132, 134, 135, 138, 164, 191
young women, 133

The Science of Medical Cannabis

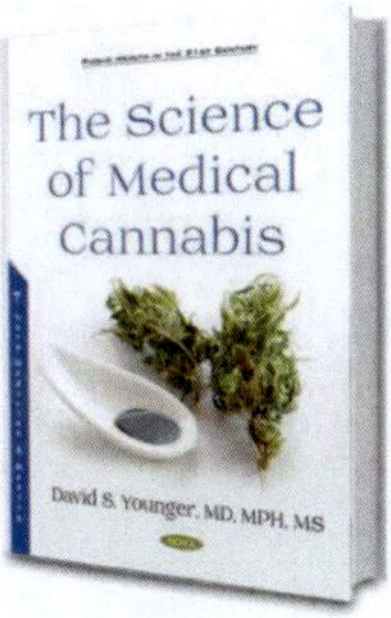

Author: David Steven Younger, M.D. (Department of Neurology, New York University Langone Medical Center, New York, NY, US)

Series: Public Health in the 21st Century

Book Description: *The Science of Medical Cannabis* evolved out of the need for a definitive book on the scientific and public health aspects of medical cannabis.

Softcover ISBN: 978-1-53614-566-3
Retail Price: $95

An Outline of Asbestos-Related Health Effects

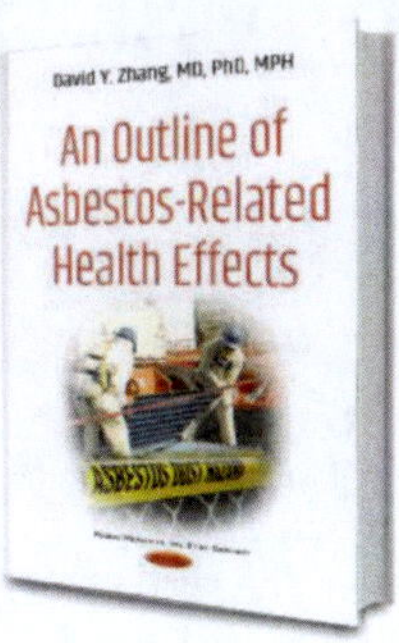

Author: David Y. Zhang, M.D., Ph.D. (Departments of Pathology and Public Health, Icahn School of Medicine at Mount Sinai, New York, NY, USA

Series: Public Health in the 21st Century

Book Description: This book summarizes the historical background, current knowledge and advancements concerning asbestos and its related diseases in a simple, easy to understand and concise format.

Softcover ISBN: 978-1-53610-961-0
Retail Price: $82

Health and Freedom in the Balance: Exploring the Tensions among Public Health, Individual Liberty, and Governmental Authority

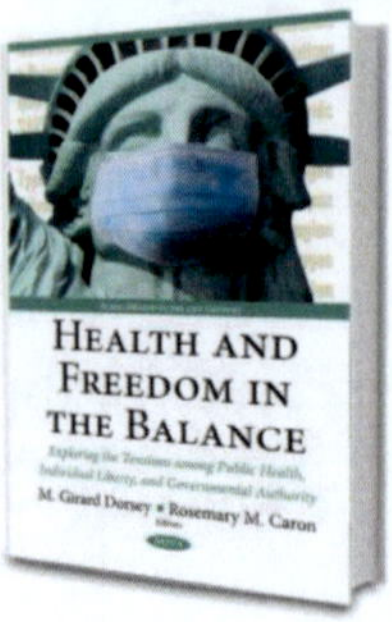

Editors: M. Girard Dorsey (Justice Studies Program, University of New Hampshire, Durham, USA); Rosemary M. Caron (University of New Hampshire, Durham, NH, USA)

Series: Public Health in the 21st Century

Book Description: The clash between individual liberties and the protection of the greater population is an ongoing conflict between core principles held dear by Americans for centuries.

Hardcover ISBN: 978-1-53612-201-5
Retail Price: $160

Advances in Health and Natural Sciences

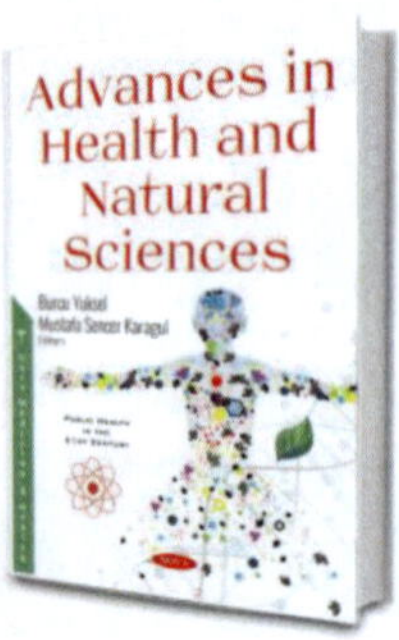

Editors: Burcu Yuksel (Kocaeli University, Vocational School of Health Sciences, Kocaeli, Turkey); Mustafa Sencer Karagul (Kocaeli University, Kartepe Vocational School of Equine Science, Kocaeli, Turkey)

Series: Public Health in the 21st Century

Book Description: The edited book aims at highlighting the state of the art research and recent findings in of agricultural, environmental, biological, marine and medical sciences and biotechnology, and bridging theoretical research with current applications.

Hardcover ISBN: 978-1-53614-639-4
Retail Price: $230